T0263205

Hepatitis C Virus: The Next Epidemic

Editor

K. RAJENDER REDDY

GASTROENTEROLOGY CLINICS OF NORTH AMERICA

www.gastro.theclinics.com

Consulting Editor
GARY W. FALK

December 2015 • Volume 44 • Number 4

ELSEVIER

1600 John F. Kennedy Boulevard • Suite 1800 • Philadelphia, Pennsylvania, 19103-2899
http://www.theclinics.com

GASTROENTEROLOGY CLINICS OF NORTH AMERICA Volume 44, Number 4
December 2015 ISSN 0889-8553, ISBN-13: 978-0-323-40248-4

Editor: Kerry Holland
Developmental Editor: Alison Swety

Gastroenterology Clinics of North America (ISSN 0889-8553) is published quarterly by Elsevier Inc., 360 Park
Avenue South, New York, NY 10010-1710. Months of issue are March, June, September, and December. Busi-
ness and Editorial Offices: 1600 John F. Kennedy Blvd., Suite 1800, Philadelphia, PA 19103-2899. Customer
Service Office: 6277 Sea Harbor Drive, Orlando, FL 32887-4800. Periodicals postage paid at New York, NY
and additional mailing offices. Subscription prices are $320.00 per year (US individuals), $160.00 per year
(US students), $530.00 per year (US institutions), $350.00 per year (Canadian individuals), $651.00 per year
(Canadian institutions), $445.00 per year (international individuals), $220.00 per year (international students),
and $651.00 per year (international institutions). Foreign air speed delivery is included in all *Clinics* subscription
prices. All prices are subject to change without notice. **POSTMASTER**: Send address changes to *Gastroenterology Clinics of North America*, Elsevier Health Sciences Division, Subscription Customer Service, 3251 Riverport
Lane, Maryland Heights, MO 63043. **Telephone: 1-800-654-2452 (U.S. and Canada); 314-447-8871 (outside
U.S. and Canada). Fax: 314-447-8029. E-mail: journalscustomerservice-usa@elsevier.com (for print
support); journalsonlinesupport-usa@elsevier.com (for online support)**.

Reprints. For copies of 100 or more, of articles in this publication, please contact the Commercial Reprints
Department, Elsevier Inc., 360 Part Avenue South, New York, New York 10010-1710. Tel. 212-633-3874,
Fax: 212-633-3820, E-mail: reprints@elsevier.com.

Gastroenterology Clinics of North America is also published in Italian by Il Pensiero Scientifico Editore, Rome,
Italy; and in Portuguese by Interlivros Edicoes Ltda., Rua Commandante Coelho 1085, 21250 Cordovil, Rio de
Janeiro, Brazil.

Gastroenterology Clinics of North America is covered in *MEDLINE/PubMed (Index Medicus)*, *Excerpta Medica*,
Current Contents/Clinical Medicine, *Science Citation Index*, *ISI/BIOMED*, and *BIOSIS*.

Contributors

CONSULTING EDITOR

GARY W. FALK, MD, MS
Professor of Medicine, Division of Gastroenterology, Hospital of the University of Pennsylvania, University of Pennsylvania Perelman School of Medicine, Philadelphia, Pennsylvania

EDITOR

K. RAJENDER REDDY, MD, FACP, FACG, FRCP (UK), FAASLD
Ruimy Family President's Distinguished Professor of Medicine, Professor of Medicine in Surgery, Director of Hepatology, Director, Viral Hepatitis Center, Medical Director of Liver Transplantation, University of Pennsylvania, Philadelphia, Pennsylvania

AUTHORS

JOSEPH AHN, MD, MS
Associate Professor of Medicine, Director of Hepatology, Oregon Health and Sciences University, Portland, Oregon

SALEH ALQAHTANI, MD
Director of Clinical Liver Research, The Johns Hopkins Hospital, Baltimore, Maryland

JAVIER AMPUERO, MD, PhD
Unit for the Clinical Management of Digestive Diseases and CIBERehd, Virgen Macarena - Virgen del Rocio University Hospitals, Sevilla, Spain

TARIK ASSELAH, MD, PhD
Department of Hepatology, Beaujon Hospital, UNITY, INSERM, UMR1149, Team Viral Hepatitis, Centre de Recherche sur l'inflammation, Labex INFLAMEX, Université Denis Diderot Paris 7, Clichy, France

MARC BOURLIÈRE, MD
Saint Joseph Hospital, Marseilles, France

CHALERMRAT BUNCHORNTAVAKUL, MD
Assistant Professor, Division of Gastroenterology and Hepatology, Department of Internal Medicine, Rajavithi Hospital, College of Medicine, Rangsit University, Bangkok, Thailand

MASSIMO COLOMBO, MD
Division of Gastroenterology and Hepatology, "A. M. and A. Migliavacca" Center for Liver Disease, Fondazione IRCCS Ca' Granda Ospedale Maggiore Policlinico, Università degli Studi di Milano, Milan, Italy

YOCK YOUNG DAN, MBBS, PhD, MRCP, MMed, FAMS
Associate Professor, Chair, University Medical Cluster; Head, Department of Medicine, Yong Loo Lin School of Medicine, National University of Singapore; Division of Gastroenterology and Hepatology, National University Health System; Cancer Science Institute, National University of Singapore, Singapore, Singapore

GEORG DULTZ, MD
Medizinische Klinik 1, Schwerpunkt Gastroenterologie und Hepatologie, Universitätsklinikum Frankfurt, Goethe-Universität, Frankfurt am Main, Germany

MARC G. GHANY, MD, MHSc
Liver Diseases Branch, National Institute of Diabetes and Digestive and Kidney Diseases, National Institutes of Health, Bethesda, Maryland

MAUREEN M. JONAS, MD
Professor of Pediatrics, Division of Gastroenterology, Hepatology and Nutrition, Boston Children's Hospital, Boston, Massachusetts

DAVID E. KAPLAN, MD, MSc, FACP
Medicine and Research Services, Philadelphia VA Medical Center; Assistant Professor, Division of Gastroenterology, Department of Medicine, University of Pennsylvania, Philadelphia, Pennsylvania

CHRISTINE K. LEE, MD
Instructor in Pediatrics, Division of Gastroenterology, Hepatology and Nutrition, Boston Children's Hospital, Boston, Massachusetts

SENG GEE LIM, MBBS, FRACP, FRCP, FAMS, MD, Cert Immunology
Professor, Director of Hepatology, Division of Gastroenterology and Hepatology, National University Health System; Department of Medicine, Yong Loo Lin School of Medicine, National University of Singapore; Institute of Molecular and Cell Biology, Agency for Science, Technology and Research, Singapore, Singapore

SHILPA LINGALA, MD
Liver Diseases Branch, National Institute of Diabetes and Digestive and Kidney Diseases, National Institutes of Health, Bethesda, Maryland

MINDIE H. NGUYEN, MD, MAS
Associate Professor of Medicine, Liver Transplant Program, Division of Gastroenterology and Hepatology, Stanford University Medical Center, Palo Alto, California

NGHIA H. NGUYEN, MD, MAS
School of Medicine, University of California, San Diego, La Jolla, California; Division of Gastroenterology and Hepatology, Stanford University Medical Center, Palo Alto, California

MANUEL ROMERO-GÓMEZ, MD, PhD
Head of Unit for the Clinical Management of Digestive Diseases and CIBERehd, Virgen Macarena - Virgen del Rocio University Hospitals, Sevilla, Spain

KENNETH E. SHERMAN, MD, PhD
Director, Division of Digestive Diseases, University of Cincinnati College of Medicine, University of Cincinnati, Cincinnati, Ohio

NORAH J. SHIRE, PhD, MPH
Director, Epidemiology, AstraZeneca Pharmaceuticals LLC, Gaithersburg, Maryland

MARK SULKOWSKI, MD
Professor of Medicine, Medical Director of Viral Hepatitis Center, The Johns Hopkins Hospital, Baltimore, Maryland

TAWESAK TANWANDEE, MD
Associate Professor, Division of Gastroenterology and Hepatology, Department of Internal Medicine, Faculty of Medicine Siriraj Hospital, Mahidol University, Bangkok, Thailand

DANIELLE M. THOLEY, MD
Fellow, Gastroenterology and Hepatology, Oregon Health and Sciences University, Portland, Oregon

MAURO VIGANÒ, MD, PhD
Hepatology Division, Ospedale San Giuseppe, Università degli Studi di Milano, Milan, Italy

STEFAN ZEUZEM, MD, PhD
Medizinische Klinik 1, Schwerpunkt Gastroenterologie und Hepatologie, Universitätsklinikum Frankfurt, Goethe-Universität, Frankfurt am Main, Germany

Contents

The hepatitis C virus (HCV) is a leading cause of liver-related morbidity and mortality in the United States and other parts of the world. The epidemiology of the disease is highly variable between and within countries, and strategies to deal with HCV identification and treatment must be tailored to the geographic location and the political and economic environment of the region. Although great strides have been made in improving HCV transmission risk in blood supply products, new challenges related to changing patterns of disease incidence continue to require fresh evaluation and new approaches to disease prevention.

Hepatitis C infection is a common cause of cirrhosis and indication for liver transplantation in the United States. The incidence of chronic hepatitis C has been declining, but rates of cirrhosis and hepatocellular carcinoma are projected to increase. The outcome of chronic hepatitis C is variable. It is estimated that 20% to 25% will develop cirrhosis over a 25-year to 30-year period. The rate of disease progression is influenced by many host, viral, and environmental factors. Few can be modified.

Despite advances in therapy, hepatitis C virus infection remains a major global health issue with 3 to 4 million incident cases and 170 million prevalent chronic infections. Complex, partially understood, host-virus interactions determine whether an acute infection with hepatitis C resolves, as occurs in approximately 30% of cases, or generates a persistent hepatic infection, as occurs in the remainder. Once chronic infection is established, the velocity of hepatocyte injury and resultant fibrosis is significantly modulated by immunologic as well as environmental factors. Immunomodulation has been the backbone of antiviral therapy despite poor understanding of its mechanism of action.

GASTROENTEROLOGY
CLINICS OF NORTH AMERICA

RELATED INTEREST

Clinics in Liver Disease
November 2015 (Vol. 19, Issue 4)
Current Management of Hepatitis C Virus
Fred Poordad, *Editor*

THE CLINICS ARE AVAILABLE ONLINE!
Access your subscription at:
www.theclinics.com

Foreword
Hepatitis C Virus

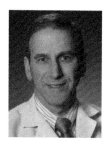

Gary W. Falk, MD, MS
Consulting Editor

The evolution of knowledge and treatment of hepatitis C (HCV) over the past three decades has been nothing short of breathtaking. HCV is now a well-characterized disease that is global in reach with significant implications regarding treatment, progression, and outcome. Furthermore, the last several years have witnessed an exciting explosion of therapies that have the potential to cure this disease. In this issue of *Gastroenterology Clinics of North America*, my associate, K. Rajender Reddy, a world-renowned expert in HCV, has assembled a superb group of authors to address all aspects of HCV infection, from global epidemiology and natural history to pathogenesis, implications for chronic liver disease, and the rapid advances in therapy. This state-of-the-art update on HCV should serve as a valuable resource for the readership as we reach the end of 2015.

Gary W. Falk, MD, MS
Division of Gastroenterology
University of Pennsylvania
Perelman School of Medicine
PCAM South Pavilion, 7th Floor
3400 Civic Center Boulevard
Philadelphia, PA 19104-4311, USA

E-mail address:
gary.falk@uphs.upenn.edu

Gastroenterol Clin N Am 44 (2015) xiii
http://dx.doi.org/10.1016/j.gtc.2015.09.002
0889-8553/15/$ – see front matter © 2015 Published by Elsevier Inc.

gastro.theclinics.com

Preface

Hepatitis C: Unfolding the Challenges

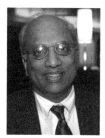

K. Rajender Reddy, MD, FACP, FACG, FRCP (UK), FAASLD
Editor

There are over 180 million people with chronic hepatitis C (HCV) infection worldwide with between 2.7 and 3.9 million people in the United States alone. HCV most significantly affects Asia and Africa, with rates up to 15% in countries such as Egypt and up to 30% in certain regions such as Punjab, Pakistan. HCV places a significant burden on the public health infrastructure, as it remains the leading cause of chronic liver disease, accounting for 50% to 75% of primary liver cancers and being responsible for 30% of all liver transplantations. It was estimated to have cost the United States $5.5 billion in 1997, comparable to the national cost of asthma of $5.8 billion in 1994. This number is only expected to grow as the current HCV population ages, increasing overall rates of end-stage liver disease and of primary liver cancer.

The evolution of directly acting antivirals has ushered in a new era for chronic HCV. The main mechanism of action of most DAAs is the inhibition of an enzyme (protease or polymerase), although others inhibit the assembly of the replication complex (NS5A inhibitors). Such all-oral therapy regimens are very well tolerated and achieve high response rates even without the backbone of pegylated interferon. NS3/4A is a serine protease essential for viral replication. Inhibitors of NS3/4A have a high potency but a low barrier to resistance and are not effective against all HCV genotypes. NS5A is a zinc-binding phosphoprotein that plays an important but currently unclear role in HCV replication. NS5B is an HCV RNA-dependent RNA polymerase, which plays a crucial role in HCV replication. Nucleotide inhibitors have been found to be pan-genotypic and possess high potency and a high barrier to resistance, as the active site of NS5B is highly conserved across all HCV genotypes. Nonnucleoside inhibitors allosterically target the NS5B region and inhibit the initiation stage of RNA synthesis. This class of inhibitors displays a low barrier to resistance, mild potency, and limited effectiveness across all HCV genotypes.

Ongoing drug development strategy has involved targeting several replication steps of the virus, and the drugs that act at various steps of the viral replication have been

Gastroenterol Clin N Am 44 (2015) xv–xvi
http://dx.doi.org/10.1016/j.gtc.2015.09.001
0889-8553/15/$ – see front matter © 2015 Published by Elsevier Inc.

gastro.theclinics.com

additive or even synergistic in their antiviral effects and have led to high SVR rates with much better tolerability than interferon-based regimens. Currently, as it stands, the role of ribavirin appears unclear in the therapeutic landscape of chronic HCV.

This issue of *Gastroenterology Clinics of North America* has a diverse range of topics and a highly recognized international author representation. Thus, it provides a global perspective on HCV infection. There are challenges unique to the various regions of the world and among these include the heterogeneity in host and viral factors, and, most importantly, the difficulty with access to expensive therapy. The issue has diverse topics of epidemiology, natural history, pathogenesis, and treatment options for the various populations, including those with the various genotypes, advanced liver disease, and other special populations, including children. I hope you find this issue useful in your understanding of the current status of HCV and also in your day-to-day practice.

K. Rajender Reddy, MD, FACP, FACG, FRCP (UK), FAASLD
Liver Transplant Office
Hospital of the
University of Pennsylvania
2 Dulles, 3400 Spruce Street
Philadelphia, PA 19104, USA

E-mail address:
Rajender.reddy@uphs.upenn.edu

Epidemiology of Hepatitis C Virus
A Battle on New Frontiers

Norah J. Shire, PhD, MPH[a],*, Kenneth E. Sherman, MD, PhD[b]

KEYWORDS

• HCV epidemiology • Incidence • Prevalence • Acute HCV • Co-infection

KEY POINTS

- HCV remains a leading cause of liver-related morbidity and mortality across the globe.
- Incidence, prevalence, and transmission risk factors vary considerably within and between countries.
- New infection risk in developed nations is generally caused by injection drug use and unsafe sexual practices but may be caused by medical procedures or other local parenteral or iatrogenic routes in developing nations.
- Regional politics, economic situations, and immigration add to changing patterns of HCV epidemiology.
- Continued evaluation and disease prevention strategies are needed to keep virus transmission in check.

INTRODUCTION

Hepatitis C viral infection (HCV) represents a significant public health burden, chronically infecting between 2.7 and 4.1 million people in the United States civilian population[1,2] and at least 150 million individuals worldwide.[3] Most of those initially infected with HCV develop chronic infection, with clearance rates mediated by sex, transmission route, and other concomitant infections such as HIV.[4] Chronic HCV can lead to progression to liver cirrhosis in 15% to 20% of those infected within 20 years,[5] resulting in severe outcomes such as end-stage liver disease and hepatocellular carcinoma (HCC). At least 35% of individuals on the wait list for liver transplant in the United

Disclosure Statement: Dr N.J. Shire is an employee of AstraZeneca Pharmaceuticals, LLC, and a former employee of Merck and owns stock in both companies. Dr K.E. Sherman has served as a member of an advisory board for Merck and MedImmune. He also is a member of Data Safety Monitoring Boards for Janssen, MedPace, and SynteractHCR.
[a] Epidemiology, AstraZeneca Pharmaceuticals LLC, 1 MedImmune Way, Gaithersburg, MD 20878, USA; [b] Division of Digestive Diseases, University of Cincinnati College of Medicine, University of Cincinnati, 231 Albert B Sabin Way, Cincinnati, OH 45267-0595, USA
* Corresponding author.
E-mail address: norah.shire@astrazeneca.com

States are infected with HCV,[6] and global HCV-associated mortality estimates are close to 500,000 deaths per year.[7] Although the advent of oral direct-acting antiviral therapy (DAA) has generated considerable enthusiasm for vastly improved control of the virus, diagnosis and treatment of populations in resource-poor settings and marginalized populations have not improved in tandem, suggesting an urgent need for continued refinement of epidemiology, cost-utility models, and targeted diagnostic strategies.

HEPATITIS C VIRUS EPIDEMIOLOGY: THE FIRST 20 YEARS (1975–1995)
Hepatitis C Virus Unmasked

Early evidence of a hepatitis virus other than hepatitis A or B was described in patients undergoing blood transfusion in the 1970s as assays for identification of hepatitis A and B became available.[8–11] This non-A, non-B hepatitis was further described in patients who had not received blood products, such as families in hepatitis-endemic regions in Costa Rica[12] and drug users in Milan.[13] Extensive analyses of blood donors were performed to identify factors associated with disease transmission. Serum alanine aminotransferase levels and the presence of hepatitis B anti-core antibody were linked to non-A, non-B transmission and by 1986 all blood in the United States was screened for these markers, despite questions about the overall efficacy.[14] It was estimated that this antigen and its parent virus were responsible for up to 89% of post-transfusion hepatitis[8,15] and it was identified as the causative agent in chronic liver disease in people with hemophilia (PWH) and other clotting disorders.[16] It was demonstrated to be transmissible even from patients without active disease.[17] However, it was not until a decade later that Choo and colleagues[18] isolated the genetic material of the virus, opening the door for vastly improved methods of viral identification[19] and eventual assignment to the Flaviviridae family. The development and application of both an enzyme-linked immunoassay (ELISA) for detection of anti-HCV antibodies[20,21] and the refinement of the polymerase chain reaction to quickly identify and sequence the genetic material of HCV during 1990s enabled accurate observational research and genotypic characterization of the virus[22,23]; thus, the field of HCV epidemiology was born during this decade.

Hepatitis C Virus Epidemic: the Early Days

Once rapid and accessible screening methods for HCV were available, a tsunami of epidemiologic research began to emerge, describing the high prevalence and blood-borne transmission patterns of HCV in various patient types and cohorts. An early study reported that more than 80% of patients with nonalcoholic liver disease who were previously diagnosed with cryptogenic hepatitis were actually positive for HCV antibodies.[24] Similarly, nearly 75% of patients at the New England hemophilia center were found to have anti-HCV antibodies.[25] By 1993, nearly 90% of hemophiliacs in the United States were infected with HCV from exposure to contaminated clotting factor concentrates received before 1987.[26] These patients experienced recurrent exposure to concentrates made from plasma pools prepared from 20,000 or more blood donors at a time when just a single-unit risk of infection approached 5%. Moreover, HCV-infected patients with clotting disorders were also at greater risk for other parentally acquired infections, such as human immunodeficiency virus (HIV) and hepatitis B virus (HBV).[27,28] HCV was detected in other settings as well, such as renal dialysis centers.[29,30] Risk factors such as injection drug use (IDU) and unsafe sexual practices were also implicated in infection; seroprevalence of anti-HCV antibodies reached 100% in an Australian population with long-term use[31] and were similarly high in drug users in Amsterdam.[32] Sexual spread of the virus was also posited as rates were higher in sex workers without known injection drug use than controls,[33] although some studies demonstrated low rates of HCV among HIV-infected sex workers in countries with low IDU, including Uganda and the Democratic Republic of Congo.[34,35]

In the United States, a 7-year study of non-A, non-B hepatitis surveyed 4 sentinel counties with the recently developed immunoassay.[36] This pivotal study revealed that although the incidence of HCV was stable over 7 years, primary modes of transmission changed from transfusion to use of injection drugs over this period. This early report solidified IDU as an important risk factor for HCV transmission in the United States, and sounded a warning for the health epidemic yet to arrive. The link between HCV and HCC was also confirmed, with the relative risk for HCC ranging from 4.8 to 7.3 if positive for anti-HCV antibodies.[37–39] From 1985 to 1987, solvent/detergent treatment of donor blood was implemented for coagulation factors, effectively eliminating transmission to patients with clotting disorders.[40] Recommendations for donor screening for HCV antibodies followed,[41] which limited viral spread from contaminated blood transfusion products. From this point on, HCV was and continues to be primarily transmitted through other blood-borne routes including IDU, unsafe or traumatic sexual activity, nasal cocaine use resulting in mucosal damage, and practices such as unsanitary tattooing.

HEPATITIS C VIRUS EPIDEMIOLOGY: 1995 TO 2015

Current HCV distribution is highly variable, both intercountry and intracountry and region (**Fig. 1**). In developed nations, such as North America, Western Europe, and Australia, the overall prevalence is less than 1.25%, according to a recent literature synthesis,[42] but this review excluded studies focusing on special populations including people who inject drugs (PWID), PWH, HIV-positive, incarcerated, military veterans, and men who have sex with men (MSM). In developing nations, the population-based prevalence of anti-HCV may reach as high as 11% (Mongolia) to 15% (Egypt), although rates of viremia may be lower. Furthermore, poorer nations are less likely to be able to afford screening and DAA therapy. The public health threat posed by HCV is not limited to developing nations, however, as fluid immigration patterns may continue to facilitate the spread of HCV globally. A comparison of age-specific 2012 HCV prevalence for selected developed and developing nations is shown in **Fig. 2**.

Current Hepatitis C Virus Epidemiology in Developed Nations

Generally, countries with a low prevalence of HCV (<2%) are developed nations where the population has access to sanitary conditions, less crowding, and adequate health care. However, variability in risk and transmission factors between these countries has led to differences in HCV epidemics, even among relatively similar countries.[43]

For example, the most recent analysis of the National Health and Nutrition Examination Surveys (NHANES) for the years 2003 to 2010 in the United States estimated HCV prevalence of 1%, corresponding to approximately 2.7 million individuals.[1] Previous NHANES analyses reported HCV prevalence of 1.6% between 1999 and 2003[2] and 1.8% between 1988 and 1994.[44] These data and others suggest that peak incidence in the United States occurred during the 1970s and 1980s. Age-specific modeling has demonstrated that the greatest risk of infection for the US population is in those born between 1940 and 1965,[2] and a recent analysis of US veterans revealed an HCV infection prevalence of 10.3% for those born between 1945 and 1965 versus 1.2% for those born after 1965.[45]

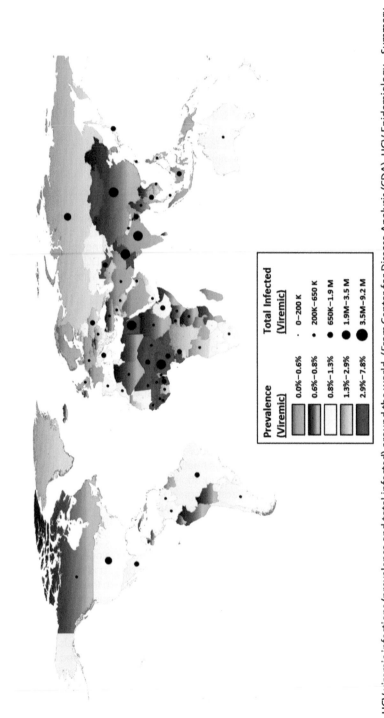

Fig. 1. HCV viremic infections (prevalence and total infected) around the world. (*From* Center for Disease Analysis (CDA). HCV Epidemiology – Summary Slides. Available at: http://www.centerforda.com/downloads.htm. Accessed July 9, 2015.)

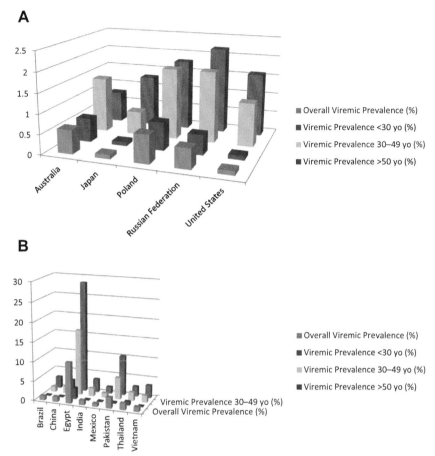

Fig. 2. 2012 HCV prevalence rates overall and by age group among selected developed (A) and developing (B) nations. yo, years old. (*Data from* Center for Disease Analysis (CDA). HepC Map. Available at: http://www.centerforda.com/HepC/HepMap.html. Accessed July 9, 2015.)

A critical limitation of all of these studies, however, is that incarcerated and homeless individuals, who may be at high risk of infection from IDU or unsafe sexual practices, are excluded. Chak and colleagues[46] conducted a comprehensive literature review to estimate the numbers of HCV-infected individuals from populations that were not accounted for in the NHANES surveys. They reported a revised estimate of between 5.2 and 7.1 million infected individuals in the United States. It is likely that age-specific prevalence would differ in some of these populations because of different risk factors than those in the 1945 to 1965 birth cohort, and that ongoing risk factors such as IDU and unsafe sexual practices may result in stable, rather than declining, incidence in these populations. Indeed, the current most frequent transmission route of HCV in the United States is IDU.[47,48]

Japan has an overall prevalence of HCV infection comparable with the United States, but different transmission patterns have resulted in different age-specific prevalence. Most of the HCV burden in Japan was caused by contaminated blood products and unsafe medical procedures during the first half of the 1900s; molecular clock analyses have suggested that peak infection rates occurred as early as the

1920s.[49] The highest age-specific prevalence in the general population is 2%, occurring in those more than 60 years of age.[50] In contrast, prevalence in those less than 40 years of age is less than 0.5%. Risk factors in younger adults include IDU and tattooing,[51] and this shift in transmission routes has led to alterations in genotype distribution in Japan.[52] Although IDU is increasing in Japan, it is still relatively rare and is not expected to increase the overall burden of HCV or HCC. Low incidence and declining prevalence of HCV has resulted in a decrease in HCC in Japan between 1990 and 2003, from a peak of 41.5 cases per 100,000 persons in 1995 to 24 cases per 100,000 in 2003.[53] Aggressive screening and treatment has largely contained the HCV epidemic in Japan.

Accurate HCV incidence and prevalence rates and genotype distributions in Europe are difficult to attain because of large differences in diagnosis rates and reporting among European nations. With this caveat in mind, HCV prevalence in Western Europe as defined by HCV viremia ranges from 0.4% (Austria, Cyprus, Germany, Denmark, France, United Kingdom) to 1.5% (Israel, Italy), totaling 2.2 million individuals[42] **(Fig. 3)**. Central and Eastern Europe have fewer available data on viremic individuals, but anti-HCV rates range from 0.7% (Czech Republic) to 4.5% (Moldova), yielding approximately 7.8 million anti-HCV-positive individuals. In general, IDU is the leading cause of transmission across Europe, although immigration from regions of higher prevalence, such as Egypt, have added to infection rates.[54–59] A 2011 review of the literature regarding anti-HCV prevalence in PWID suggests that prevalence in that population is greater than 60% in nearly every European country; incidence rates up to 66/100 person-years have been reported.[60] Cornberg and colleagues[61] undertook a comprehensive systematic review of the literature on the epidemiology of HCV in Europe, Canada, and Israel. They describe decreasing HCV incidence in most countries in Western Europe. This decrease is partially the result of the changes in transmission routes, and partially a result of effective public awareness and health campaigns. For example, Denmark has a national centralized registry; some nations such as France have implemented national surveillance and prevention programs; and there is mandatory reporting of HCV infection in countries such as Sweden, Switzerland, and Poland. However, increasing incidence in many Eastern and Central European countries, including the Czech Republic, Poland, and particularly Russia, remains a serious concern, particularly with ease of travel and immigration throughout Europe. Romania in particular also merits attention. Epidemics of HIV, HBV, and HCV have been documented in Romanian children caused by the practice of whole-blood injections in orphanages in an attempt to improve nutritional status and re-use of needles and syringes. In 1993, 17% of children aged 0 to 3 years from Bucharest orphanages were HCV positive.[62]

Australia also has implemented mandatory notification for HCV infection and has been reported to have HCV prevalence comparable with that of the United States (~1%).[63] Again, IDU is the primary mode of transmission.[64] An elegant model of the Australian epidemic demonstrates a steady increase in incidence from 1960 to 2000, which was the peak of the epidemic (a decline after 2000 is attributed to a sharp decrease in heroin availability).[65] Since 2004, prevalence has continued to decline among all adult age groups, but incidence is stable with the highest rates (between 6 and 8 notifications per year per 100,000 individuals) reported in those aged 20 to 29 years.[63] Thus, the birth cohort experiencing the greatest HCV prevalence is younger than that in the United States, and the health burden from HCV can be expected to crest a decade later. Two-to three-fold increases in the numbers of HCV-positive individuals progressing through fibrosis to cirrhosis, HCC, and end-stage liver disease have been observed from 2003 to 2013. It is hoped that the advent of the DAA era for HCV will prevent further disease progression in patients who are successfully treated.

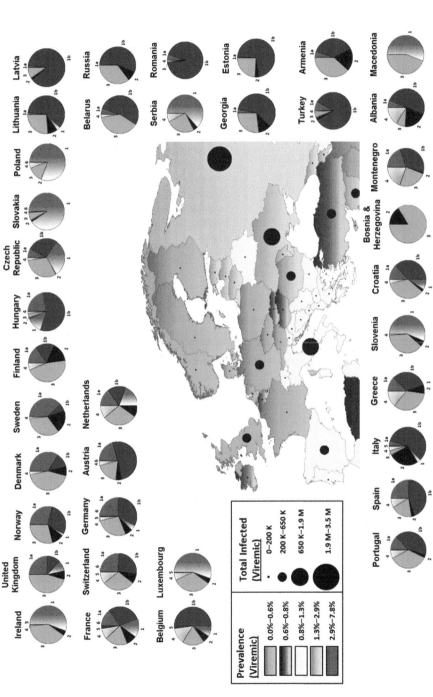

Fig. 3. HCV prevalence and genotype distribution across Europe. (*From* Center for Disease Analysis (CDA). HCV Epidemiology – Summary Slides. Available at: http://www.centerforda.com/downloads.htm. Accessed July 9, 2015.)

Current Hepatitis C Virus Epidemiology in Developing Nations

Given the challenges to gathering accurate epidemiology data in developed countries, it is not a surprise that the difficulties are even greater in developing nations. Many of these countries have little national health infrastructure for HCV screening or reporting, and limited resources for access to health care and treatment. Based on available data, prevalence varies greatly by country and within country. China, the largest by population size, has generally a low overall HCV prevalence, less than 1% in blood donors and the general population,[66,67] as a result of stringent screening of blood product donors. However, pockets of high infection rates remain, particularly in older populations.[68,69] Transmission seems to be primarily iatrogenic; dental work, cosmetic work, and blood transfusions have all been identified as risk factors. Family transmission, suggesting sexual transmission between spouses, has also been linked to infection risk. And as is the case with many countries, PWID and sex workers and clients remain at much higher risk for HCV infection.[70–73] One study found an adjusted odds ratio of 60 for HCV positivity for female sex workers who had ever injected drugs,[73] and prevalence in HIV-infected PWID is nearly universal.[70] With a population size of 1.35 billion, even a conservative estimate of 0.5% HCV prevalence would yield 6.75 million infected individuals, and other reviews have estimated nearly double that number[74]; thus, HCV remains a primary health concern in China.

India is another developing nation with a population-based HCV prevalence rate of less than 2%, but a large population of nearly 1.3 billion individuals. Data from India are highly heterogeneous and generalizability is poor. Study populations tend to be either local or blood-bank donors, and donor screening data do not provide good estimates for an overall population as donors tend to be young and healthy. Currently there is no national surveillance or reporting system for HCV. The recent Consensus Statement of the HCV Task Force of the Indian National Association for Study of the Liver (INASL) has estimated overall prevalence of HCV between 0.5% and 1.5%, and has recommended the initiation of large-scale epidemiology studies to help fill this knowledge gap.[75] Transmission in India has been primarily attributed to contaminated blood products, as mandatory blood product screening was not initiated until 2001. Unsafe injection practices have also been implicated. Puri and colleagues[75] report that injections for common ailments are more frequent in India than in the developed world and inadequate sterilization is frequent; up to nearly 40% of cases of HCV in India has been attributed to unsafe medical injections.

Pakistan, although smaller than India and China, also has a sizable population and has higher estimated HCV prevalence of 4.7%.[76] Hepatitis A infection is universal and hepatitis E is endemic, compounding the risk of liver disease. As in India, injections are popular remedies for illnesses and frequently used during medical procedures. Medical injection is the most commonly reported risk factor for HCV.[77] A hepatitis sentinel surveillance system was implemented in 2011 to track all forms of viral hepatitis, with the aim of understanding the burden of liver disease caused by each. Local initiatives to improve awareness of HCV and the association with unsanitary injections may lower or stabilize the epidemic over the next several years.[78]

Egypt has been reported to have the highest population-based prevalence of HCV, nearly 15% in individuals aged 15 to 59 years, and varies by region and age.[79] Prevalence in Egypt has been shown to increase with lower education level, greater poverty, and with the number of household inhabitants. Nearly half of people aged 50 to 59 years are infected, and modeled incidence rates project more than 500,000 new cases in Egypt each year, stemming from a rate of ~6.9 cases/1000 persons per year.[80] Transmission in Egypt has primarily been attributed to a national anti-schistosomiasis campaign from the 1920s to the 1980s during which 3- to 4-month regimens of parenteral injections were given to children and young adults in parasite-infested areas.[81,82] Although this practice was discontinued in the 1980s after the availability of oral anti-schistosomiasis therapies, iatrogenic transmission of HCV in Egypt remains a significant source of new infections. In 1 recent analysis of acute HCV in 4 Egyptian hospitals, hospital admissions were highly associated with risk of acute HCV.[83] Vaginal or cesarean delivery, gum surgery, intravenous infusions, and injections all independently increased risk. However, this study was among nondrug users. In a recent meta-analysis of risk factors of HCV in Egypt, El-Ghitany and colleagues[84] demonstrate that the highest odds of acquiring HCV are with IDU. Given the incidence and prevalence of HCV in Egypt and the health risks that infection poses, particularly superimposed on other infections such as schistosomiasis and endemic hepatitis viruses, prevention and treatment must be improved in this region.

Sub-Saharan Africa deserves discussion as it may contribute to as much as 20% of the global burden of HCV.[85] High rates of seropositivity have been reported, up to greater than 8% in Nigeria,[42] but wide variation in viremia has led to speculation of a high false-positive rate from immunoassays. However, a recent report has confirmed rates of viremia between 75% and 88% in a blood donor population in Ghana.[86] It is possible that pockets of high transmission exist as a result of specific risk factors such as home births, tribal scarring, and traditional (versus hospital) circumcision.

Overall, HCV epidemiology in developing nations is highly heterogeneous. Different countries have idiosyncratic histories that mediate the risk of HCV transmission (**Table 1**). Data are sparse and centralized screening, reporting, and treatments for

Table 1
Top risk factors for HCV and regions/populations most affected

Risk Factor	Region Most Affected	Population at Risk
Injection drug use	North America; Western, Central, and Eastern Europe; South Asia/South Pacific	US veterans, particularly from the Vietnam War (1970s) Injection drug users, especially youth
Unsafe/unprotected sexual practices	North America; Western, Central, and Eastern Europe; South Asia/South Pacific	MSM with or without HIV who practice unprotected sex, particularly with mucosal trauma Sex workers and their clients Rape victims, particularly in regions with high prevalence
Iatrogenic procedures (injections, surgery, intravenous lines, dental work)	Asia/Pacific, Sub-Saharan Africa	Persons undergoing procedures in Pakistan, India, Sub-Saharan Africa, and Western Africa
Contaminated blood products	Global, particularly Japan, United States, Italy, China	Those receiving blood products before ~1990 (United States, Japan, Europe) or ~2002 (China)
Parenteral antiparasitic treatment	Egypt, Nile River region	Individuals receiving injections for schistosomiasis
Home births, tribal customs such as scarring and circumcision	Sub-Saharan Africa	Persons born at home rather than in hospital; persons undergoing tribal customs involving scarring

HCV are largely absent. Diagnosis rates in countries such as India and the Slovak Republic are estimated to be as low as 5%, whereas in developed countries with registries such as Finland and Norway, most of their infected population has been diagnosed.[87] Current unrest in many of these parts of the world is likely to contribute to factors that facilitate HCV spread: iatrogenic transmission from trauma; IDU; unsanitary conditions caused by poor water and electric supply; overcrowding; and lack of financial resources and infrastructure. India and Egypt combined are projected to result in nearly half a million cases of end-stage liver disease or HCC by 2030 (**Fig. 4**).[88] Public health measures are imperative to stem the flow of HCV both within and from these countries and resource allocation will be required to screen, diagnose, and treat patients early in the infection for prevention of a larger health burden over the next 2 decades.

ACUTE HEPATITIS C VIRUS: AN EMERGING THREAT

Acute HCV is defined as the initial 6-month phase after infection. When symptoms occur during this phase, they are typically mild, fairly transient, and nonspecific. In contrast to this standard definition, the past several years have given rise to clusters of acute HCV outbreaks, particularly in HIV-positive MSM,[47,89–93] although HIV-negative MSM are also at risk.[94] In some cases, this acute infection has progressed rapidly through fibrosis stages, resulting in severe liver disease.[95,96] Transmission may be a result of unsafe sexual practices involving mucosal trauma or may be mixed with IDU.[97,98] Group sex and noninjection drug use, including nasal cocaine use, have also been implicated as risk factors.[99] Moreover, reinfection is possible; reinfection rates of nearly 30% have been reported.[100–102] Although increased risk for HCV infection in HIV-positive individuals[103] and more rapid progression of liver fibrosis in those with HCV/HIV has been known for some time,[104] the specter of acute HCV epidemics as a source of continued transmission and potential morbidity must be considered as an ongoing and important threat.

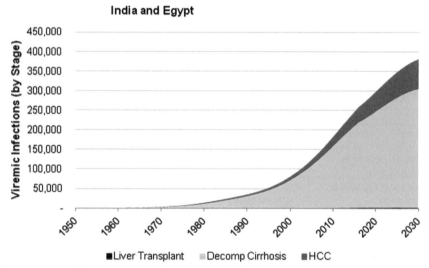

Fig. 4. Burden of liver transplant, decompensated cirrhosis, and hepatocellular carcinoma projected through 2030 in India and Egypt. (*From* Center for Disease Analysis (CDA). HCV Epidemiology – Summary Slides. Available at: http://www.centerforda.com/downloads. htm. Accessed July 9, 2015.)

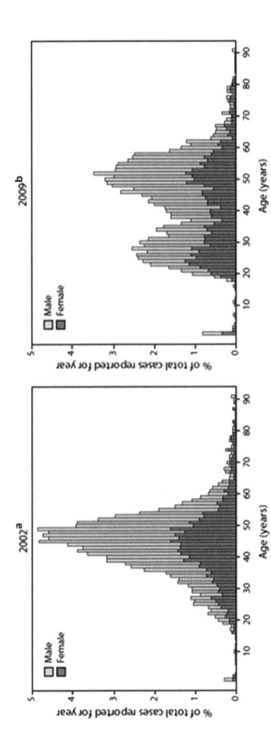

Fig. 5. Age distribution of newly reported confirmed cases of hepatitis C infection: Massachusetts, 2002 and 2009. (*A*) N = 6,281; excludes 35 cases with missing age or sex information. (*B*) N = 3,904; excludes 346 cases with missing age or sex information. (*From* Centers for Disease Control and Prevention (CDC). Hepatitis C virus infection among adolescents and young adults: Massachusetts, 2002–2009. MMWR Morb Mortal Wkly Rep 2011;60(17):539.)

In some areas of the United States, acute HCV is an emerging epidemic among young adults as a result of a significant shift in recreational drug use behavior that has seen the re-introduction of heroin into populations where this was previously uncommon.[105] This change from a unimodal to a bimodal age distribution (**Fig. 5**) has serious implications for current policies related to surveillance, including reliance on birth cohort testing alone for detection of HCV. Similar findings have been seen elsewhere in the Appalachian Ridge region, including Ohio and Kentucky.[106]

SUMMARY

The HCV is a leading cause of liver-related morbidity and mortality in the United States and other parts of the world. The epidemiology of the disease is highly variable between and within countries, and strategies to deal with HCV identification and treatment must be tailored to the geographic location and the political and economic environment of the region. Although great strides have been made in improving HCV transmission risk in blood supply products, new challenges related to changing patterns of disease incidence continue to require fresh evaluation and new approaches to disease prevention.

REFERENCES

1. Denniston MM, Jiles RB, Drobeniuc J, et al. Chronic hepatitis C virus infection in the United States, National Health and Nutrition Examination Survey 2003 to 2010. Ann Intern Med 2014;160(5):293–300.
2. Armstrong GL, Wasley A, Simard EP, et al. The prevalence of hepatitis C virus infection in the United States, 1999 through 2002. Ann Intern Med 2006; 144(10):705–14.
3. World Health Organization. Hepatitis C fact sheet. 2014. Available at: http://www.who.int/mediacentre/factsheets/fs164/en/. Accessed April 14, 2015.
4. Micallef JM, Kaldor JM, Dore GJ. Spontaneous viral clearance following acute hepatitis C infection: a systematic review of longitudinal studies. J Viral Hepat 2006;13(1):34–41.
5. Thein HH, Yi Q, Dore GJ, et al. Estimation of stage-specific fibrosis progression rates in chronic hepatitis C virus infection: a meta-analysis and meta-regression. Hepatology 2008;48(2):418–31.
6. Wong RJ, Aguilar M, Cheung R, et al. Nonalcoholic steatohepatitis is the second leading etiology of liver disease among adults awaiting liver transplantation in the United States. Gastroenterology 2015;148(3):547–55.
7. Lozano R, Naghavi M, Foreman K, et al. Global and regional mortality from 235 causes of death for 20 age groups in 1990 and 2010: a systematic analysis for the global burden of disease study 2010. Lancet 2012;380(9859):2095–128.
8. Alter HJ, Holland PV, Morrow AG, et al. Clinical and serological analysis of transfusion-associated hepatitis. Lancet 1975;2(7940):838–41.
9. Dienstag JL, Purcell HR, Alter HJ, et al. Non-A, non-B post-transfusion hepatitis. Lancet 1977;1(8011):560–2.
10. Hoofnagle JH, Gerety RJ, Tabor E, et al. Transmission of non-A, non-B hepatitis. Ann Intern Med 1977;87(1):14–20.
11. Aach RD, Szmuness W, Mosley JW, et al. Serum alanine aminotransferase of donors in relation to the risk of non-A,non-B hepatitis in recipients: the transfusion-transmitted viruses study. N Engl J Med 1981;304(17):989–94.
12. Villarejos VM, Visona KA, Eduarte CA, et al. Evidence for viral hepatitis other than type A or type B among persons in Costa Rica. N Engl J Med 1975; 293(26):1350–2.

13. Caredda F, d'Arminio Monforte A, Rossi E, et al. Non-A, non-B hepatitis in Milan. Lancet 1981;2(8236):48.

14. Hornbrook MC, Dodd RY, Jacobs P, et al. Reducing the incidence of non-A, non-B post-transfusion hepatitis by testing donor blood for alanine aminotransferase: economic considerations. N Engl J Med 1982;307(21):1315–21.

15. Seeff LB, Zimmerman HJ, Wright EC, et al. A randomized, double blind controlled trial of the efficacy of immune serum globulin for the prevention of post-transfusion hepatitis. A Veterans Administration cooperative study. Gastroenterology 1977;72(1):111–21.

16. Kim HC, Saidi P, Ackley AM, et al. Prevalence of type B and non-A, non-B hepatitis in hemophilia: relationship to chronic liver disease. Gastroenterology 1980; 79(6):1159–64.

17. Tabor E, Seeff LB, Gerety RJ. Chronic non-A, non-B hepatitis carrier state: transmissible agent documented in one patient over a six-year period. N Engl J Med 1980;303(3):140–3.

18. Choo QL, Kuo G, Weiner AJ, et al. Isolation of a cDNA clone derived from a blood-borne non-A, non-B viral hepatitis genome. Science 1989;244(4902): 359–62.

19. Takeuchi K, Kubo Y, Boonmar S, et al. Nucleotide sequence of core and envelope genes of the hepatitis C virus genome derived directly from human healthy carriers. Nucleic Acids Res 1990;18(15):4626.

20. Kuo G, Choo QL, Alter HJ, et al. An assay for circulating antibodies to a major etiologic virus of human non-A, non-B hepatitis. Science 1989; 244(4902):362–4.

21. Miyamura T, Saito I, Katayama T, et al. Detection of antibody against antigen expressed by molecularly cloned hepatitis C virus cDNA: application to diagnosis and blood screening for posttransfusion hepatitis. Proc Natl Acad Sci U S A 1990;87(3):983–7.

22. Weiner AJ, Kuo G, Bradley DW, et al. Detection of hepatitis C viral sequences in non-A, non-B hepatitis. Lancet 1990;335(8680):1–3.

23. Kato N, Yokosuka O, Omata M, et al. Detection of hepatitis C virus ribonucleic acid in the serum by amplification with polymerase chain reaction. J Clin Invest 1990;86(5):1764–7.

24. Sanchez-Tapias JM, Barrera JM, Costa J, et al. Hepatitis C virus infection in patients with nonalcoholic chronic liver disease. Ann Intern Med 1990;112(12): 921–4.

25. Brettler DB, Alter HJ, Dienstag JL, et al. Prevalence of hepatitis C virus antibody in a cohort of hemophilia patients. Blood 1990;76(1):254–6.

26. Troisi CL, Hollinger FB, Hoots WK, et al. A multicenter study of viral hepatitis in a United States hemophilic population. Blood 1993;81(2):412–8.

27. Makris M, Preston FE, Triger DR, et al. Hepatitis C antibody and chronic liver disease in haemophilia. Lancet 1990;335(8698):1117–9.

28. Eyster ME, Schaefer JH, Ragni MV, et al. Changing causes of death in Pennsylvania's hemophiliacs 1976 to 1991: impact of liver disease and acquired immunodeficiency syndrome. Blood 1992;79(9):2494–5.

29. Jeffers LJ, Perez GO, de Medina MD, et al. Hepatitis C infection in two urban hemodialysis units. Kidney Int 1990;38(2):320–2.

30. Ha SK, Park JH, Choi WC, et al. Hepatitis C infection in hemodialysis units. Korean J Intern Med 1990;5(2):83–6.

31. Bell J, Batey RG, Farrell GC, et al. Hepatitis C virus in intravenous drug users. Med J Aust 1990;153(5):274–6.

32. van den Hoek JA, van Haastrecht HJ, Goudsmit J, et al. Prevalence, incidence, and risk factors of hepatitis C virus infection among drug users in Amsterdam. J Infect Dis 1990;162(4):823–6.

33. Sanchez-Quijano A, Rey C, Aguado I, et al. Hepatitis C virus infection in sexually promiscuous groups. Eur J Clin Microbiol Infect Dis 1990;9(8):610–2.

34. Laurent C, Henzel D, Mulanga-Kabeya C, et al. Seroepidemiological survey of hepatitis C virus among commercial sex workers and pregnant women in Kinshasa, Democratic Republic of Congo. Int J Epidemiol 2001;30(4):872–7.

35. Hadush H, Gebre-Selassie S, Mihret A. Hepatitis C virus and human immunodeficiency virus coinfection among attendants of voluntary counseling and testing centre and HIV follow up clinics in Mekelle hospital. Pan Afr Med J 2013;14:107.

36. Alter MJ, Hadler SC, Judson FN, et al. Risk factors for acute non-A, non-B hepatitis in the United States and association with hepatitis C virus infection. JAMA 1990;264(17):2231–5.

37. Yu MC, Tong MJ, Coursaget P, et al. Prevalence of hepatitis B and C viral markers in black and white patients with hepatocellular carcinoma in the United States. J Natl Cancer Inst 1990;82(12):1038–41.

38. Di Bisceglie AM, Order SE, Klein JL, et al. The role of chronic viral hepatitis in hepatocellular carcinoma in the United States. Am J Gastroenterol 1991;86(3): 335–8.

39. Saito I, Miyamura T, Ohbayashi A, et al. Hepatitis C virus infection is associated with the development of hepatocellular carcinoma. Proc Natl Acad Sci U S A 1990;87(17):6547–9.

40. Soucie JM, Richardson LC, Evatt BL, et al. Risk factors for infection with HBV and HCV in a large cohort of hemophiliac males. Transfusion 2001;41(3): 338–43.

41. Stevens CE, Taylor PE, Pindyck J, et al. Epidemiology of hepatitis C virus. A preliminary study in volunteer blood donors. JAMA 1990;263(1):49–53.

42. Gower E, Estes C, Blach S, et al. Global epidemiology and genotype distribution of the hepatitis C virus infection. J Hepatol 2014;61(1 Suppl):S45–57.

43. Alter MJ. Epidemiology of hepatitis C virus infection. World J Gastroenterol 2007;13(17):2436–41.

44. Alter MJ, Kruszon-Moran D, Nainan OV, et al. The prevalence of hepatitis C virus infection in the United States, 1988 through 1994. N Engl J Med 1999;341(8): 556–62.

45. Backus LI, Belperio PS, Loomis TP, et al. Impact of race/ethnicity and gender on HCV screening and prevalence among U.S. veterans in Department of Veterans Affairs care. Am J Public Health 2014;104(Suppl 4):S555–61.

46. Chak E, Talal AH, Sherman KE, et al. Hepatitis C virus infection in USA: an estimate of true prevalence. Liver Int 2011;31(8):1090–101.

47. Williams IT, Bell BP, Kuhnert W, et al. Incidence and transmission patterns of acute hepatitis C in the United States, 1982-2006. Arch Intern Med 2011; 171(3):242–8.

48. Suryaprasad AG, White JZ, Xu F, et al. Emerging epidemic of hepatitis C virus infections among young nonurban persons who inject drugs in the United States, 2006-2012. Clin Infect Dis 2014;59(10):1411–9.

49. Tanaka Y, Hanada K, Mizokami M, et al. A comparison of the molecular clock of hepatitis C virus in the United States and Japan predicts that hepatocellular carcinoma incidence in the United States will increase over the next two decades. Proc Natl Acad Sci U S A 2002;99(24):15584–9.

50. Tanaka J, Koyama T, Mizui M, et al. Total numbers of undiagnosed carriers of hepatitis C and B viruses in Japan estimated by age- and area-specific prevalence on the national scale. Intervirology 2011;54(4):185–95.
51. Chung H, Ueda T, Kudo M. Changing trends in hepatitis C infection over the past 50 years in Japan. Intervirology 2010;53(1):39–43.
52. Toyoda H, Kumada T, Takaguchi K, et al. Changes in hepatitis C virus genotype distribution in Japan. Epidemiol Infect 2014;142(12):2624–8.
53. Tanaka H, Imai Y, Hiramatsu N, et al. Declining incidence of hepatocellular carcinoma in Osaka, Japan, from 1990 to 2003. Ann Intern Med 2008;148(11): 820–6.
54. Palmateer N, Hutchinson S, McAllister G, et al. Risk of transmission associated with sharing drug injecting paraphernalia: analysis of recent hepatitis C virus (HCV) infection using cross-sectional survey data. J Viral Hepat 2014;21(1): 25–32.
55. Hahne SJ, Veldhuijzen IK, Wiessing L, et al. Infection with hepatitis B and C virus in Europe: a systematic review of prevalence and cost-effectiveness of screening. BMC Infect Dis 2013;13:181.
56. Spada E, Mele A, Mariano A, et al, SEIEVA Collaborating Group. Risk factors for and incidence of acute hepatitis C after the achievement of blood supply safety in Italy: results from the national surveillance system. J Med Virol 2013;85(3): 433–40.
57. Vermehren J, Schlosser B, Domke D, et al. High prevalence of anti-HCV antibodies in two metropolitan emergency departments in Germany: a prospective screening analysis of 28,809 patients. PLoS One 2012;7(7):e41206.
58. Hope V, Parry JV, Marongui A, et al. Hepatitis C infection among recent initiates to injecting in England 2000-2008: is a national hepatitis C action plan making a difference? J Viral Hepat 2012;19(1):55–64.
59. Flisiak R, Halota W, Horban A, et al. Prevalence and risk factors of HCV infection in Poland. Eur J Gastroenterol Hepatol 2011;23(12):1213–7.
60. Wiessing L, Ferri M, Grady B, et al. Hepatitis C virus infection epidemiology among people who inject drugs in Europe: a systematic review of data for scaling up treatment and prevention. PLoS One 2014;9(7):e103345.
61. Cornberg M, Razavi HA, Alberti A, et al. A systematic review of hepatitis C virus epidemiology in Europe, Canada and Israel. Liver Int 2011;31(Suppl 2):30–60.
62. Paquet C, Babes VT, Drucker J, et al. Viral hepatitis in Bucharest. Bull World Health Organ 1993;71(6):781–6.
63. The Kirby Institute. HIV, viral hepatitis and sexually transmissible infections in Australia annual surveillance report 2014. Sydney (Australia): The Kirby Institute, UNSW; 2014. p. 2052.
64. Maher L, Jalaludin B, Chant KG, et al. Incidence and risk factors for hepatitis C seroconversion in injecting drug users in Australia. Addiction 2006;101(10): 1499–508.
65. Topp L, Day C, Degenhardt L. Changes in patterns of drug injection concurrent with a sustained reduction in the availability of heroin in Australia. Drug Alcohol Depend 2003;70(3):275–86.
66. Song Y, Bian Y, Petzold M, et al. Prevalence and trend of major transfusion-transmissible infections among blood donors in Western China, 2005 through 2010. PLoS One 2014;9(4):e94528.
67. Huang P, Zhu LG, Zhai XJ, et al. Hepatitis C virus infection and risk factors in the general population: a large community-based study in Eastern China, 2011-2012. Epidemiol Infect 2015;1–10 [Epub ahead of print].

68. Kuang YQ, Yan J, Li Y, et al. Molecular epidemiologic characterization of a clustering HCV infection caused by inappropriate medical care in Heyuan city of Guangdong, China. PLoS One 2013;8(12):e82304.

69. Piao HX, Yang AT, Sun YM, et al. Increasing newly diagnosed rate and changing risk factors of HCV in Yanbian Prefecture, a high endemic area in China. PLoS One 2014;9(1):e86190.

70. Dong Y, Qiu C, Xia X, et al. Hepatitis B virus and hepatitis C virus infection among HIV-1-infected injection drug users in Dali, China: prevalence and infection status in a cross-sectional study. Arch Virol 2015;160(4):929–36.

71. Xiaoli W, Lirong W, Xueliang W, et al. Risk factors of hepatitis C virus infection in drug users from eleven methadone maintenance treatment clinics in Xi'an, China. Hepat Mon 2014;14(11):e19601.

72. Zhou W, Wang X, Zhou S, et al. Hepatitis C seroconversion in methadone maintenance treatment programs in Wuhan, China. Addiction 2015;110(5):796–802.

73. Chen Y, Shen Z, Morano JP, et al. Bridging the epidemic: a comprehensive analysis of prevalence and correlates of HIV, hepatitis C, and syphilis, and infection among female sex workers in Guangxi province, China. PLoS One 2015;10(2): e0115311.

74. Sievert W, Altraif I, Razavi HA, et al. A systematic review of hepatitis C virus epidemiology in Asia, Australia and Egypt. Liver Int 2011;31(Suppl 2):61–80.

75. Puri P, Anand AC, Saraswat VA, et al. Consensus statement of HCV task force of the Indian National Association for Study of the Liver (INASL). Part I: status report of HCV infection in India. J Clin Exp Hepatol 2014;4(2):106–16.

76. Umar M, Bushra HT, Ahmad M, et al. Hepatitis C in Pakistan: a review of available data. Hepat Mon 2010;10(3):205–14.

77. Centers for Disease Control and Prevention (CDC). Establishment of a viral hepatitis surveillance system–Pakistan, 2009-2011. MMWR Morb Mortal Wkly Rep 2011;60(40):1385–90.

78. Altaf A, Shah SA, Shaikh K, et al. Lessons learned from a community based intervention to improve injection safety in Pakistan. BMC Res Notes 2013;6:159.

79. Guerra J, Garenne M, Mohamed MK, et al. HCV burden of infection in Egypt: results from a nationwide survey. J Viral Hepat 2012;19(8):560–7.

80. Miller FD, Abu-Raddad LJ. Evidence of intense ongoing endemic transmission of hepatitis C virus in Egypt. Proc Natl Acad Sci U S A 2010;107(33):14757–62.

81. Frank C, Mohamed MK, Strickland GT, et al. The role of parenteral antischistosomal therapy in the spread of hepatitis C virus in Egypt. Lancet 2000; 355(9207):887–91.

82. Derbala M, Chandra P, Amer A, et al. Reexamination of the relationship between the prevalence of hepatitis C virus and parenteral antischistosomal therapy among Egyptians resident in Qatar. Clin Exp Gastroenterol 2014;7:427–33.

83. Mohsen A, Bernier A, LeFouler L, et al. Hepatitis C virus acquisition among Egyptians: analysis of a 10-year surveillance of acute hepatitis C. Trop Med Int Health 2015;20(1):89–97.

84. El-Ghitany EM, Abdel Wahab MM, Abd El-Wahab EW, et al. A comprehensive hepatitis C virus risk factors meta-analysis (1989-2013): do they differ in Egypt? Liver Int 2015;35(2):489–501.

85. Layden JE, Phillips R, Opare-Sem O, et al. Hepatitis C in sub-Saharan Africa: urgent need for attention. Open Forum Infect Dis 2014;1(2):ofu065.

86. Layden JE, Phillips RO, Owusu-Ofori S, et al. High frequency of active HCV infection among seropositive cases in West Africa and evidence for multiple transmission pathways. Clin Infect Dis 2015;60(7):1033–41.

87. Hatzakis A, Chulanov V, Gadano AC, et al. The present and future disease burden of hepatitis C virus (HCV) infections with today's treatment paradigm - volume 2. J Viral Hepat 2015;22(Suppl 1):26–45.
88. Center for Disease Analysis. Hep C epidemiology–summary slides. 2015. Available at: http://www.centerforda.com/downloads.htm. Accessed April 7, 2015.
89. van de Laar TJ, Matthews GV, Prins M, et al. Acute hepatitis C in HIV-infected men who have sex with men: an emerging sexually transmitted infection. AIDS 2010;24(12):1799–812.
90. Obermeier M, Ingiliz P, Weitner L, et al. Acute hepatitis C in persons infected with the human immunodeficiency virus (HIV): the "real-life setting" proves the concept. Eur J Med Res 2011;16(5):237–42.
91. Lambers FA, Prins M, Thomas X, et al. Alarming incidence of hepatitis C virus re-infection after treatment of sexually acquired acute hepatitis C virus infection in HIV-infected MSM. AIDS 2011;25(17):F21–7.
92. Urbanus AT, van de Laar TJ, Stolte IG, et al. Hepatitis C virus infections among HIV-infected men who have sex with men: an expanding epidemic. AIDS 2009; 23(12):F1–7.
93. Centers for Disease Control and Prevention (CDC). Sexual transmission of hepatitis C virus among HIV-infected men who have sex with men–New York city, 2005-2010. MMWR Morb Mortal Wkly Rep 2011;60(28):945–50.
94. McFaul K, Maghlaoui A, Nzuruba M, et al. Acute hepatitis C infection in HIV-negative men who have sex with men. J Viral Hepat 2015;22(6):535–8.
95. Fierer DS, Uriel AJ, Carriero DC, et al. Liver fibrosis during an outbreak of acute hepatitis C virus infection in HIV-infected men: a prospective cohort study. J Infect Dis 2008;198(5):683–6.
96. Osinusi A, Kleiner D, Wood B, et al. Rapid development of advanced liver fibrosis after acquisition of hepatitis C infection during primary HIV infection. AIDS Patient Care STDS 2009;23(6):403–6.
97. Ward C, Lee V. Experience of acute hepatitis C and HIV co-infection in an inner city clinic in the UK. J Int AIDS Soc 2014;17(4 Suppl 3):19639.
98. Orsetti E, Staffolani S, Gesuita R, et al. Changing characteristics and risk factors of patients with and without incident HCV infection among HIV-infected individuals. Infection 2013;41(5):987–90.
99. Schmidt AJ, Rockstroh JK, Vogel M, et al. Trouble with bleeding: risk factors for acute hepatitis C among HIV-positive gay men from Germany–a case-control study. PLoS One 2011;6(3):e17781.
100. Vanhommerig JW, Thomas XV, van der Meer JT, et al. Hepatitis C virus (HCV) antibody dynamics following acute HCV infection and reinfection among HIV-infected men who have sex with men. Clin Infect Dis 2014; 59(12):1678–85.
101. Ingiliz P, Krznaric I, Stellbrink HJ, et al. Multiple hepatitis C virus (HCV) reinfections in HIV-positive men who have sex with men: no influence of HCV genotype switch or interleukin-28B genotype on spontaneous clearance. HIV Med 2014; 15(6):355–61.
102. Martin TC, Martin NK, Hickman M, et al. Hepatitis C virus reinfection incidence and treatment outcome among HIV-positive MSM. AIDS 2013;27(16): 2551–7.
103. Sherman KE, Rouster SD, Chung RT, et al. Hepatitis C virus prevalence among patients infected with human immunodeficiency virus: a cross-sectional analysis of the US adult AIDS Clinical Trials Group. Clin Infect Dis 2002;34(6): 831–7.

104. Benhamou Y, Bochet M, Di Martino V, et al. Liver fibrosis progression in human immunodeficiency virus and hepatitis C virus coinfected patients. The Multivirc Group. Hepatology 1999;30(4):1054–8.
105. Centers for Disease Control and Prevention (CDC). Hepatitis C virus infection among adolescents and young adults: Massachusetts, 2002-2009. MMWR Morb Mortal Wkly Rep 2011;60(17):537–41.
106. Jennings CL, Sherman KE. Hepatitis C and HIV co-infection: new drugs in practice and in the pipeline. Curr HIV/AIDS Rep 2012;9(3):231–7.

Natural History of Hepatitis C

Shilpa Lingala, MD, Marc G. Ghany, MD, MHSc*

KEYWORDS

- Natural history • Hepatitis C virus • Chronic hepatitis C • Fibrosis • Cirrhosis
- Decompensated liver disease

KEY POINTS

- The incidence of chronic hepatitis C is declining in the United States but rates of cirrhosis and hepatocellular carcinoma are projected to increase over the next decade.
- Approximately 20% to 25% of patients with chronic hepatitis C progress to cirrhosis over 25 to 30 years.
- The outcome of chronic hepatitis C is highly variable and influenced by many host, viral, and environmental factors, many of which cannot be modified.

INTRODUCTION

Hepatitis C virus (HCV) infection is an important cause of cirrhosis and hepatocellular carcinoma (HCC) worldwide.[1] It is also a common cause of chronic liver disease in the United States and the leading indication for liver transplantation in the adult US population. The incidence of chronic hepatitis C (CHC) is declining in the United States, but rates of cirrhosis and HCC are expected to increase.[2] Recent data estimate that approximately 1% of the noninstitutionalized US population have chronic HCV infection, corresponding to 2.7 million persons.[3] HCV is primarily transmitted through parental exposure to blood and other bodily fluids. After exposure, an acute hepatitis with jaundice occurs in about 20% of persons, although fulminant hepatitis is rare, occurring in less than 1% of persons. In most cases, the acute infection goes unnoticed. Spontaneous resolution may occur in 15% to 45% of persons and usually

Disclosures: The authors have nothing to disclose.
Financial Support: This work was supported by the Intramural Program of the National Institute of Diabetes and Digestive and Kidney Diseases, National Institutes of Health (ZIA DK075009 09).
Liver Diseases Branch, National Institute of Diabetes and Digestive and Kidney Diseases, National Institutes of Health, Building 10, Room 9B-16, 10 Center Drive, MSC 1800, Bethesda, MD 20892-1800, USA
* Corresponding author. Liver Diseases Branch, National Institute of Diabetes and Digestive and Kidney Diseases, National Institutes of Health, Building 10, Room 9B-16, 10 Center Drive, MSC 1800, Bethesda, MD 20892-1800.
E-mail address: marcg@intra.niddk.nih.gov

occurs in the first 6 months of exposure. The remainder develop a chronic hepatitis that has an unpredictable course. Approximately 20% to 30% of persons with chronic hepatitis progress to cirrhosis over a 25-year to 30-year period. The natural history study of CHC is greatly influenced by host, viral, and environmental factors, most of which are not modifiable (**Table 1**).[4] In this article, the natural history of CHC is reviewed and the factors that influence its outcome are discussed.

ACUTE HEPATITIS C

The incidence of acute hepatitis C had been declining in the United States but a marked increase in cases was noted between 2010 and 2013, from 850 in 2010 to 2138 in 2013, representing a 152% increase in cases of acute hepatitis C. This sharp increase has been attributed to an increase in injection drug use among the suburban population in the Eastern and Midwestern states.

The most common symptoms of acute hepatitis C include jaundice, nausea, abdominal pain, and flulike symptoms. In most individuals, HCV RNA is usually detectable within 2 weeks and anti-HCV antibodies within 12 weeks of exposure to HCV. Serum alanine aminotransferase (ALT) levels usually increase within 8 to 10 weeks, with a peak ALT level of 10 to 20 times the upper limit of normal. Serum HCV RNA levels may fluctuate widely during the acute phase and even become negative transiently, only to reappear again. This finding is seen only in the acute phase and may be a clinical clue to the diagnosis of acute HCV infection. Spontaneous resolution occurs in 15% to 25% of individuals and may be up to 45% in persons who present with jaundice, children, and young women. Higher rates of spontaneous clearance were also observed in persons with certain polymorphisms (the rs12979860-C,[5] rs8099917-T,[6] and the ss469415590 TT[7]) near to the IL28B gene (interferon λ [IFN-λ]). HLA class II alleles may play a role in spontaneous clearance. Less genetic diversity of the viral E1 and E2 envelope genes was observed in individuals with spontaneous recovery compared with those who progressed to chronic infection.[8]

NATURAL HISTORY OF CHRONIC HEPATITIS C

CHC is defined as persistence of HCV RNA in the blood for more than 6 months after the onset of acute infection. About 55% to 85% of patients with acute hepatitis C transition to CHC (**Fig. 1**). Once the infection becomes chronic, spontaneous resolution is

Table 1
Factors that affect the natural history of CHC

Host Factors	Viral Factors	Environmental Factors
Age at infection	Viral load	Alcohol
Gender	Genotype	Smoking
Race	Coinfection with HBV	Cannabis use
Obesity	Coinfection with HIV	Caffeine
Steatosis	—	—
Insulin resistance	—	—
Diabetes	—	—
Genetics	—	—
ALT levels	—	—
Exercise	—	—

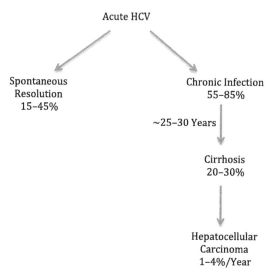

Fig. 1. Natural history of hepatitis C virus infection. After exposure to hepatitis C virus, an acute hepatitis ensues. About 20% present with jaundice but most are asymptomatic. Spontaneous resolution occurs in 15% to 45%. The remainder develop a chronic hepatitis with a variable course. Cirrhosis develops in approximately 20% to 30% of patients over a 25-year to 30-year period. Once cirrhosis develops, patients are at risk for hepatic decompensation, hepatocellular carcinoma, and liver-related death.

rare. CHC can subsequently lead to progressive fibrosis and cirrhosis, end-stage liver disease, and HCC (see **Fig. 1**).

It is estimated that 20% to 30% patients with CHC progress to cirrhosis. However, this rate is highly variable and dependent on the methodology used to define the natural history of the disease, whether prospective, retrospective, or retrospective-prospective study designs, and the population studied. This factor was highlighted in an analysis of 57 studies undertaken to estimate progression to cirrhosis. Studies were broadly classified as those from tertiary-care liver clinics, posttransfusion cohorts, blood donors, and community-based cohorts. Estimates of progression to cirrhosis after 20 years of CHC varied widely from a high of 24% for posttransfusion cohorts and 22% for tertiary-care liver clinics, to a low of 7% for community-based cohorts and 4% for blood donors.[9] Selection bias, recall bias, and short duration of follow-up probably account for differences in the estimated rate. Community-based cohort studies are likely to provide the best evidence for estimating disease progression at a population level.

Monitoring progression of fibrosis is another way of estimating the outcome of CHC. Because progression of fibrosis is the precursor of cirrhosis, following its progression should reflect the course of the disease. Fibrosis stage was shown to be a good predictor of development of cirrhosis and clinical outcomes, need for liver transplantation, and liver-related death, confirming the importance of fibrosis as a surrogate for outcome of CHC.[10–12] Cross-sectional biopsy studies estimate a period of 30 years to develop cirrhosis. However, because fibrosis progression is unlikely to be linear, performing repeated liver biopsies in patients should provide a more accurate determination of the rate of progression of fibrosis. Paired liver biopsy studies suggest a time to cirrhosis of 30 to 40 years.[11,13–15]

NATURAL HISTORY OF CIRRHOSIS

The development of cirrhosis is an important milestone in the natural history of CHC. Once cirrhosis develops, patients are at risk for decompensation, including the development of ascites, spontaneous bacterial peritonitis, variceal hemorrhage, and hepatic encephalopathy. Occurrence of any of these events heralds an increased risk of death or need for liver transplantation. Information on the natural history of hepatitis C after development of cirrhosis has been mostly derived from studies conducted at tertiary referral centers, which may not be representative of all persons with CHC. With this caveat, survival of patients with cirrhosis in the short-term and medium-term is good. Five-year survival ranges from 85% to 91% with a 10-year survival of 60% to 79%. The rate of clinical decompensation is approximately 2% to 5% per year and the development of HCC 1% to 4% per year.[16]

The HALT-C (Hepatitis C Antiviral Long-Term Treatment Against Cirrhosis) trial provided important data on the natural history of patients with advanced fibrosis and cirrhosis.[17] The study treated previous IFN nonresponders with 6 months of peginterferon and ribavirin. Failures to this intervention were then randomized to low-dose peginterferon or observation for the next 3.5 years. After 4 years of follow-up, outcomes occurred at a similar rate between the treated group (34.1%) and the control group (33.8%). The most common clinical outcome was an increase of 2 or more points in the Child-Turcotte-Pugh score (documented on 2 consecutive visits), which occurred in 109 patients (10.4%). Ascites was the most common clinical decompensation event and occurred in 59 patients (5.6%). HCC occurred in 29 patients (2.8%): 13 (2.1%) in the patients without and 16 (3.7%) in those with cirrhosis. Fifty-three patients (5.0%) died, 31 in the treatment group (15 of liver-related causes) and 22 in the control group (12 of liver-related causes). At 3.8 years, the overall death rate was 6.6% in patients who received peginterferon and 4.6% in control patients.

Once decompensation develops, there is an increased risk of death or need for liver transplant. One study followed 200 patients with HCV-related cirrhosis without known HCC after hospitalization for their first hepatic decompensation.[18] During a mean follow-up of approximately 3 years, HCC developed in 33 (16.5%) patients, and death occurred in 85 patients (42.5%). The probability of survival after diagnosis of decompensated cirrhosis was 82% and 51% at 1 and 5 years, respectively.[18] Development of hepatic encephalopathy or ascites as the first hepatic decompensation event was associated with a lower survival rate.

FACTORS THAT INFLUENCE THE OUTCOME OF CHRONIC HEPATITIS C
Host Factors

Age at infection
Age plays a major role in the progression of fibrosis. Multiple studies have shown that older age at infection was associated with more rapid progression of fibrosis.[19–22] In 1 study, 9 host, viral, and environmental factors were correlated with fibrosis progression among 2235 untreated patients who underwent liver biopsy. Fibrosis progression per year was defined as the ratio between fibrosis stage in Metavir units and duration of infection in years. Older age at infection greater than 40 years was independently associated with a faster rate of fibrosis progression.[19]

The reasons for the age-related differences in fibrosis progression are not clear. Alteration in physiologic or immunologic status with increasing age may be important. For example, a decline in liver volume and liver blood flow with aging or decreased immunologic response might contribute to fibrogenesis or fibrinolysis.[16,23] Alternatively, older individuals may have a greater prevalence of or exposure to factors associated with fibrosis progression. Based on these data, persons older than 50 years should be monitored more closely for disease progression and considered for treatment earlier in the course of their infection.

Gender

Many studies have shown that women have a higher rate of spontaneous resolution of acute HCV infection.[24–28] Among young women who acquired hepatitis C from receipt of contaminated Rh immune globulin, 45% cleared the infection spontaneously. Similarly, studies of acute hepatitis C among drug users have shown that spontaneous clearance was higher among women compared with men.[29–32]

Gender also influences the outcome of chronic infection. Men have a higher risk of progression to advanced liver disease, cirrhosis, and HCC when compared with women. Differences in sex hormones have been proposed to explain the gender differences in the progression of the disease. Higher serum testosterone levels were shown to be associated with greater severity of fibrosis. For each 1-ng/mL increase in total serum testosterone, there was a 25% increase in risk of advanced fibrosis.[33] In contrast, estrogen has been proposed to play a protective role in women.[34] In cross-sectional studies, postmenopausal women (with presumed reduced estrogen levels) had higher rates of fibrosis progression compared with premenopausal women, and nulliparous women had higher rates of fibrosis progression compared with multiparous women.[35] In vitro data suggest that estrogen can modify extracellular matrix production and attenuate hepatic stellate cell activation, resulting in less collagen production.

Race

CHC is approximately 3 times more common among non-Hispanic blacks compared with non-Hispanic whites.[3] The prevalence of hepatitis C was similar among Latinos and non-Hispanic whites. African Americans were more likely to be infected with genotype 1,[36–38] have lower baseline serum ALT levels,[36–38] less piecemeal necrosis,[36–38] and less fibrosis,[36–38] but higher rates of HCC.[39] Latinos were reported to have more severe necroinflammatory activity compared with non-Hispanic whites and a higher prevalence of cirrhosis and HCC compared with African Americans and non-Hispanic whites.[40–42] A higher prevalence of the metabolic syndrome, insulin resistance (IR), and hepatic steatosis as well as genetic differences among Hispanics are likely important contributing factors.[41]

African Americans and Latinos have lower response rates to IFN-based therapy compared with non-Hispanic whites.[43–45] A lower prevalence of the favorable IL28b C allele among African Americans and Latinos compared with whites and Asians partially accounts for the lower response rates.[5] Differences in HLA class II alleles influencing host immune response to the virus may also contribute to the racial differences in viral clearance.[46,47]

Obesity

Obesity, defined as a body mass index (BMI, calculated as weight in kilograms divided by the square of height in meters) greater than 30 kg/m^2, is an independent risk factor for fibrosis progression and development of cirrhosis. In 1 study, patients undergoing liver biopsy were classified as rapid or nonrapid progressors based on a fibrosis progression rate of greater than 0.2 fibrosis units/y. It was shown that a BMI greater than 25 kg/m^2 was predictive of rapid fibrosis progression.[48] Steatohepatitis associated with obesity and increasing circulating insulin levels are believed to be contributing factors responsible for fibrosis progression in CHC irrespective of the genotype.[49] Obesity is also found to be a risk factor for nonresponse to antiviral therapy independent of steatosis, genotype, and the presence of cirrhosis. Obese individuals have an 80% lower chance of a sustained response to IFN-based therapy compared with normal or overweight patients.[50]

Steatosis

Hepatic steatosis is a common finding among the general population, ranging from 10% to 24%. Using the presence of fat on ultrasonography as a surrogate for steatosis, the prevalence of steatosis was 21% in NHANES-3 (the third National Health and Nutrition Examination Survey) study of the noninstitutionalized US population.[51] The prevalence of steatosis is approximately 2 to 3 times more common in persons with CHC, ranging from 42% to 70%.[52–56] The cause of steatosis in patients with hepatitis C is multifactorial, resulting from metabolic derangements in the host because of obesity but also because of HCV infection itself. Hepatic steatosis has been suggested to promote the development of fibrosis and hasten progression to cirrhosis, increase the risk for HCC, and lower the response to IFN-based therapy. Nonalcoholic steatohepatitis (NASH) represents a more advanced form of steatosis and has been associated with progressive liver disease and cirrhosis. Therefore, coexistent NASH and CHC may result in more rapid progression of liver disease. Given these adverse consequences of steatosis and NASH, patients with hepatitis C should try to maintain an ideal body weight.

Insulin resistance/diabetes

Diabetes mellitus is a common comorbidity in patients with CHC, ranging from 24% to 62%.[57,58] The development of IR/diabetes in patients with CHC is complex and seems to be related to presence of the metabolic syndrome as well as a result of the viral infection, both of which may independently lead to the development of cirrhosis. Two meta-analyses[59,60] have suggested a strong association between CHC and the development of IR. However, some studies have found no association between CHC and prediabetes or diabetes. Rather an association was found with increased ALT and γ glutamyl transpeptidase levels, suggesting that inflammation per se may lead to IR and diabetes.[61] Eradication of HCV has been associated with improvement and even reversal of IR[62–64] and diabetes.[65]

IR and diabetes are associated with faster progression of fibrosis, increased risk of cirrhosis and its complications (including HCC), and lower response to therapy in patients with CHC. In 1 study of patients with cirrhosis, the presence of diabetes was an independent risk factor for decompensation, liver transplantation, and death. A population-based study from Taiwan reported that new-onset diabetes was an independent predictor of cirrhosis and hepatic decompensation. These findings suggest but do not prove that better control of diabetes or IR could lead to better outcomes among patients with CHC, including those with cirrhosis.

Genetics

Although several host, viral, and environmental factors have been linked with outcome of CHC, they do not completely explain the variable outcome of the disease. A strong host immune response against HCV favors viral clearance. Therefore, variability in genes involved in the immune response may contribute to viral clearance. In a landmark study, a genetic polymorphism near the IL28B gene, encoding IFN-λ3, was shown to be strongly associated with response to treatment with IFN and spontaneous clearance of HCV.[5] The C allele of rs12979860 and G allele of rs8099917 were associated with an almost 2-fold change in treatment-related clearance of HCV compared with the T allele at both loci.[5] This observation was true for individuals of both European and African ancestry. In another study of 1015 patients with chronic infection and 347 who spontaneously cleared the infection, the minor allele (G) of the single nuclear polymorphism at position rs8099917 was associated with a greater than 2-fold progression to chronic HCV infection.[66] The IL28B CC genotype was also shown to be associated with greater hepatic necroinflammation, higher ALT level, and worse clinical outcomes in patients with CHC.[67] Other genetic factors also play a role in outcome of HCV infection but are beyond the scope of this review.

Alanine aminotransferase levels

In population studies, increasing ALT levels were shown to be associated with a progressive increase in death from all causes and in particular liver-related death.[68] Persistently normal ALT levels are found in approximately 20% to 30% of patients with chronic hepatitis.[69,70] Patients with persistently normal ALT levels are more likely to have mild liver fibrosis on liver biopsy. In a review of 23 studies with more than 1100 patients, 80% of patients with a normal ALT level had mild fibrosis, whereas only 20% had advanced fibrosis.[71] In addition, patients with normal ALT levels progress at a slower rate compared with those with increased ALT levels.[72–75]

In cross-sectional biopsy studies, serum ALT level was not predictive of severity of fibrosis. However, in paired liver biopsies, increased ALT levels were associated with progression of fibrosis.[11,13,14] Serum ALT level was not predictive of development of clinical outcomes; however, the aspartate aminotransferase(AST)/ALT ratio was predictive.[76] Patients with increased serum ALT levels are also found to have increased risk for HCC. In a large Taiwanese study, the cumulative risk for HCC was 1.7% for ALT levels 15 U/L or lower and increased to 4.2% for levels between 15 and 45 U/L and to 13.8% for ALT levels 45 U/L or greater.[77] Therefore, monitoring of ALT levels is useful in managing CHC.

Exercise

Weight loss and exercise are known to cause reduction in steatosis, obesity, diabetes, and IR, leading to improvement in serum ALT levels and fibrosis, despite the persistence of the HCV RNA. The potential benefits of exercise in patients with CHC were shown in a study of 16 obese patients with CHC. Dietary intervention and increased exercise were associated with reduction in BMI, improved insulin sensitivity and serum ALT and AST levels, suggesting that dietary and exercise intervention may improve hepatic and metabolic status in obese IR CHC.[78] The intensity and type of exercise may be important to derive the beneficial effects. High-intensity aerobic exercise training was shown to improve hepatic enzymes and also psychological well-being in patients with CHC. Aerobic exercise has also been shown to improve psychological well-being and quality of life in overweight and obese patients with CHC.[79,80] Therefore, recommending exercise should be an important component in the management of CHC.

VIRAL FACTORS
Hepatitis C Virus RNA Level

Unlike human immunodeficiency virus (HIV) infection, there is little evidence to support the notion that HCV viral load affects outcome of CHC. The viral load observed among persons with CHC usually ranges from 10^4 to 10^8 copies/mL, with an average HCV RNA level of approximately 10^6 copies/mL.[81] HCV RNA levels tend to remain relatively stable when serial determinations were made over time and rarely fluctuate above or below 1 log of the baseline. HCV viral load does not differ among viral genotypes.[82] Most studies have shown no correlation between HCV RNA level and histologic outcome.[83–85] Therefore, there is no role for serially assessing viral load in a patient.

Viral load is predictive of response to treatment, with lower viral load being associated with higher response rates.

Hepatitis C Virus Quasispecies/Genotype

The HCV polymerase lacks proofreading capacity, as a result many errors are introduced during replication. Consequently, the virus circulates as a viral swarm or quasispecies. Viral quasispecies were shown to affect spontaneous viral clearance.[8] Lower genetic diversity of the envelope region was associated with a higher rate of spontaneous clearance.

Six major genotypes have been identified based on a sequence divergence of 30% among isolates. HCV genotypes have a geographic distribution, with genotype 1 being the most common worldwide, accounting for 46% of all HCV cases, approximately one-third of which are in East Asia. Genotype 3 is the next most prevalent globally, at 30%. Genotypes 2, 4, and 6 are responsible for a total 23% of all cases, and the remaining cases comprise genotype 5.[86] The association between HCV genotype and disease progression is not clear. A meta-analysis of 16 studies[87] suggested that HCV genotype 3 was associated with accelerated fibrosis progression in single biopsy studies but not paired biopsy studies. It is possible that steatosis associated with genotype 3, an independent predictor of fibrosis progression, might be the cause of the fibrosis progression rather than the HCV genotype 3 itself. The most important clinical usefulness of HCV genotype is as a predictor of response to therapy. The development of HCV regimens with pangenotypic activity may preclude the need for genotyping altogether.

Coinfection with Hepatitis B Virus

HCV shares similar routes of transmission to hepatitis B virus (HBV), so coinfection with these viruses is not uncommon. The prevalence of HBV/HCV coinfection is about 2% to 10%, but there is significant geographic variation.[88–95] Most studies of HBV-HCV-coinfected patients show that usually only a single virus predominates, although which one was unpredictable.[96,97] Several studies have shown that coinfected patients are at substantially higher risk for cirrhosis, HCC, and overall mortality compared with HCV-monoinfected patients. In a large US cohort study, a significantly increased risk of cirrhosis ($\sim$89% increase), HCC ($\sim$112% increase), and death ($\sim$62% increase) were seen in HBV/HCV-coinfected patients who were HBV DNA positive compared with monoinfected patients, whereas the absence of HBV replication was associated with a clinical course similar to that of HCV-monoinfected patients.[98] Therefore, patients with HBV and HCV coinfection require close monitoring for the development of cirrhosis and may warrant more intensive HCC screening.

Coinfection with Human Immunodeficiency Virus

HCV and HIV share similar routes of transmission. The overall burden of HIV/HCV coinfection is estimated at 4 to 5 million people worldwide.[99] The prevalence of HIV/HCV varies geographically and by mode of transmission. The highest rates are seen in injection drug users and men who have sex with men. HCV infection is not associated with an increased rate of AIDS-defining events or deaths.[100] However, HIV has several adverse consequences on the outcome of HCV infection. HIV has been shown to increase the rate of chronic HCV infection,[101,102] to increase HCV RNA levels,[81,101,103,104] and is associated with faster progression of fibrosis and development of cirrhosis. Response rates to IFN-based treatment are also lower among coinfected persons. Before highly active antiretroviral therapy (HAART) therapy, most coinfected individuals died of complications of HIV infection. However, in the post-HAART era, HCV-related liver disease (primarily end-stage liver disease) is a major cause of death among coinfected persons.[105,106] HIV has been shown to accelerate progression of fibrosis among persons with CHC, including those with persistently normal ALT levels.[107,108] Approximately one-third of persons with HIV-HCV coinfection progress to cirrhosis over a 20-year period and about 50% progress to cirrhosis over a 30-year period compared with 25% over a 25-year to 30-year period among monoinfected patients.[109]

ENVIRONMENTAL FACTORS
Alcohol

There are limited data on the prevalence of alcohol use among persons with CHC. A large meta-analysis of 111 studies which included 33,121 patients,[110] conducted to examine progression of fibrosis, reported that 19% of patients consumed alcohol ranging from 20 g/d to 80 g/d. The prevalence of CHC seems to be 5-fold to 10-fold higher among persons with a history of alcohol abuse. Alcohol consumption is known to adversely affect the outcome of HCV infection: it has been associated with faster progression of liver fibrosis, higher frequency of cirrhosis, and increased incidence of HCC. Patients with HCV who abuse alcohol have decreased survival compared with patients with either alcohol abuse or HCV liver injury alone. Alcohol consumption may be the single most important factor affecting disease progression in patients with CHC. Seeff and colleagues[4] have reported that more than two-thirds of deaths with end-stage liver disease secondary to non-A, non-B hepatitis occurred in alcoholic patients.

An alcohol intake between 30 and 80 g/d has been shown to cause progression of liver disease.[111] In one study, mean fibrosis stage was significantly higher and progression of fibrosis higher in patients whose daily alcohol consumption was 50 g or more than in those who consumed less than 50 g, irrespective of age or duration of infection.[19] A large meta-analysis[112] conducted to explore the relationship between advanced liver disease and alcohol use, taking into account the different definitions of heavy alcohol consumption across many studies, including more than 15,000 patients with HCV infection, showed that heavy intake between 210 and 560 g/wk was associated with a 2.3-fold increased risk of cirrhosis. It was also shown that even moderate alcohol consumption, as low as 31 to 50 g/d in men and 21 to 50 g/d in women, might worsen histologic activity and fibrosis in HCV-infected patients.[113] The mechanism by which alcohol causes the progression of the disease is not clear. Immune dysfunction, increased viral replication, emergence of HCV quasispecies, apoptosis, steatosis, and increased iron overload have been proposed.[113] There is insufficient evidence to determine a safe amount of alcohol use. Therefore, despite the beneficial cardiovascular effects of light alcohol use (10–20 g/d), given the uncertainty on the effects of this amount of alcohol on liver disease progression, patients should be counseled about the adverse effects of alcohol on outcome of CHC and advised to refrain from alcohol use.

Smoking

Whether smoking has any effect on outcome of CHC is uncertain. Smoking for greater than 15 pack-years was shown to be an independent predictor of liver fibrosis, but this association was lost when disease activity was controlled for in a multivariate analysis.[114] Tobacco use higher than 15 cigarettes/d was associated with more severe histologic activity in patients with CHC. In 1 study,[115] the proportion of patients with moderate and marked activity (Metavir A2–A3) increased gradually from 62% in patients who did not smoke to 82% in patients who smoked more than 15 cigarettes/d 6 months before biopsy. Release of proinflammatory cytokines, lipid peroxidation, oxidative stress, steatosis, and iron overload from secondary polycythemia are believed to be the mechanisms by which smoking causes progression of liver disease.[116] Tobacco use is also known to independently contribute to the development of HCC. Alcohol, smoking, and obesity act synergistically in the development of HCC.[117] Although the evidence for smoking on outcome of HCV infection is weak, patients with CHC should be advised to not smoke.

Cannabis

There is both clinical and experiment evidence indicating that daily cannabis use is a cofactor modulating disease progression in patients with CHC. Several studies have reported a strong association between cannabis use and significant fibrosis ($\geq$Metavir F3). In one study from France, 270 consecutive patients with CHC undergoing liver biopsy were studied. Categorizing cannabis use as none, occasional, or daily, daily cannabis use was associated with severe fibrosis on biopsy and a faster rate of fibrosis progression.[118] The CB_1 receptor is widely expressed in the human liver and its upregulation is associated with steatosis and advanced fibrosis.[118–120] Furthermore, daily cannabis use and moderate to heavy alcohol use have additive effects in fibrosis progression.[120] Therefore, patients with CHC should abstain from use of cannabis.

Caffeine

Multiple epidemiologic studies from different geographic regions have reported an association between daily caffeine consumption and lower risk of an increased ALT level in persons without liver disease or at high risk for liver disease.[121–123] Coffee consumption has also been associated with a lower risk of advanced liver disease, cirrhosis, and HCC in patients with chronic liver disease. In 1 study,[124] 177 patients scheduled to undergo liver biopsy were asked to complete a detailed caffeine questionnaire on 3 occasions over a 6-month period. Caffeine intake was correlated with severity of liver disease. A daily caffeine consumption greater than 308 (equivalent to 2.25 cups/d) was associated with less severe hepatic fibrosis. Caffeine from other sources such as tea or caffeinated beverages was not associated with stage of liver fibrosis.[124] Although the evidence of the protective effects of coffee/caffeine on liver disease is growing, no prospective trials have been conducted on the use of caffeine/coffee to improve liver disease. In addition, because the amount of caffeine varies considerably from cup to cup of coffee, the amount of caffeine that is required for a beneficial effect is unknown. Until more data are forthcoming, we cannot recommend that patients with CHC use caffeine/coffee excessively.

Herbals

In the United States, silymarin (an extract of milk thistle) is the most popular herbal product used by persons with liver disease. The HALT-C trial examined the frequency and the potential effects of herbal supplements in a large cohort of patients with advanced CHC. Silymarin was found to be the most frequently used herbal supplement. Silymarin had no beneficial effect on ALT or HCV RNA levels, but users reported fewer and milder symptoms of liver disease and better overall quality of life. Silymarin users had similar ALT and HCV levels to those of nonusers.[125] Further analysis of the HALT-C trial dataset[126] reported that silymarin use was associated with reduced progression to cirrhosis but had no impact on clinical outcomes. Silymarin was also evaluated in a randomized controlled trial to improve disease activity using serum ALT level as a surrogate in patients who had previously failed IFN-based therapy. Higher than usual doses of silymarin had no benefit on reducing serum ALT levels in persons who failed to respond to previous IFN-based therapy and its use cannot be recommended in this population.[127] Another herbal compound, glycyrrhizin, used in Japan, was reported to decrease ALT levels and also prevent carcinogenesis.[128] There is little evidence to support the use of herbals to improve outcome of CHC.

SUMMARY

The natural history of HCV is influenced by a wide variety of host, viral, and environmental factors. Physicians should seek to identify these factors to risk stratify patients. In addition, patients should be counseled to improve modifiable ones to limit disease progression.

REFERENCES

1. Lozano R, Naghavi M, Foreman K, et al. Global and regional mortality from 235 causes of death for 20 age groups in 1990 and 2010: a systematic analysis for the Global Burden of Disease Study 2010. Lancet 2012;380(9859):2095–128.
2. Davis GL, Alter MJ, El-Serag H, et al. Aging of hepatitis C virus (HCV)-infected persons in the United States: a multiple cohort model of HCV prevalence and disease progression. Gastroenterology 2010;138(2):513–21, 521.e1–6.
3. Denniston MM, Jiles RB, Drobeniuc J, et al. Chronic hepatitis C virus infection in the United States, National Health and Nutrition Examination Survey 2003 to 2010. Ann Intern Med 2014;160(5):293–300.
4. Seeff LB. The natural history of chronic hepatitis C virus infection. Clin Liver Dis 1997;1(3):587–602.
5. Ge D, Fellay J, Thompson AJ, et al. Genetic variation in IL28B predicts hepatitis C treatment-induced viral clearance. Nature 2009;461(7262):399–401.
6. Tanaka Y, Nishida N, Sugiyama M, et al. Genome-wide association of IL28B with response to pegylated interferon-alpha and ribavirin therapy for chronic hepatitis C. Nat Genet 2009;41(10):1105–9.
7. Prokunina-Olsson L, Muchmore B, Tang W, et al. A variant upstream of IFNL3 (IL28B) creating a new interferon gene IFNL4 is associated with impaired clearance of hepatitis C virus. Nat Genet 2013;45(2):164–71.
8. Farci P, Shimoda A, Coiana A, et al. The outcome of acute hepatitis C predicted by the evolution of the viral quasispecies. Science 2000;288(5464):339–44.
9. Freeman AJ, Dore GJ, Law MG, et al. Estimating progression to cirrhosis in chronic hepatitis C virus infection. Hepatology 2001;34(4 Pt 1):809–16.
10. Yano M, Kumada H, Kage M, et al. The long-term pathological evolution of chronic hepatitis C. Hepatology 1996;23(6):1334–40.
11. Ghany MG, Kleiner DE, Alter H, et al. Progression of fibrosis in chronic hepatitis C. Gastroenterology 2003;124(1):97–104.
12. Everhart JE, Wright EC, Goodman ZD, et al. Prognostic value of Ishak fibrosis stage: findings from the hepatitis C antiviral long-term treatment against cirrhosis trial. Hepatology 2010;51(2):585–94.
13. Boccato S, Pistis R, Noventa F, et al. Fibrosis progression in initially mild chronic hepatitis C. J Viral Hepat 2006;13(5):297–302.
14. Marcellin P, Asselah T, Boyer N. Fibrosis and disease progression in hepatitis C. Hepatology 2002;36(5 Suppl 1):S47–56.

15. Ryder SD, Irving WL, Jones DA, et al. Progression of hepatic fibrosis in patients with hepatitis C: a prospective repeat liver biopsy study. Gut 2004;53(3):451–5.
16. Fattovich G, Giustina G, Degos F, et al. Morbidity and mortality in compensated cirrhosis type C: a retrospective follow-up study of 384 patients. Gastroenterology 1997;112(2):463–72.
17. Di Bisceglie AM, Shiffman ML, Everson GT, et al. Prolonged therapy of advanced chronic hepatitis C with low-dose peginterferon. N Engl J Med 2008;359(23):2429–41.
18. Planas R, Balleste B, Alvarez MA, et al. Natural history of decompensated hepatitis C virus-related cirrhosis. A study of 200 patients. J Hepatol 2004;40(5):823–30.
19. Poynard T, Bedossa P, Opolon P. Natural history of liver fibrosis progression in patients with chronic hepatitis C. The OBSVIRC, METAVIR, CLINIVIR, and DOSVIRC groups. Lancet 1997;349(9055):825–32.
20. Minola E, Prati D, Suter F, et al. Age at infection affects the long-term outcome of transfusion-associated chronic hepatitis C. Blood 2002;99(12):4588–91.
21. Pradat P, Voirin N, Tillmann HL, et al. Progression to cirrhosis in hepatitis C patients: an age-dependent process. Liver Int 2007;27(3):335–9.
22. Wright M, Goldin R, Fabre A, et al. Measurement and determinants of the natural history of liver fibrosis in hepatitis C virus infection: a cross sectional and longitudinal study. Gut 2003;52(4):574–9.
23. Kanwal F, Hoang T, Kramer JR, et al. Increasing prevalence of HCC and cirrhosis in patients with chronic hepatitis C virus infection. Gastroenterology 2011;140(4):1182–8.e1.
24. Bakr I, Rekacewicz C, El Hosseiny M, et al. Higher clearance of hepatitis C virus infection in females compared with males. Gut 2006;55(8):1183–7.
25. Wang CC, Krantz E, Klarquist J, et al. Acute hepatitis C in a contemporary US cohort: modes of acquisition and factors influencing viral clearance. J Infect Dis 2007;196(10):1474–82.
26. Guadagnino V, Stroffolini T, Rapicetta M, et al. Prevalence, risk factors, and genotype distribution of hepatitis C virus infection in the general population: a community-based survey in southern Italy. Hepatology 1997;26(4):1006–11.
27. Cox AL, Netski DM, Mosbruger T, et al. Prospective evaluation of community-acquired acute-phase hepatitis C virus infection. Clin Infect Dis 2005;40(7):951–8.
28. Alter MJ, Kruszon-Moran D, Nainan OV, et al. The prevalence of hepatitis C virus infection in the United States, 1988 through 1994. N Engl J Med 1999;341(8):556–62.
29. van den Berg CH, Grady BP, Schinkel J, et al. Female sex and IL28B, a synergism for spontaneous viral clearance in hepatitis C virus (HCV) seroconverters from a community-based cohort. PLoS One 2011;6(11):e27555.
30. Page K, Hahn JA, Evans J, et al. Acute hepatitis C virus infection in young adult injection drug users: a prospective study of incident infection, resolution, and reinfection. J Infect Dis 2009;200(8):1216–26.
31. Grebely J, Page K, Sacks-Davis R, et al. The effects of female sex, viral genotype, and IL28B genotype on spontaneous clearance of acute hepatitis C virus infection. Hepatology 2014;59(1):109–20.
32. Mosley JW, Operskalski EA, Tobler LH, et al. The course of hepatitis C viraemia in transfusion recipients prior to availability of antiviral therapy. J Viral Hepat 2008;15(2):120–8.
33. White DL, Tavakoli-Tabasi S, Kuzniarek J, et al. Higher serum testosterone is associated with increased risk of advanced hepatitis C-related liver disease in males. Hepatology 2012;55(3):759–68.

34. White DL, Liu Y, Garcia J, et al. Sex hormone pathway gene polymorphisms are associated with risk of advanced hepatitis C-related liver disease in males. Int J Mol Epidemiol Genet 2014;5(3):164–76.
35. Di Martino V, Lebray P, Myers RP, et al. Progression of liver fibrosis in women infected with hepatitis C: long-term benefit of estrogen exposure. Hepatology 2004;40(6):1426–33.
36. Wiley TE, Brown J, Chan J. Hepatitis C infection in African Americans: its natural history and histological progression. Am J Gastroenterol 2002;97(3):700–6.
37. Sterling RK, Stravitz RT, Luketic VA, et al. A comparison of the spectrum of chronic hepatitis C virus between Caucasians and African Americans. Clin Gastroenterol Hepatol 2004;2(6):469–73.
38. Crosse K, Umeadi OG, Anania FA, et al. Racial differences in liver inflammation and fibrosis related to chronic hepatitis C. Clin Gastroenterol Hepatol 2004;2(6): 463–8.
39. El-Serag HB. Hepatocellular carcinoma and hepatitis C in the United States. Hepatology 2002;36(5 Suppl 1):S74–83.
40. Bonacini M, Groshen MD, Yu MC, et al. Chronic hepatitis C in ethnic minority patients evaluated in Los Angeles County. Am J Gastroenterol 2001;96(8): 2438–41.
41. Rodriguez-Torres M. Latinos and chronic hepatitis C: a singular population. Clin Gastroenterol Hepatol 2008;6(5):484–90.
42. El-Serag HB, Kramer J, Duan Z, et al. Racial differences in the progression to cirrhosis and hepatocellular carcinoma in HCV-infected veterans. Am J Gastroenterol 2014;109(9):1427–35.
43. Conjeevaram HS, Fried MW, Jeffers LJ, et al. Peginterferon and ribavirin treatment in African American and Caucasian American patients with hepatitis C genotype 1. Gastroenterology 2006;131(2):470–7.
44. Muir AJ, Hu KQ, Gordon SC, et al. Hepatitis C treatment among racial and ethnic groups in the IDEAL trial. J Viral Hepat 2011;18(4):e134–43.
45. Rodriguez-Torres M, Jeffers LJ, Sheikh MY, et al. Peginterferon alfa-2a and ribavirin in Latino and non-Latino whites with hepatitis C. N Engl J Med 2009;360(3): 257–67.
46. Thio CL, Thomas DL, Goedert JJ, et al. Racial differences in HLA class II associations with hepatitis C virus outcomes. J Infect Dis 2001;184(1):16–21.
47. Sugimoto K, Stadanlick J, Ikeda F, et al. Influence of ethnicity in the outcome of hepatitis C virus infection and cellular immune response. Hepatology 2003; 37(3):590–9.
48. Ortiz V, Berenguer M, Rayon JM, et al. Contribution of obesity to hepatitis C-related fibrosis progression. Am J Gastroenterol 2002;97(9):2408–14.
49. Hickman IJ, Powell EE, Prins JB, et al. In overweight patients with chronic hepatitis C, circulating insulin is associated with hepatic fibrosis: implications for therapy. J Hepatol 2003;39(6):1042–8.
50. Bressler BL, Guindi M, Tomlinson G, et al. High body mass index is an independent risk factor for nonresponse to antiviral treatment in chronic hepatitis C. Hepatology 2003;38(3):639–44.
51. Lazo M, Hernaez R, Eberhardt MS, et al. Prevalence of nonalcoholic fatty liver disease in the United States: the Third National Health and Nutrition Examination Survey, 1988-1994. Am J Epidemiol 2013;178(1):38–45.
52. Hourigan LF, Macdonald GA, Purdie D, et al. Fibrosis in chronic hepatitis C correlates significantly with body mass index and steatosis. Hepatology 1999; 29(4):1215–9.

53. Adinolfi LE, Gambardella M, Andreana A, et al. Steatosis accelerates the progression of liver damage of chronic hepatitis C patients and correlates with specific HCV genotype and visceral obesity. Hepatology 2001;33(6):1358–64.

54. Monto A, Alonzo J, Watson JJ, et al. Steatosis in chronic hepatitis C: relative contributions of obesity, diabetes mellitus, and alcohol. Hepatology 2002; 36(3):729–36.

55. Perumalswami P, Kleiner DE, Lutchman G, et al. Steatosis and progression of fibrosis in untreated patients with chronic hepatitis C infection. Hepatology 2006;43(4):780–7.

56. Leandro G, Mangia A, Hui J, et al. Relationship between steatosis, inflammation, and fibrosis in chronic hepatitis C: a meta-analysis of individual patient data. Gastroenterology 2006;130(6):1636–42.

57. Grimbert S, Valensi P, Levy-Marchal C, et al. High prevalence of diabetes mellitus in patients with chronic hepatitis C. A case-control study. Gastroenterol Clin Biol 1996;20(6–7):544–8.

58. Mehta SH, Brancati FL, Sulkowski MS, et al. Prevalence of type 2 diabetes mellitus among persons with hepatitis C virus infection in the United States. Ann Intern Med 2000;133(8):592–9.

59. White DL, Ratziu V, El-Serag HB. Hepatitis C infection and risk of diabetes: a systematic review and meta-analysis. J Hepatol 2008;49(5):831–44.

60. Naing C, Mak JW, Ahmed SI, et al. Relationship between hepatitis C virus infection and type 2 diabetes mellitus: meta-analysis. World J Gastroenterol 2012; 18(14):1642–51.

61. Ruhl CE, Menke A, Cowie CC, et al. Relationship of hepatitis C virus infection with diabetes in the US population. Hepatology 2014;60(4):1139–49.

62. Kim HJ, Park JH, Park DI, et al. Clearance of HCV by combination therapy of pegylated interferon alpha-2a and ribavirin improves insulin resistance. Gut Liver 2009;3(2):108–15.

63. Delgado-Borrego A, Jordan SH, Negre B, et al. Reduction of insulin resistance with effective clearance of hepatitis C infection: results from the HALT-C trial. Clin Gastroenterol Hepatol 2010;8(5):458–62.

64. Butt AA, Umbleja T, Andersen JW, et al. Impact of peginterferon alpha and ribavirin treatment on lipid profiles and insulin resistance in hepatitis C virus/HIV-coinfected persons: the AIDS Clinical Trials Group A5178 study. Clin Infect Dis 2012;55(5):631–8.

65. Romero-Gomez M, Fernandez-Rodriguez CM, Andrade RJ, et al. Effect of sustained virological response to treatment on the incidence of abnormal glucose values in chronic hepatitis C. J Hepatol 2008;48(5):721–7.

66. Rauch A, Kutalik Z, Descombes P, et al. Genetic variation in IL28B is associated with chronic hepatitis C and treatment failure: a genome-wide association study. Gastroenterology 2010;138(4):1338–45, 1345.e1–7.

67. Noureddin M, Wright EC, Alter HJ, et al. Association of IL28B genotype with fibrosis progression and clinical outcomes in patients with chronic hepatitis C: a longitudinal analysis. Hepatology 2013;58(5):1548–57.

68. Kim HC, Nam CM, Jee SH, et al. Normal serum aminotransferase concentration and risk of mortality from liver diseases: prospective cohort study. BMJ 2004; 328(7446):983.

69. McOmish F, Chan SW, Dow BC, et al. Detection of three types of hepatitis C virus in blood donors: investigation of type-specific differences in serologic reactivity and rate of alanine aminotransferase abnormalities. Transfusion 1993;33(1): 7–13.

70. Conry-Cantilena C, VanRaden M, Gibble J, et al. Routes of infection, viremia, and liver disease in blood donors found to have hepatitis C virus infection. N Engl J Med 1996;334(26):1691–6.
71. Alberti A, Benvegnu L, Boccato S, et al. Natural history of initially mild chronic hepatitis C. Dig Liver Dis 2004;36(10):646–54.
72. Hui CK, Belaye T, Montegrande K, et al. A comparison in the progression of liver fibrosis in chronic hepatitis C between persistently normal and elevated transaminase. J Hepatol 2003;38(4):511–7.
73. Persico M, Persico E, Suozzo R, et al. Natural history of hepatitis C virus carriers with persistently normal aminotransferase levels. Gastroenterology 2000;118(4):760–4.
74. Nunnari G, Pinzone MR, Cacopardo B. Lack of clinical and histological progression of chronic hepatitis C in individuals with true persistently normal ALT: the result of a 17-year follow-up. J Viral Hepat 2013;20(4):e131–7.
75. Mathurin P, Moussalli J, Cadranel JF, et al. Slow progression rate of fibrosis in hepatitis C virus patients with persistently normal alanine transaminase activity. Hepatology 1998;27(3):868–72.
76. Ghany MG, Lok AS, Everhart JE, et al. Predicting clinical and histologic outcomes based on standard laboratory tests in advanced chronic hepatitis C. Gastroenterology 2010;138(1):136–46.
77. Lee MH, Yang HI, Lu SN, et al. Hepatitis C virus seromarkers and subsequent risk of hepatocellular carcinoma: long-term predictors from a community-based cohort study. J Clin Oncol 2010;28(30):4587–93.
78. Pattullo V, Duarte-Rojo A, Soliman W, et al. A 24-week dietary and physical activity lifestyle intervention reduces hepatic insulin resistance in the obese with chronic hepatitis C. Liver Int 2013;33(3):410–9.
79. Abd El-Kader SM, Al-Jiffri OH, Al-Shreef FM. Liver enzymes and psychological well-being response to aerobic exercise training in patients with chronic hepatitis C. Afr Health Sci 2014;14(2):414–9.
80. McKenna O, Cunningham C, Gissane C, et al. Management of the extrahepatic symptoms of chronic hepatitis C: feasibility of a randomized controlled trial of exercise. Am J Phys Med Rehabil 2013;92(6):504–12.
81. Thomas DL, Astemborski J, Vlahov D, et al. Determinants of the quantity of hepatitis C virus RNA. J Infect Dis 2000;181(3):844–51.
82. Yamada M, Kakumu S, Yoshioka K, et al. Hepatitis C virus genotypes are not responsible for development of serious liver disease. Dig Dis Sci 1994;39(2):234–9.
83. Yeo AE, Ghany M, Conry-Cantilena C, et al. Stability of HCV-RNA level and its lack of correlation with disease severity in asymptomatic chronic hepatitis C virus carriers. J Viral Hepat 2001;8(4):256–63.
84. De Moliner L, Pontisso P, De Salvo GL, et al. Serum and liver HCV RNA levels in patients with chronic hepatitis C: correlation with clinical and histological features. Gut 1998;42(6):856–60.
85. Gervais A, Martinot M, Boyer N, et al. Quantitation of hepatic hepatitis C virus RNA in patients with chronic hepatitis C. Relationship with severity of disease, viral genotype and response to treatment. J Hepatol 2001;35(3):399–405.
86. Messina JP, Humphreys I, Flaxman A, et al. Global distribution and prevalence of hepatitis C virus genotypes. Hepatology 2015;61(1):77–87.
87. Probst A, Dang T, Bochud M, et al. Role of hepatitis C virus genotype 3 in liver fibrosis progression–a systematic review and meta-analysis. J Viral Hepat 2011;18(11):745–59.

88. Crespo J, Lozano JL, de la Cruz F, et al. Prevalence and significance of hepatitis C viremia in chronic active hepatitis B. Am J Gastroenterol 1994;89(8):1147–51.

89. Kaur S, Rybicki L, Bacon BR, et al. Performance characteristics and results of a large-scale screening program for viral hepatitis and risk factors associated with exposure to viral hepatitis B and C: results of the National Hepatitis Screening Survey. National Hepatitis Surveillance Group. Hepatology 1996; 24(5):979–86.

90. Liang TJ, Bodenheimer HC Jr, Yankee R, et al. Presence of hepatitis B and C viral genomes in US blood donors as detected by polymerase chain reaction amplification. J Med Virol 1994;42(2):151–7.

91. Caccamo G, Saffioti F, Raimondo G. Hepatitis B virus and hepatitis C virus dual infection. World J Gastroenterol 2014;20(40):14559–67.

92. Tyson GL, Kramer JR, Duan Z, et al. Prevalence and predictors of hepatitis B virus coinfection in a United States cohort of hepatitis C virus-infected patients. Hepatology 2013;58(2):538–45.

93. Sato S, Fujiyama S, Tanaka M, et al. Coinfection of hepatitis C virus in patients with chronic hepatitis B infection. J Hepatol 1994;21(2):159–66.

94. Di Marco V, Lo Iacono O, Camma C, et al. The long-term course of chronic hepatitis B. Hepatology 1999;30(1):257–64.

95. Fattovich G, Tagger A, Brollo L, et al. Hepatitis C virus infection in chronic hepatitis B virus carriers. J Infect Dis 1991;163(2):400–2.

96. Zarski JP, Bohn B, Bastie A, et al. Characteristics of patients with dual infection by hepatitis B and C viruses. J Hepatol 1998;28(1):27–33.

97. Fong TL, Di Bisceglie AM, Waggoner JG, et al. The significance of antibody to hepatitis C virus in patients with chronic hepatitis B. Hepatology 1991;14(1): 64–7.

98. Kruse RL, Kramer JR, Tyson GL, et al. Clinical outcomes of hepatitis B virus coinfection in a United States cohort of hepatitis C virus-infected patients. Hepatology 2014;60(6):1871–8.

99. Alter MJ. Epidemiology of viral hepatitis and HIV co-infection. J Hepatol 2006; 44(1 Suppl):S6–9.

100. Hernando V, Perez-Cachafeiro S, Lewden C, et al. All-cause and liver-related mortality in HIV positive subjects compared to the general population: differences by HCV co-infection. J Hepatol 2012;57(4):743–51.

101. Daar ES, Lynn H, Donfield S, et al. Relation between HIV-1 and hepatitis C viral load in patients with hemophilia. J Acquir Immune Defic Syndr 2001;26(5): 466–72.

102. Messick K, Sanders JC, Goedert JJ, et al. Hepatitis C viral clearance and antibody reactivity patterns in persons with haemophilia and other congenital bleeding disorders. Haemophilia 2001;7(6):568–74.

103. Eyster ME, Fried MW, Di Bisceglie AM, et al. Increasing hepatitis C virus RNA levels in hemophiliacs: relationship to human immunodeficiency virus infection and liver disease. Multicenter Hemophilia Cohort Study. Blood 1994;84(4): 1020–3.

104. Ghany MG, Leissinger C, Lagier R, et al. Effect of human immunodeficiency virus infection on hepatitis C virus infection in hemophiliacs. Dig Dis Sci 1996; 41(6):1265–72.

105. Rosenthal E, Pialoux G, Bernard N, et al. Liver-related mortality in human-immunodeficiency-virus-infected patients between 1995 and 2003 in the French GERMIVIC Joint Study Group Network (MORTAVIC 2003 Study). J Viral Hepat 2007;14(3):183–8.

106. Weber R, Sabin CA, Friis-Moller N, et al. Liver-related deaths in persons infected with the human immunodeficiency virus: the D:A:D study. Arch Intern Med 2006; 166(15):1632–41.
107. Martin-Carbonero L, de Ledinghen V, Moreno A, et al. Liver fibrosis in patients with chronic hepatitis C and persistently normal liver enzymes: influence of HIV infection. J Viral Hepat 2009;16(11):790–5.
108. Martinez-Sierra C, Arizcorreta A, Diaz F, et al. Progression of chronic hepatitis C to liver fibrosis and cirrhosis in patients coinfected with hepatitis C virus and human immunodeficiency virus. Clin Infect Dis 2003;36(4):491–8.
109. Thein HH, Yi Q, Dore GJ, et al. Natural history of hepatitis C virus infection in HIV-infected individuals and the impact of HIV in the era of highly active antiretroviral therapy: a meta-analysis. AIDS 2008;22(15):1979–91.
110. Thein HH, Yi Q, Dore GJ, et al. Estimation of stage-specific fibrosis progression rates in chronic hepatitis C virus infection: a meta-analysis and meta-regression. Hepatology 2008;48(2):418–31.
111. Seeff LB, Buskell-Bales Z, Wright EC, et al. Long-term mortality after transfusion-associated non-A, non-B hepatitis. The National Heart, Lung, and Blood Institute Study Group. N Engl J Med 1992;327(27):1906–11.
112. Hutchinson SJ, Bird SM, Goldberg DJ. Influence of alcohol on the progression of hepatitis C virus infection: a meta-analysis. Clin Gastroenterol Hepatol 2005; 3(11):1150–9.
113. Hezode C, Lonjon I, Roudot-Thoraval F, et al. Impact of moderate alcohol consumption on histological activity and fibrosis in patients with chronic hepatitis C, and specific influence of steatosis: a prospective study. Aliment Pharmacol Ther 2003;17(8):1031–7.
114. Pessione F, Ramond MJ, Njapoum C, et al. Cigarette smoking and hepatic lesions in patients with chronic hepatitis C. Hepatology 2001;34(1):121–5.
115. Hezode C, Lonjon I, Roudot-Thoraval F, et al. Impact of smoking on histological liver lesions in chronic hepatitis C. Gut 2003;52(1):126–9.
116. El-Zayadi AR, Selim O, Hamdy H, et al. Heavy cigarette smoking induces hypoxic polycythemia (erythrocytosis) and hyperuricemia in chronic hepatitis C patients with reversal of clinical symptoms and laboratory parameters with therapeutic phlebotomy. Am J Gastroenterol 2002;97(5):1264–5.
117. Marrero JA, Fontana RJ, Fu S, et al. Alcohol, tobacco and obesity are synergistic risk factors for hepatocellular carcinoma. J Hepatol 2005;42(2):218–24.
118. Hezode C, Roudot-Thoraval F, Nguyen S, et al. Daily cannabis smoking as a risk factor for progression of fibrosis in chronic hepatitis C. Hepatology 2005;42(1): 63–71.
119. Hezode C, Zafrani ES, Roudot-Thoraval F, et al. Daily cannabis use: a novel risk factor of steatosis severity in patients with chronic hepatitis C. Gastroenterology 2008;134(2):432–9.
120. Ishida JH, Peters MG, Jin C, et al. Influence of cannabis use on severity of hepatitis C disease. Clin Gastroenterol Hepatol 2008;6(1):69–75.
121. Casiglia E, Spolaore P, Ginocchio G, et al. Unexpected effects of coffee consumption on liver enzymes. Eur J Epidemiol 1993;9(3):293–7.
122. Honjo S, Kono S, Coleman MP, et al. Coffee consumption and serum aminotransferases in middle-aged Japanese men. J Clin Epidemiol 2001;54(8): 823–9.
123. Ruhl CE, Everhart JE. Coffee and caffeine consumption reduce the risk of elevated serum alanine aminotransferase activity in the United States. Gastroenterology 2005;128(1):24–32.

124. Modi AA, Feld JJ, Park Y, et al. Increased caffeine consumption is associated with reduced hepatic fibrosis. Hepatology 2010;51(1):201–9.
125. Seeff LB, Curto TM, Szabo G, et al. Herbal product use by persons enrolled in the hepatitis C antiviral long-term treatment against cirrhosis (HALT-C) trial. Hepatology 2008;47(2):605–12.
126. Freedman ND, Curto TM, Morishima C, et al. Silymarin use and liver disease progression in the Hepatitis C Antiviral Long-Term Treatment against Cirrhosis trial. Aliment Pharmacol Ther 2011;33(1):127–37.
127. Fried MW, Navarro VJ, Afdhal N, et al. Effect of silymarin (milk thistle) on liver disease in patients with chronic hepatitis C unsuccessfully treated with interferon therapy: a randomized controlled trial. JAMA 2012;308(3):274–82.
128. Arase Y, Ikeda K, Murashima N, et al. The long term efficacy of glycyrrhizin in chronic hepatitis C patients. Cancer 1997;79(8):1494–500.

Immunopathogenesis of Hepatitis C Virus Infection

David E. Kaplan, MD, MSc[a,b,*]

KEY WORDS

- Hepatitis C • Human • Innate immunity • Adaptive immunity • Regulatory T cells

KEY POINTS

- Disruption of the generation of type I and III interferons (IFN), such as IFN-α, IFN-β, and IFN-λ, is critical for establishment of persistent infection of hepatocytes. As such, the specific viral particles specifically inhibit several pathways required for generation of and response to secreted interferons.
- The efficacy of dendritic cell antigen presentation to adaptive B- and T-cell effectors determines whether brisk and effective response resolves acute infection or delayed and weak responses allow chronic infection.
- Multiple nonparenchymal cells in the liver can either contribute to antiviral effects or induce tolerance by T cells.
- Regulatory T cells play a fundamental role in suppressing early antiviral responses by T and B cells but may play a critical protective role against rapid liver injury in chronic infection.
- Neutralizing antibodies produced by B cells do not universally resolve early infection nor protect against reinfection and can even facilitate viral entry into hepatocytes.

INTRODUCTION

Despite advances in therapy, hepatitis C virus (HCV) infection remains a major global health issue with 3 to 4 million incident cases and 170 million prevalent chronic infections.[1] Complex, partially understood, host-virus interactions determine whether an acute infection with hepatitis C resolves, as occurs in approximately 30% of cases, or generates a persistent hepatic infection, as occurs in the remainder. Once chronic infection is established, the velocity of hepatocyte injury and resultant fibrosis is significantly modulated by immunologic as well as environmental factors. Although the

[a] Medicine and Research Services, Corporal Michael J. Crescenz VA Medical Center, 3900 Woodland Avenue, Philadelphia, PA 19104, USA; [b] Division of Gastroenterology, Department of Medicine, University of Pennsylvania, BRB II/III, 9th Floor, 415 Curie Boulevard, Philadelphia, PA 19104, USA
* Divisions of Gastroenterology and Hepatology, Perelman School of Medicine, University of Pennsylvania, BRB II/III, 9th Floor, 415 Curie Boulevard, Philadelphia, PA 19104.
E-mail address: dakaplan@mail.med.upenn.edu

Gastroenterol Clin N Am 44 (2015) 735–760
http://dx.doi.org/10.1016/j.gtc.2015.07.004
0889-8553/15/$ – see front matter Published by Elsevier Inc.

backbone of antiviral therapy for most of the past 15 years has consisted of innate immune stimulation with interferon-α (IFN-α), more recent data regarding of the role of T-cell exhaustion and antigen-presenting cell defects have encouraged early-phase clinical trials of several novel immunomodulators with modest initial effects. An appreciation of the complexity, redundancy, and interdependence of the regulatory mechanisms involved in maintaining chronic infection may inform future approaches to restore immunoreactivity to HCV as feasible antiviral therapy. This review focuses on virus-induced immunologic dysfunction that allows the establishment of persistent infection as well as the impact of these immunologic defects on disease progression during chronic infection.

INTRAHEPATOCYTIC SENSING AND SIGNALING

HCV is a highly mutable, hepatotropic, enveloped single-stranded RNA virus of the Flaviviridae family.[2] The 9.5-kB genome encodes for a single polyprotein of 3011 amino acids flanked by 5′ and 3′ noncoding regions essential for viral replication.[3] The viral polyprotein is translated in toto and then processed by host cell- and virus-encoded proteases into structural (Core, E1, E2) and nonstructural proteins (p7, NS2, NS3, NS4A, NS4B, NS5A, NS5B). The Core protein forms the viral nucleocapsid.[4] E1 and E2 are the viral envelope glycoproteins that interact with various surface receptors, including claudin-1, CD81, DC-SIGN, scavenger receptor B I (SR-BI), and the LDL receptor, to mediate viral entry into target cells.[5–11] The remainder of the nonstructural proteins creates a membrane-associated viral replication complex critical for establishment for persistent, and along with structural proteins, modulates host cell function to disrupt intracellular and extracellular antiviral pathways (**Table 1**).

The induction of type I (IFN-α and IFN-β), II (IFN-γ), and III (interleukin [IL]-28A/IFN-λ2, IL-28B/IFN-λ3, IL-29/IFN-λ1, and IFN-λ4) interferons is critical for host-defense against intracellular pathogens. Type I, II, and III IFNs signals in autocrine and paracrine manners through their respective heterodimeric receptors (IFNAR, IFNGR, IFNLR) to phosphorylate STAT-1 and STAT-2, leading to the formation of the transcription factor ISGF3 (consisting of pSTAT-1, pSTAT-2, and Interferon Response

Table 1 Selected immunoregulatory effects of viral proteins	
Core	Activation of PKR[283]
	Inhibition of TLR3-mediated secretion of type I and III interferon[43]
	Inhibition of STAT1 activation[46,49]
	Inhibition of ISGFR3 nuclear translocation[47]
	Impairment of dendritic cell maturation and antigen presentation[89,90,92,93,284,287]
	Blockade of IL-1β production in macrophages[43]
	Stabilization of HLA-E[124]
	C1q-mediated T-cell inhibition[189,190]
E2	Activation of PKR and elongation initiation factor 2a (eIF2a)[30]
	Stimulation of CD81 on B cells[274]
NS2	Inhibition of TBK1 and IKKe[285]
NS3/4A	Cleavage of MAVS[32–38]
	Inhibition of TBK1 and IKKe[41]
	Cleavage of TRIF[40]
	Suppression of CXCL8 and CXCL10 chemokines[42,286]
NS5A	Activation of PKR[29]
NS5B	Viral mutations leading to escape or inhibition of T-cell function[168,188]

Factor [IRF] 9) that translocates to the nucleus to modulate the production of hundreds of IFN-stimulated antiviral genes (ISGs).[12] Specific ISGs suppress viral replication and sensitize infected cells to apoptosis.[13] Critical to the development of adaptive immune responses, type I interferons also stimulate immunoproteasome formation critical for presentation of antigen by hepatocytes to CD8 T cells.[14] Although IFNAR and IFNGR expression is ubiquitous, the heterodimeric IFNLR (consisting of IFN-λR1 and IL-10R2 chains) is restricted to epithelial cells, hepatocytes, and dendritic cells (DCs).[15] Although there is significant overlap in the number and types of genes induced by type I, II, and III interferons, IFN-α and IFN-λ do have subtle differences in gene expression profiles and kinetics.[16–18] Notably, the permissiveness of hepatocyte cell lines to support HCV infection in vitro appears critically dependent on defects in type I and III interferon signaling.[19,20]

After viral entry and uncoating, hepatocytes sense intracellular HCV infection to generate type I and III interferons both by toll-like receptors (TLRs) and by retinoic-acid-inducible gene-like receptors, a family of proteins that includes retinoic acid-inducible gene I (RIG-I), melanoma differentiation-associated gene 5 (MDA-5), and laboratory of genetics and physiology gene 2 (Lgp2), in the cytoplasm. TLR3 recognizes double-stranded RNA replication intermediates on the cell membrane or within endosomes to activate Toll/interleukin-1 receptor-domain-containing adapter-inducing interferon-β (TRIF), which in turn phosphorylates IRF3, the transcription factor critical for generating type I and III interferon production. Binding of specific viral dsRNA and ssRNA motifs by RIG-I and MDA-5[19,21–23] triggers a signaling cascade that similarly includes TRIF but also stimulates Mitochondrial AntiViral Signaling protein (MAVS, also known as Cardif, IPS-1, or VISA) to activate IKK-related kinases (IKKε and TBK-1), which also phosphorylate IRF3 and IRF7 to trigger the production of type I and III interferons. Intracellular sensing mechanisms are initially preserved in HCV-infected hepatocytes. Type I IFN and ISGs are rapidly induced in vivo in experimentally infected chimpanzees.[24] In humans, HCV predominantly produces a type III IFN response, predominantly with IFN-λ4 transcripts,[25–27] that induces multiple ISGs that potentially could inhibit HCV viral replication by suppressing primary translation of viral RNA.[28]

Therefore, disruption of these antiviral pathways is critical for establishment of viral persistence. Early after infection, the viral E2 and NS5A proteins both induce phosphorylation of protein kinase R (PKR) and elongation initiation factor 2a, which suppress general cellular mRNA translation without negatively impacting translation of HCV proteins.[29–31] Subsequently, the NS3/4A protease cleaves MAVS, preventing its dimerization, resulting in its disassociation from mitochondrial membranes and disruption of its signaling through IKKε to activate IRF3.[32–39] The NS3/4A protease may also degrade TRIF,[40] blocking TLR3 signaling, as well as directly interacting with TBK1 and IKKε.[41] In addition to suppressing type I and III interferon production, MAVS inactivation reduces the production of the chemokines CXCL8 and CXCL10 critical for recruitment of inflammatory cells to the liver.[42] HCV Core also interferes with TLR3-mediated secretion of interferons,[43] which may particularly impair TLR3-dependent type III IFN production.[44,45] Furthermore, to block cellular responses to type I and III interferons that are produced, HCV Core protein upregulates SOCS3, a negative regulator of STAT phosphorylation[46] and also directly inhibits ISGF3 activity.[47–49] Thus, HCV has evolved multiple strategies not only to disrupt the generation of antiviral type I and III interferons but also to interrupt interferon-induced gene expression to maintain viral replication.

Genome-wide association studies have identified 3 polymorphisms on chromosome 19 near the IFN-λ3 gene (rs12979860, rs8099917, and ss469415590/

rs368234815) that are associated with spontaneous resolution of acute infection[50–52] and sensitivity to interferon-based antiviral therapy.[27,50,51,53–59] The rs8099917 TT or rs12979860 CC polymorphisms are associated with a stronger induction of IFN-λ2 on stimulation.[15] The ss469415590 polymorphism (TT → ΔG) causes a frameshift mutation that creates IFN-λ4, protein that binds to IFNLR to induce STAT1 and STAT2 phosphorylation, ISGF3, and ISG expression.[56] The TT polymorphism abrogates IFN-λ4 production, which, somewhat counterintuitively, improves spontaneous resolution and antiviral treatment outcome.[56,60] Paradoxically, IFN-λ4 exerts strong antiviral activity in vitro,[61,62] and it remains unexplained how the presence of this highly functional antiviral protein impairs antiviral responses in HCV. In human liver, the apparent paradox appears to be relevant because intrahepatic expression of IFN-λ4 is positively rather than negatively associated with intrahepatic HCV RNA and ISG induction.[26,27] Other genetic polymorphisms that impact viral sensing and ISG expression, such as the rs3747517 MDA-5 H843/T946 variant, also appear to impact the likelihood of spontaneous resolution of acute infection.[63] IL-28B polymorphisms associated with greater clearance rates have variably been associated with more active necroinflammation and rapid fibrosis progression in chronic infection,[64–67] suggesting impact of these genetic markers throughout the natural history of HCV disease.

In chronic infection, IFN-λ polymorphisms associated with viral persistence are associated with chronic upregulation of ISGs made ineffective by concurrent upregulation of inhibitory ISGs, such as USP18.[68,69] Because of maximal upregulation, IFN-α therapy cannot upregulate ISGs further.[69–76] Type III interferon induction of STAT1 phosphorylation does not appear to be impaired by type I interferon-induced USP18,[70] leading to interest in the use of IFN-λ as an alternative therapeutic approach,[77] but although better tolerated, pegylated IFN-λ to date has not shown superior antiviral efficacy. In vitro, NS3/4A protease inhibitors used as antiviral therapy can restore IFN-β secretion but at concentrations greater than 100-fold higher than the EC_{50},[78] suggesting that restoration of type I interferon production constitutes a minor effect of protease inhibitor-based direct acting antiviral regimens.

INDUCTION OF CELLULAR AND ADAPTIVE IMMUNE RESPONSES

Once hepatocytes are productively infected with HCV, cellular defenses become activated. Type I and III interferons and stress signals from hepatocytes trigger resident DC, hepatic stellate cells (HSC), and Kupffer cells (KC) to produce cytokines, such as MIP-1α, IL-12, IL-15 and IL-18, to recruit IFN-γ-producing natural killer (NK) cells to the liver. Type I and III interferons activate liver sinusoidal endothelial cells (LSEC) to produce chemokines, such as CXCL10 and MIG, to attract T cells (reviewed in[79]). HCV has evolved mechanisms to disrupt several of these steps for critical efficient induction of cellular immune responses.

Dendritic Cell Dysfunction

DCs resident in tissues survey for pathogen infections, and pon detection, activate, mature, and migrate to lymphoid tissue to present antigens and induce B- and T-cell responses. Human DCs are subdivided into 3 main subtypes: CD11c+ myeloid DC (mDC1), BDCA3+ (CD141+) myeloid DC (mDC2), and CD11c-CD123+ plasmacytoid DC (pDC).[80] Although pDC typically traffic in lymphoid organs, mDC preferentially home to peripheral tissues. On recognition of pathogens through pattern-recognition receptor (eg, TLRs),[81–83] DCs increase class I and II HLA expression, upregulate costimulation ligands, and produce immunostimulatory cytokines, such as IL-12 (mDC1), IFN-λ (mDC2), and IFN-α plus IFN-λ (pDC).[15,45,84–87] Circulating numbers of mDC and pDC are reduced in chronic HCV infection (reviewed in[85,88]), possibly because of enhanced homing of activated mDC1 and mDC2 to the liver.[15,80]

That DC function is impaired in HCV is fairly well established, but the critical mechanisms remain controversial. Some studies indicate that HCV infection is associated with impaired DC maturation and antigen-presenting function,[88–93] possibly mediated by the HCV core protein[90–92] and possibly due to upregulation of indoleamine-2,3,-deoxygenase.[93] A few studies suggest the impairment may preferentially affect pDC subset[94] possibly by inducing pDC apoptosis.[95] Other studies suggest that DC phagocytic function, expression of costimulation ligands, expression of class I and II HLA molecules, and cytokine function are preserved, but that antigen processing by proteasomal subunits is dysregulated.[85] DC migration to lymphoid tissue may also be impaired because of unresponsiveness to the chemokine CCL21.[96] Downregulation of HCV-sensing TLRs or critical adaptor molecules, such as TRIF and TRAF6, have been implicated in the reduced activation of pDC[97] and mDC[98] in vitro. Two key effects of impaired DC function in early HCV infection include reduced cytokine-dependent NK cell maturation[44,99] and defective priming of CD4 and CD8 T cells with a resultant IL-10-secreting regulatory T-cell (Treg) phenotype.[88,90–92,100]

Antiviral Effect of Nonparenchymal Liver Cells

HSC are pericytes that reside in the space of Disse between LSEC and hepatocytes, making up 5% to 8% of total human liver cells. During normal physiology, HSC store vitamin A, but once activated, HSC deposit extracellular matrix, resulting in liver. HSC themselves do not appear to be permissive to HCV infection or replication.[101] HSC express TLR3 and may exert an antiviral effect by producing IFN-λ, which could suppress HCV replication in infected neighboring hepatocytes.[102] However, to date, this effect has been demonstrated only in vitro. LSEC constitute approximately half of nonparenchymal liver cells. Human LSEC endocytose HCV but do not support replication. However, translated HCV RNA induces TLR7 and RIG-I-dependent production of IFN-α, IFN-β, and IFN-λ[103] with potential antiviral effects. LSEC also may present antigen to T cells.[104] The importance of this effect in vivo remains poorly characterized. KC are a heterogeneous group of liver-resident macrophages that line hepatic sinusoids that are critical for phagocytosing translocated bacterial products and iron reutilization. In vitro, HCV Core protein, a ligand for TLR2 present in KC, blocks TLR3-mediated production of IL-1β by macrophages,[43] a cytokine that is thought to enhance the antiviral effects of IFN-α,[105] suggesting that inhibition of KC activation may be critical to viral persistence. However, in chronic HCV infections, KC retain normal activation, producing high levels of IL-1β in a TLR7- and NLRP3 inflammasone-dependent manner,[106] particularly in individuals with chronic infection and advanced fibrosis.[106] KC also produce galectin-9, which has potent regulatory affects on HCV-specific T cells.[107]

Innate Cellular Responses to Hepatitis C Virus Infection

NK cells are critical early antiviral effectors that kill infected target cells by secretion of perforin or through death receptor ligands, such as FasL or TRAIL, and also potently produce of IFN-γ and chemokines, such as MIP1α, MIP1β, RANTES, and granulocyte-macrophage colony-stimulating factor, needed to recruit T and B cells to infected tissues. NK cells are typically activated by stress-induced molecules, such as MHC I-like proteins (MICA, MICB, ULBP), as well as by cytokines such as IL-12, IL-15, IL-18, and IL-21. NK cell activation is intricately controlled by the balance of activating and inhibitory signals including Killer Inhibitory Receptors (KIR) (which may be activating or inhibitory despite the nomenclature) that bind HLA-C, NKG2 family receptors that bind nonclassical HLA ligands, such as HLA-E, MICA, and MICB, and activating receptors, such as NKp30, NKp44, and NKp46. Two classic subsets can be defined based on the expression of CD16 (FcγRIII, which binds IgG) and CD56; $CD16^+CD56^{dim}$ (90% of NK cells) have a cytotoxic phenotype, and $CD16^-CD56^{bright}$ produce greater cytokine responses. There is critical cross-talk between DCs and NK cells. DC activate NK cells by binding to NKp30 and secreting IL-12. In turn, NK cells secrete IFN-γ and TNF-α to foster DC maturation and antigen-presenting function.[108]

Certain aspects of NK cell function in acute hepatitis C infection are genetically determined. Specifically, genetic homozygosity for a weakly inhibitor KIR gene (KIR2DL3), when coexisting with homozygosity for the strongly activating HLA-C1 gene, is strongly associated with early viral clearance.[109,110] The strong impact of NK cell activation on viral clearance creates context for the evolutionary priority for HCV to dysregulate NK cell function. Highly active cytotoxic NK cells are associated with the absence of infection in highly exposed injection drug users.[111] However, studies of acute hepatitis C patients do not universally indicate that the magnitude of NK cell cytotoxicity and IFN-γ production clearly is associated with virological outcome, with both $CD16^+CD56^{dim}$ and $CD16^-CD56^{bright}$ subsets showing activation.[112–114] Controversy exists about the impact of chronic HCV infection of NK cell cytotoxicity.[115,116] Although the frequency of peripheral NK cells appears to be decreased in chronic HCV, particularly among $CD16^+CD56^{dim}$ NK cells, no difference in NK cell cytotoxicity appears to be present between chronic HCV patients and healthy donors or resolved patients.[117–120]

Possible mechanisms of NK cell inhibition in chronic HCV infection in the literature include but are not limited to HCV E2 interaction with CD81, which has largely been disproven; HCV core-induced stabilization of HLA-E, which would inhibit NK cells; altered NK cell activation receptor expression; and altered NK cell cytokine production leading to impaired activation of DCs.[121] In 2002, 2 groups showed that plate-bound HCV E2 protein interacting with CD81 reduces NK cell function in vitro.[122,123] These findings have been since contradicted by studies using intact viral particles in which no inhibition occurred.[118,120] In vitro, an HCV $Core_{35–44}$ peptide sequence has been shown to bind to HLA-E and stabilizes it on cell surfaces, inhibiting NK activation.[124] The expression of HLA-E on multiple intrahepatic cell subsets including expression on HCV-infected hepatocytes was demonstrated,[124] indicating possible in vivo relevance. Furthermore, hepatocyte HLA-E expression might skew NK cells to produce the immunosuppressive cytokines IL-10 and transforming growth factor-β (TGF-β), which inhibit DC maturation.[121] Monocyte-derived IL-10 and TGF-β also downregulate NK cell expression of the NKG2D receptor that might reduce NK cell sensitivity to MICA and MICB on infected hepatocytes.[125,126] Controversy exists about the expression of other activating receptors, such as NKp30 and NKp46, on NK cells in chronic HCV infection, with some studies showing decreases[127] and others showing increases.[118]

In established chronic infection, the balance of cytolytic and cytokine-producing NK cells in the liver may be associated with fibrosis progression. Intrahepatic compartmentalization of activated cytotoxic NK cells (NKG2D+, inhibitory KIR^{lo}, $CD16^+CD56^{dim}$, NKp44+, or TRAIL+ NK cells) with reduced IFN-γ secretion correlates with liver injury.[128–130] By contrast, NK cell IFN-γ production may attenuate fibrosis by HSC.[131] Recent work suggests that contact with HCV-infected hepatocytes reduces NK cell expression of microRNA-155, which upregulates the transcription factor T-bet and the inhibitory receptor Tim-3 and was associated with reversible inhibition of NK cell IFN-γ production.[132] Modulation of NK cell function also seems to impact response to IFN-α-based antiviral therapy with higher expression levels of inhibitory

NK receptors in treatment nonresponders[133] and increased expression of activating receptors in responders.[134,135]

In addition to NK cells, natural killer T (NKT) cells are also overrepresented in liver. NKT cells are a heterogenous population of lymphocytes including invariant NKT cells that express NK cell markers, such as CD56, CD161, KIR, and NKG2 receptors, as well as a T-cell receptor. Subpopulations include invariant NKT that express a specific CD-1d-reactive T-cell receptor (most commonly Vα24Jα18/Vβ11), variant NKT cells, Vδ3 γδ T cells, and general cytolytic NKT cells (reviewed in[136]). The relative frequencies of NKT cells are variable in HCV-infected livers[137–139] and blood.[140] Peripheral CD56+ NKT levels are reduced early in acute HCV infection,[141] but whether this is due to compartmentalization to the liver is not known, an effect suggested by the association of intrahepatic activated NKT cells and spontaneous recovery.[141] In chronic infection, there appears to be a regulatory effect of NKT cells that prime naive antigen-specific CD8+ T cells to produce IL-10.[142]

Adaptive Cellular Response to Hepatitis C Virus Infection

After activation, mDC and pDC migrate to lymphoid tissue to stimulate the generation of antigen-specific B- and T-cell responses. Early adaptive immune responses are critical in the outcome of viral infections. CD8+ T cells are the immune effectors that directly eliminate virus-infected cells by both cytolytic and noncytolytic mechanisms,[143] whereas CD4+ T cells play a key regulatory role, providing help for CD8+ T cells and B cells.

The strength and scope of HCV-specific T-cell response are strongly associated with the outcome of acute HCV infection. In humans with acute hepatitis C, sustained vigorous and multispecific CD4+ and CD8+ IFN-γ+ T-cell responses to HCV (particularly to nonstructural antigens) in peripheral blood are associated with resolution of acute infection, whereas weak, focused, or transient responses are associated with viral persistence.[144–151] In experimentally infected chimpanzees, HCV-specific T-cell responses in the liver correlate with virological outcome, validating the observations made with peripheral blood in patients.[152–154] Cell depletion experiments in chimpanzees confirm that both CD4+ and CD8+ T cells are needed for efficient viral clearance.[155–157] During very early phases of acute hepatitis infection, the capacity of CD4+ T cells to proliferate in response to viral antigens[146,150,158–163] is associated with conversion of hyporeactive "stunned" HCV-specific CD8+ T cells into strong antiviral effectors[150,160] that can be cytotoxic to infected hepatocytes.[164,165]

The role of HCV-specific effector T cells in the long-term outcome of chronic infection is less well defined. The detection of, albeit weak, peripheral HCV-specific CD4+ T-cell IFN-γ responses has been associated with a more benign clinical course.[166,167] No consistent link between intrahepatic HCV-specific CD4+ and CD8+ T-cell IFN-γ frequencies and long-term clinical outcomes has been shown.[166,168–171] However, circumstantial evidence for the importance of effector T cells in control of HCV-related liver disease can be found in the setting of generalized T-cell defects (eg, HIV/HCV coinfection, chronic steroid use, posttransplant immunosuppression) in which immune dysregulation leads to accelerated liver disease progression and high viral titers.[172–174]

Failure of antiviral T cells to control initial HCV infection is multifactorial, likely resulting from impaired priming of T cells by DC (discussed earlier), aberrant T-cell priming by intrahepatic antigen-presenting cells (LSEC, hepatocytes, NKT),[90,104,142,175–177] viral escape mutation,[163,168,178,179] induction of various Treg subsets,[180,181] and T-cell anergy.[182–184] Specific viral sequences in founder viruses may have varying degrees of immunogenicity,[185] and certain HLA alleles are more or less likely to induce sterilizing immune responses.[110,186,187] Presentation of epitopes from viral escape variants may antagonize HCV-specific T-cell responses.[168,188] Furthermore, HCV core may suppress T-cell activation through the C1q complement receptor.[189,190] The induction of multiple subtypes of Treg and antigen-induced expression of inhibitory costimulation receptors are critical additional steps required for viral persistence.

Treg, typically defined by expression of the transcription factor foxp3 and high expression of the IL-2 receptor α chain (CD25), relevant in hepatitis C infection include natural CD304+ Tregs (nTreg) specific for self-epitopes[191,192] and induced Tregs derived from virus-specific CD4+CD25− effector T cells. Activated Tregs suppress effector T cells in a contact-dependent manner[181,193,194] within target tissues. The generation of nTregs sequence homology for self-epitopes present in the HCV Core and p7 antigens.[195,196] In vitro, CD4+ T cells cocultured with HCV-infected hepatocyte cell lines develop a Treg phenotype with increased expression of foxp3, CD25, CTLA-4, and TGF-β.[197] High-level expression of a viral antigen in hepatocytes may also be a critical factor predisposing to the development of Tregs.[198] The overall frequency of Tregs does not differ in acute resolving or persisting HCV infection, but the suppressive capacity of Tregs increases over time in persistent acute infection while decreasing in resolving infection.[199] In chronic infection, there is not only increased circulating CD4+CD25+ Tregs[180,193,200] but also significant CD4+foxp3+ Treg infiltration into the liver[201] with associated suppression of necroinflammation and fibrosis.[192,202] Several mouse models of acute and chronic hepatitis have provided strong evidence that Tregs play a fundamental role in dampening the potentially deleterious impact of activated effector T cells in the liver.[203]

HCV-specific IL-10-producing Tr1 T cells, typically not expressing foxp3 or high-level CD25, comprise an additional regulatory cell population important for HCV pathogenesis.[204–213] Although IL-10 is produced by many cell types, including DCs, macrophages, monocytes, NK, and NKT cells,[214] IL-10+foxp3− CD4+ T cells appear to be an important source of IL-10 and TGF-β, directly inhibiting effector T-cell function in both IL-10-dependent and IL-10-independent fashion.[210,212] In vitro, HCV proteins directly induce virus-specific T-cell production of IL-10[215–217] in both CD4+[218,219] and CD8+ T-cell[220,221] subsets. In acute infection, early skewing of antiviral T cells to produce IL-10, possibly influenced by polymorphisms in the IL-10 promoter,[222–226] is associated with chronic evolution.[219,227,228] Viral mutation under immune selection pressure may also reprogram T cells to produce IL-10.[179] Because of its anti-inflammatory effects, exogenous administration of IL-10 in humans reduces hepatic fibrosis.[229] The frequency of CD8+IL-10+ T cells in the liver also inversely correlates with inflammation,[221] suggesting that T-cell IL-10 production may be a critical negative feedback to prevent rapid liver injury in chronic infection.

In chronic infection, prolonged antigenic stimulation leads to the upregulation of several inhibitory coreceptors on antigen-specific CD8+ T cells that individually or in combination generate a state of functional hyporeactivity, termed anergy. The inhibitory receptors best characterized for this effect include programmed death-1 (PD-1), cytotoxic T-lymphocyte associated protein-4 (CTLA-4), T-cell immunoglobulin and mucin 3 engagement of high-mobility group box 1, NK cell receptor 2B4 (CD244), lymphocyte associated gene-3, Killer cell lectin-like receptor subfamily G member 1, and CD160.

PD-1 is 55-kDa glycoprotein member of the CD28 superfamily that contains an immunoreceptor tyrosine-based inhibitory motif and immunoreceptor switch motif that phosphorylate the kinase SHP-2, which then dephosphorylates various signal transduction kinases involved in T-cell receptor induction of IL-2 and proliferation.[230] The ligand for PD-1, PD-L1, is expressed on intrahepatic mDC, LSEC, and KC.[231,232] CTLA-4 is an immunoglobulin-like receptor that competes with CD28 for binding of CD80 and

CD86, thereby blocking T-cell costimulation. PD-1 and CTLA-4 become highly expressed on HCV-specific CD8[+] T cells and CD4[+] T cells early in acute HCV infection, remaining elevated in persistent infection but normalizing after viral clearance.[233–236] In chronic infection, HCV-specific memory CD8[+] T cells particularly within the liver express high levels of PD-1, impaired effector cytokines production, and low levels of cytolytic granules.[231,237,238] Early studies indicated that single blockade of PD-1/PD-L1 interactions ex vivo augments the expansion of peripheral CD8[+] T-cell expansion.[231,233,237] However, intrahepatic HCV-specific CD8[+] T cells from patients with cirrhosis express high levels of other costimulation inhibitory receptors such as CTLA-4 and require multiple pathway blockade to restore antigen-specific responses in some patients.[239,240] More recent studies suggest that among peripheral HCV-specific CD8[+] T cells in individual patients, various combinations of inhibitory receptors may be expressed and that responses to blockade of any single inhibitor is highly variable[241–244]; indeed, a 4-pathway blockade was required to improve HCV-specific CD8[+] T-cell function in greater than half of the patient samples in one study.[244] Other studies suggest that the anergic state is irreversible, even after curing infection through antiviral therapy[245] and that residual functional CD8[+] T cells detected ex vivo are specific for viral sequence not expressed by circulating virus.[241,245,246] Therapeutically, the use of anti-PD-1 antibody appeared to cause significant reduction of viral loads in one-third of treated chimpanzees[247] and a similar number of humans[248]; in light of the relative inefficacy of single blockade in ex vivo experiments and the rapid evolution of direct acting antivirals, the further development of this treatment strategy is unknown. Nonetheless, induction of T-cell anergy is thought to play a critical role in preventing sterilizing antiviral CD8[+] T-cell responses in both acute and chronic HCV infection.

The B-cell-mediated antibody response to HCV can be detected within 6 to 8 weeks of inoculation.[158,249–251] Neutralizing antibodies, which interfere with viral envelope binding to targets such as LDLR, SRBI, CD81, and claudin-1,[252,253] in early acute infection are associated with resolution in some[254,255] but not all studies.[158,251] However, chimpanzee cross-challenge experiments[152,256–264] and human series[265] show that HCV-specific antibodies do not universally mediate protection. Possible reasons for the lack of antibody-mediated protection include (1) the mutable quasi-species nature of HCV with rapid selection of antibody escape variants[251,266]; (2) intrinsic sequence-specific variability of the sensitivity of E1E2 proteins to neutralization[267,268]; and (3) paradoxic facilitation of viral entry by sensitivity of E1E2 protein.[267,269] In up to 40% of patients with spontaneous viral clearance, HCV antibody titers may wane after 2 to 3 decades.[270] In persistent infection, novel B-cell clones are continuously stimulated to respond to evolving viral mutations.[255,267,271–273] In addition, interactions between the HCV E2 envelope protein and B-cell CD81, an activating tetraspanin coreceptor, drive antigen-independent polyclonal B-cell stimulation,[274] predisposing to B-cell lymphoproliferative disorders. Despite chronic activation of virus-specific and non-virus-specific B cells, memory B cells do not accumulate in chronically infected patients[275–279] for reasons yet to be clearly defined. As seen with T cells, chronic viral infection creates an anergic state in some HCV-specific B cells, phenotypically defined as CD27[+]CD27[−/lo] tissue-like memory B cells with impaired proliferation[280–282] with unclear clinical significance. A clear pathogenic role for B cells in liver disease progression in chronic HCV infection has not as yet been defined.

SUMMARY

The establishment of persistent infection, resistance to interferon-based therapy, and progression of fibrosis are tightly linked with immune dysregulation induced by specific hepatitis C viral proteins or by rapid viral mutation. Genetic polymorphisms that alter either cytokine responses, antigen-independent stimulation of innate immune cells, or antigen presentation in part determine the susceptibility of an individual human host to initial infection, and the impact on the liver of a persistent infection. Other host factors, some quantifiable, such as age, gender, alcohol use, and pre-existing immunologic defects, and others poorly quantifiable, shape the complex dynamic host-virus interactions that determine permissiveness to chronic infection and disease progression rates. Critical events for the establishment of persistent infection include the disruption of type I and III interferon induction and signaling, interference with innate cellular activation, impairment and skewing of antigen-presentation to B and T cells, induction of various Treg T cell subsets, and functional inhibition of antigen-specific T- and B-cell responses. After initial failure to control infection, these processes control the magnitude of necroinflammation and resultant fibrosis progression. The complexity of interactions makes it unlikely that any therapeutic modality aimed at any single component will have universal efficacy, thus defining the critical nodes in these networks suitable for intervention remains an important endeavor despite the development of highly effective, oral therapy for chronic hepatitis C.

REFERENCES

1. Lavanchy D. The global burden of hepatitis C. Liver Int 2009;29(Suppl 1):74–81.
2. Alter HJ. To C or not to C: these are the questions. Blood 1995;85:1681–95.
3. Major ME, Feinstone SM. The molecular virology of hepatitis C. Hepatology 1997;25:1527–38.
4. Houghton M, Weiner A, Han J, et al. Molecular biology of the hepatitis C viruses: implications for diagnosis, development and control of viral disease. Hepatology 1991;14:381–8.
5. Pileri P, Uematsu Y, Campagnoli S, et al. Binding of hepatitis C virus to CD81. Science 1998;282:938–41.
6. Hsu M, Zhang J, Flint M, et al. Hepatitis C virus glycoproteins mediate pH-dependent cell entry of pseudotyped retroviral particles. Proc Natl Acad Sci U S A 2003;100:7271–6.
7. Wunschmann S, Medh JD, Klinzmann D, et al. Characterization of hepatitis C virus (HCV) and HCV E2 interactions with CD81 and the low-density lipoprotein receptor. J Virol 2000;74:10055–62.
8. Lozach PY, Lortat-Jacob H, de Lacroix de Lavalette A, et al. DC-SIGN and L-SIGN are high affinity binding receptors for hepatitis C virus glycoprotein E2. J Biol Chem 2003;278:20358–66.
9. Pohlmann S, Zhang J, Baribaud F, et al. Hepatitis C virus glycoproteins interact with DC-SIGN and DC-SIGNR. J Virol 2003;77:4070–80.
10. McKeating JA, Zhang LQ, Logvinoff C, et al. Diverse hepatitis C virus glycoproteins mediate viral infection in a CD81-dependent manner. J Virol 2004;78:8496–505.
11. Evans MJ, von Hahn T, Tscherne DM, et al. Claudin-1 is a hepatitis C virus co-receptor required for a late step in entry. Nature 2007;446:801–5.
12. Stetson DB, Medzhitov R. Type I interferons in host defense. Immunity 2006;25:373–81.
13. Metz P, Dazert E, Ruggieri A, et al. Identification of type I and type II interferon-induced effectors controlling hepatitis C virus replication. Hepatology 2012;56:2082–93.
14. Shin EC, Seifert U, Kato T, et al. Virus-induced type I IFN stimulates generation of immunoproteasomes at the site of infection. J Clin Invest 2006;116:3006–14.

15. Yoshio S, Kanto T, Kuroda S, et al. Human blood dendritic cell antigen 3 (BDCA3)(+) dendritic cells are a potent producer of interferon-lambda in response to hepatitis C virus. Hepatology 2013;57:1705–15.

16. Marcello T, Grakoui A, Barba-Spaeth G, et al. Interferons alpha and lambda inhibit hepatitis C virus replication with distinct signal transduction and gene regulation kinetics. Gastroenterology 2006;131:1887–98.

17. Kohli A, Zhang X, Yang J, et al. Distinct and overlapping genomic profiles and antiviral effects of interferon-lambda and -alpha on HCV-infected and noninfected hepatoma cells. J Viral Hepat 2012;19:843–53.

18. Dickensheets H, Sheikh F, Park O, et al. Interferon-lambda (IFN-lambda) induces signal transduction and gene expression in human hepatocytes, but not in lymphocytes or monocytes. J Leukoc Biol 2013;93:377–85.

19. Sumpter R Jr, Loo YM, Foy E, et al. Regulating intracellular antiviral defense and permissiveness to hepatitis C virus RNA replication through a cellular RNA helicase, RIG-I. J Virol 2005;79:2689–99.

20. Israelow B, Narbus CM, Sourisseau M, et al. HepG2 cells mount an effective antiviral interferon-lambda based innate immune response to hepatitis C virus infection. Hepatology 2014;60:1170–9.

21. Foy E, Li K, Sumpter R Jr, et al. Control of antiviral defenses through hepatitis C virus disruption of retinoic acid-inducible gene-I signaling. Proc Natl Acad Sci U S A 2005;102:2986–91.

22. Saito T, Gale M Jr. Principles of intracellular viral recognition. Curr Opin Immunol 2007;19:17–23.

23. Saito T, Owen DM, Jiang F, et al. Innate immunity induced by composition-dependent RIG-I recognition of hepatitis C virus RNA. Nature 2008;454:523–7.

24. Su AI, Pezacki JP, Wodicka L, et al. Genomic analysis of the host response to hepatitis C virus infection. Proc Natl Acad Sci U S A 2002;99:15669–74.

25. Thomas E, Gonzalez VD, Li Q, et al. HCV infection induces a unique hepatic innate immune response associated with robust production of type III interferons. Gastroenterology 2012;142:978–88.

26. Amanzada A, Kopp W, Spengler U, et al. Interferon-lambda4 (IFNL4) transcript expression in human liver tissue samples. PLoS One 2013;8:e84026.

27. Terczynska-Dyla E, Bibert S, Duong FH, et al. Reduced IFNlambda4 activity is associated with improved HCV clearance and reduced expression of interferon-stimulated genes. Nat Commun 2014;5:5699.

28. Schoggins JW, MacDuff DA, Imanaka N, et al. Pan-viral specificity of IFN-induced genes reveals new roles for cGAS in innate immunity. Nature 2014; 505:691–5.

29. Gale M Jr, Blakely CM, Kwieciszewski B, et al. Control of PKR protein kinase by hepatitis C virus nonstructural 5A protein: molecular mechanisms of kinase regulation. Mol Cell Biol 1998;18:5208–18.

30. Taylor DR, Shi ST, Romano PR, et al. Inhibition of the interferon-inducible protein kinase PKR by HCV E2 protein. Science 1999;285:107–10.

31. Arnaud N, Dabo S, Maillard P, et al. Hepatitis C virus controls interferon production through PKR activation. PLoS One 2010;5:e10575.

32. Meylan E, Curran J, Hofmann K, et al. Cardif is an adaptor protein in the RIG-I antiviral pathway and is targeted by hepatitis C virus. Nature 2005;437:1167–72.

33. Breiman A, Grandvaux N, Lin R, et al. Inhibition of RIG-I-dependent signaling to the interferon pathway during hepatitis C virus expression and restoration of signaling by IKKepsilon. J Virol 2005;79:3969–78.

34. Loo YM, Owen DM, Li K, et al. Viral and therapeutic control of IFN-beta promoter stimulator 1 during hepatitis C virus infection. Proc Natl Acad Sci U S A 2006; 103:6001–6.
35. Lin R, Lacoste J, Nakhaei P, et al. Dissociation of a MAVS/IPS-1/VISA/Cardif-IKKepsilon molecular complex from the mitochondrial outer membrane by hepatitis C virus NS3-4A proteolytic cleavage. J Virol 2006;80:6072–83.
36. Cheng G, Zhong J, Chisari FV. Inhibition of dsRNA-induced signaling in hepatitis C virus-infected cells by NS3 protease-dependent and -independent mechanisms. Proc Natl Acad Sci U S A 2006;103:8499–504.
37. Tasaka M, Sakamoto N, Itakura Y, et al. Hepatitis C virus non-structural proteins responsible for suppression of the RIG-I/Cardif-induced interferon response. J Gen Virol 2007;88:3323–33.
38. Baril M, Racine ME, Penin F, et al. MAVS dimer is a crucial signaling component of innate immunity and the target of hepatitis C virus NS3/4A protease. J Virol 2009;83:1299–311.
39. Ding Q, Huang B, Lu J, et al. Hepatitis C virus NS3/4A protease blocks IL-28 production. Eur J Immunol 2012;42:2374–82.
40. Li K, Foy E, Ferreon JC, et al. Immune evasion by hepatitis C virus NS3/4A protease-mediated cleavage of the Toll-like receptor 3 adaptor protein TRIF. Proc Natl Acad Sci U S A 2005;102:2992–7.
41. Otsuka M, Kato N, Moriyama M, et al. Interaction between the HCV NS3 protein and the host TBK1 protein leads to inhibition of cellular antiviral responses. Hepatology 2005;41:1004–12.
42. Wagoner J, Austin M, Green J, et al. Regulation of CXCL-8 (interleukin-8) induction by double-stranded RNA signaling pathways during hepatitis C virus infection. J Virol 2007;81:309–18.
43. Tu Z, Pierce RH, Kurtis J, et al. Hepatitis C virus core protein subverts the antiviral activities of human Kupffer cells. Gastroenterology 2010;138:305–14.
44. Ebihara T, Shingai M, Matsumoto M, et al. Hepatitis C virus-infected hepatocytes extrinsically modulate dendritic cell maturation to activate T cells and natural killer cells. Hepatology 2008;48:48–58.
45. Okamoto M, Oshiumi H, Azuma M, et al. IPS-1 is essential for type III IFN production by hepatocytes and dendritic cells in response to hepatitis C virus infection. J Immunol 2014;192:2770–7.
46. Bode JG, Ludwig S, Ehrhardt C, et al. IFN-alpha antagonistic activity of HCV core protein involves induction of suppressor of cytokine signaling-3. FASEB J 2003;17:488–90.
47. Melen K, Fagerlund R, Nyqvist M, et al. Expression of hepatitis C virus core protein inhibits interferon-induced nuclear import of STATs. J Med Virol 2004;73:536–47.
48. de Lucas S, Bartolome J, Carreno V. Hepatitis C virus core protein downregulates transcription of interferon-induced antiviral genes. J Infect Dis 2005; 191:93–9.
49. Lin W, Kim SS, Yeung E, et al. Hepatitis C virus core protein blocks interferon signaling by interaction with the STAT1 SH2 domain. J Virol 2006;80:9226–35.
50. Thomas DL, Thio CL, Martin MP, et al. Genetic variation in IL28B and spontaneous clearance of hepatitis C virus. Nature 2009;461:798–801.
51. Rauch A, Kutalik Z, Descombes P, et al. Genetic variation in IL28B is associated with chronic hepatitis C and treatment failure: a genome-wide association study. Gastroenterology 2010;138:1338–45, 1345.e1–7.
52. Hajarizadeh B, Grady B, Page K, et al. Patterns of hepatitis C virus RNA levels during acute infection: the InC3 study. PLoS One 2015;10:e0122232.

53. Ge D, Fellay J, Thompson AJ, et al. Genetic variation in IL28B predicts hepatitis C treatment-induced viral clearance. Nature 2009;461:399–401.
54. Suppiah V, Moldovan M, Ahlenstiel G, et al. IL28B is associated with response to chronic hepatitis C interferon-alpha and ribavirin therapy. Nat Genet 2009;41: 1100–4.
55. Tanaka Y, Nishida N, Sugiyama M, et al. Genome-wide association of IL28B with response to pegylated interferon-alpha and ribavirin therapy for chronic hepatitis C. Nat Genet 2009;41:1105–9.
56. Prokunina-Olsson L, Muchmore B, Tang W, et al. A variant upstream of IFNL3 (IL28B) creating a new interferon gene IFNL4 is associated with impaired clearance of hepatitis C virus. Nat Genet 2013;45:164–71.
57. Real LM, Neukam K, Herrero R, et al. IFNL4 ss469415590 variant shows similar performance to rs12979860 as predictor of response to treatment against Hepatitis C Virus genotype 1 or 4 in Caucasians. PLoS One 2014;9:e95515.
58. Stattermayer AF, Strassl R, Maieron A, et al. Polymorphisms of interferon-lambda4 and IL28B—effects on treatment response to interferon/ribavirin in patients with chronic hepatitis C. Aliment Pharmacol Ther 2014;39: 104–11.
59. Susser S, Herrmann E, Lange C, et al. Predictive value of interferon-lambda gene polymorphisms for treatment response in chronic hepatitis C. PLoS One 2014;9:e112592.
60. Bibert S, Roger T, Calandra T, et al. IL28B expression depends on a novel TT/-G polymorphism which improves HCV clearance prediction. J Exp Med 2013;210: 1109–16.
61. Hamming OJ, Terczynska-Dyla E, Vieyres G, et al. Interferon lambda 4 signals via the IFNlambda receptor to regulate antiviral activity against HCV and coronaviruses. EMBO J 2013;32:3055–65.
62. Lu YF, Goldstein DB, Urban TJ, et al. Interferon-lambda4 is a cell-autonomous type III interferon associated with pre-treatment hepatitis C virus burden. Virology 2015;476:334–40.
63. Hoffmann FS, Schmidt A, Dittmann Chevillotte M, et al. Polymorphisms in melanoma differentiation-associated gene 5 link protein function to clearance of hepatitis C virus. Hepatology 2015;61:460–70.
64. Marabita F, Aghemo A, De Nicola S, et al. Genetic variation in the interleukin-28B gene is not associated with fibrosis progression in patients with chronic hepatitis C and known date of infection. Hepatology 2011;54:1127–34.
65. Bochud PY, Bibert S, Kutalik Z, et al. IL28B alleles associated with poor hepatitis C virus (HCV) clearance protect against inflammation and fibrosis in patients infected with non-1 HCV genotypes. Hepatology 2012;55:384–94.
66. Noureddin M, Wright EC, Alter HJ, et al. Association of IL28B genotype with fibrosis progression and clinical outcomes in patients with chronic hepatitis C: a longitudinal analysis. Hepatology 2013;58:1548–57.
67. Eslam M, Leung R, Romero-Gomez M, et al. IFNL3 polymorphisms predict response to therapy in chronic hepatitis C genotype 2/3 infection. J Hepatol 2014;61:235–41.
68. Randall G, Chen L, Panis M, et al. Silencing of USP18 potentiates the antiviral activity of interferon against hepatitis C virus infection. Gastroenterology 2006; 131:1584–91.
69. Urban TJ, Thompson AJ, Bradrick SS, et al. IL28B genotype is associated with differential expression of intrahepatic interferon-stimulated genes in patients with chronic hepatitis C. Hepatology 2010;52:1888–96.

70. Makowska Z, Duong FH, Trincucci G, et al. Interferon-beta and interferon-lambda signaling is not affected by interferon-induced refractoriness to interferon-alpha in vivo. Hepatology 2011;53:1154–63.

71. Sarasin-Filipowicz M, Oakeley EJ, Duong FH, et al. Interferon signaling and treatment outcome in chronic hepatitis C. Proc Natl Acad Sci U S A 2008;105: 7034–9.

72. Feld JJ, Lutchman GA, Heller T, et al. Ribavirin improves early responses to peginterferon through improved interferon signaling. Gastroenterology 2010;139: 154–62.e4.

73. Bigger CB, Brasky KM, Lanford RE. DNA microarray analysis of chimpanzee liver during acute resolving hepatitis C virus infection. J Virol 2001;75:7059–66.

74. Bigger CB, Guerra B, Brasky KM, et al. Intrahepatic gene expression during chronic hepatitis C virus infection in chimpanzees. J Virol 2004;78:13779–92.

75. Chen L, Borozan I, Feld J, et al. Hepatic gene expression discriminates responders and nonresponders in treatment of chronic hepatitis C viral infection. Gastroenterology 2005;128:1437–44.

76. Feld JJ, Nanda S, Huang Y, et al. Hepatic gene expression during treatment with peginterferon and ribavirin: identifying molecular pathways for treatment response. Hepatology 2007;46:1548–63.

77. Muir AJ, Shiffman ML, Zaman A, et al. Phase 1b study of pegylated interferon lambda 1 with or without ribavirin in patients with chronic genotype 1 hepatitis C virus infection. Hepatology 2010;52:822–32.

78. Liang Y, Ishida H, Lenz O, et al. Antiviral suppression vs restoration of RIG-I signaling by hepatitis C protease and polymerase inhibitors. Gastroenterology 2008;135(5):1710–8.e2.

79. Ahmad A, Alvarez F. Role of NK and NKT cells in the immunopathogenesis of HCV-induced hepatitis. J Leukoc Biol 2004;76:743–59.

80. Velazquez VM, Hon H, Ibegbu C, et al. Hepatic enrichment and activation of myeloid dendritic cells during chronic hepatitis C virus infection. Hepatology 2012;56:2071–81.

81. Takahashi K, Asabe S, Wieland S, et al. Plasmacytoid dendritic cells sense hepatitis C virus-infected cells, produce interferon, and inhibit infection. Proc Natl Acad Sci U S A 2010;107:7431–6.

82. Grabski E, Wappler I, Pfaender S, et al. Efficient virus assembly, but not infectivity, determines the magnitude of hepatitis C virus-induced interferon alpha responses of plasmacytoid dendritic cells. J Virol 2015;89:3200–8.

83. Zhang S, Kodys K, Babcock GJ, et al. CD81/CD9 tetraspanins aid plasmacytoid dendritic cells in recognition of hepatitis C virus-infected cells and induction of interferon-alpha. Hepatology 2013;58:940–9.

84. Zhang S, Kodys K, Li K, et al. Human type 2 myeloid dendritic cells produce interferon-lambda and amplify interferon-alpha in response to hepatitis C virus infection. Gastroenterology 2013;144:414–25.e7.

85. Leone P, Di Tacchio M, Berardi S, et al. Dendritic cell maturation in HCV infection: altered regulation of MHC class I antigen processing-presenting machinery. J Hepatol 2014;61:242–51.

86. Murata K, Sugiyama M, Kimura T, et al. Ex vivo induction of IFN-lambda3 by a TLR7 agonist determines response to Peg-IFN/ribavirin therapy in chronic hepatitis C patients. J Gastroenterol 2014;49:126–37.

87. Marukian S, Andrus L, Sheahan TP, et al. Hepatitis C virus induces interferon-lambda and interferon-stimulated genes in primary liver cultures. Hepatology 2011;54:1913–23.

88. Ryan EJ, O'Farrelly C. The affect of chronic hepatitis C infection on dendritic cell function: a summary of the experimental evidence. J Viral Hepat 2011;18: 601–7.
89. Auffermann-Gretzinger S, Keeffe EB, Levy S. Impaired dendritic cell maturation in patients with chronic, but not resolved, hepatitis C virus infection. Blood 2001; 97:3171–6.
90. Zimmermann M, Flechsig C, La Monica N, et al. Hepatitis C virus core protein impairs in vitro priming of specific T cell responses by dendritic cells and hepatocytes. J Hepatol 2008;48:51–60.
91. Saito K, Ait-Goughoulte M, Truscott SM, et al. Hepatitis C virus inhibits cell surface expression of HLA-DR, prevents dendritic cell maturation, and induces interleukin-10 production. J Virol 2008;82:3320–8.
92. O'Beirne J, Mitchell J, Farzaneh F, et al. Inhibition of major histocompatibility complex class I antigen presentation by hepatitis C virus core protein in myeloid dendritic cells. Virology 2009;389:1–7.
93. Schulz S, Landi A, Garg R, et al. Indolamine 2,3-dioxygenase expression by monocytes and dendritic cell populations in hepatitis C patients. Clin Exp Immunol 2015;180(3):484–98.
94. Shiina M, Rehermann B. Cell culture-produced hepatitis C virus impairs plasmacytoid dendritic cell function. Hepatology 2008;47:385–95.
95. Dolganiuc A, Chang S, Kodys K, et al. Hepatitis C virus (HCV) core protein-induced, monocyte-mediated mechanisms of reduced IFN-alpha and plasmacytoid dendritic cell loss in chronic HCV infection. J Immunol 2006;177:6758–68.
96. Nattermann J, Zimmermann H, Iwan A, et al. Hepatitis C virus E2 and CD81 interaction may be associated with altered trafficking of dendritic cells in chronic hepatitis C. Hepatology 2006;44:945–54.
97. Gondois-Rey F, Dental C, Halfon P, et al. Hepatitis C virus is a weak inducer of interferon alpha in plasmacytoid dendritic cells in comparison with influenza and human herpesvirus type-1. PLoS One 2009;4:e4319.
98. Miyazaki M, Kanto T, Inoue M, et al. Impaired cytokine response in myeloid dendritic cells in chronic hepatitis C virus infection regardless of enhanced expression of Toll-like receptors and retinoic acid inducible gene-I. J Med Virol 2008; 80:980–8.
99. Gerosa F, Gobbi A, Zorzi P, et al. The reciprocal interaction of NK cells with plasmacytoid or myeloid dendritic cells profoundly affects innate resistance functions. J Immunol 2005;174:727–34.
100. Niesen E, Schmidt J, Flecken T, et al. Suppressive effect of interleukin 10 on priming of naive hepatitis C virus-specific CD8+ T cells. J Infect Dis 2015; 211:821–6.
101. Florimond A, Chouteau P, Bruscella P, et al. Human hepatic stellate cells are not permissive for hepatitis C virus entry and replication. Gut 2015;64(6):957–65.
102. Wang Y, Li J, Wang X, et al. Induction of interferon-lambda contributes to Toll-like receptor-3-activated hepatic stellate cell-mediated hepatitis C virus inhibition in hepatocytes. J Viral Hepat 2013;20:385–94.
103. Giugliano S, Kriss M, Golden-Mason L, et al. Hepatitis C virus infection induces autocrine interferon signaling by human liver endothelial cells and release of exosomes, which inhibits viral replication. Gastroenterology 2015;148: 392–402.e13.
104. Knolle PA, Kremp S, Hohler T, et al. Viral and host factors in the prediction of response to interferon-alpha therapy in chronic hepatitis C after long-term follow-up. J Viral Hepat 1998;5:399–406.

105. Ramos HJ, Lanteri MC, Blahnik G, et al. IL-1beta signaling promotes CNS-intrinsic immune control of West Nile virus infection. PLoS Pathog 2012;8: e1003039.
106. Negash AA, Ramos HJ, Crochet N, et al. IL-1β production through the NLRP3 inflammasome by hepatic macrophages links hepatitis C virus infection with liver inflammation and disease. PLoS Pathog 2013;9:e1003330.
107. Mengshol JA, Golden-Mason L, Arikawa T, et al. A crucial role for Kupffer cell-derived galectin-9 in regulation of T cell immunity in hepatitis C infection. PLoS One 2010;5:e9504.
108. Lunemann S, Schlaphoff V, Cornberg M, et al. NK cells in hepatitis C: role in disease susceptibility and therapy. Dig Dis 2012;30(Suppl 1):48–54.
109. Khakoo SI, Thio CL, Martin MP, et al. HLA and NK cell inhibitory receptor genes in resolving hepatitis C virus infection. Science 2004;305:872–4.
110. Romero V, Azocar J, Zuniga J, et al. Interaction of NK inhibitory receptor genes with HLA-C and MHC class II alleles in hepatitis C virus infection outcome. Mol Immunol 2008;45:2429–36.
111. Golden-Mason L, Cox AL, Randall JA, et al. Increased natural killer cell cytotoxicity and NKp30 expression protects against hepatitis C virus infection in high-risk individuals and inhibits replication in vitro. Hepatology 2010;52:1581–9.
112. Amadei B, Urbani S, Cazaly A, et al. Activation of natural killer cells during acute infection with hepatitis C virus. Gastroenterology 2010;138:1536–45.
113. Pelletier S, Drouin C, Bedard N, et al. Increased degranulation of natural killer cells during acute HCV correlates with the magnitude of virus-specific T cell responses. J Hepatol 2010;53:805–16.
114. Kokordelis P, Kramer B, Korner C, et al. An effective interferon-gamma-mediated inhibition of hepatitis C virus replication by natural killer cells is associated with spontaneous clearance of acute hepatitis C in human immunodeficiency virus-positive patients. Hepatology 2014;59:814–27.
115. Corado J, Toro F, Rivera H, et al. Impairment of natural killer (NK) cytotoxic activity in hepatitis C virus (HCV) infection. Clin Exp Immunol 1997;109:451–7.
116. Kaser A, Enrich B, Ludwiczek O, et al. Interferon-alpha (IFN-alpha) enhances cytotoxicity in healthy volunteers and chronic hepatitis C infection mainly by the perforin pathway. Clin Exp Immunol 1999;118:71–7.
117. Morishima C, Paschal DM, Wang CC, et al. Decreased NK cell frequency in chronic hepatitis C does not affect ex vivo cytolytic killing. Hepatology 2006; 43:573–80.
118. De Maria A, Fogli M, Mazza S, et al. Increased natural cytotoxicity receptor expression and relevant IL-10 production in NK cells from chronically infected viremic HCV patients. Eur J Immunol 2007;37:445–55.
119. Golden-Mason L, Madrigal-Estebas L, McGrath E, et al. Altered natural killer cell subset distributions in resolved and persistent hepatitis C virus infection following single source exposure. Gut 2008;57:1121–8.
120. Yoon JC, Shiina M, Ahlenstiel G, et al. Natural killer cell function is intact after direct exposure to infectious hepatitis C virions. Hepatology 2009;49: 12–21.
121. Jinushi M, Takehara T, Tatsumi T, et al. Negative regulation of NK cell activities by inhibitory receptor CD94/NKG2A leads to altered NK cell-induced modulation of dendritic cell functions in chronic hepatitis C virus infection. J Immunol 2004;173:6072–81.
122. Tseng CT, Klimpel GR. Binding of the hepatitis C virus envelope protein E2 to CD81 inhibits natural killer cell functions. J Exp Med 2002;195:43–9.

123. Crotta S, Stilla A, Wack A, et al. Inhibition of natural killer cells through engagement of CD81 by the major hepatitis C virus envelope protein. J Exp Med 2002;195:35–41.
124. Nattermann J, Nischalke HD, Hofmeister V, et al. The HLA-A2 restricted T cell epitope HCV core 35-44 stabilizes HLA-E expression and inhibits cytolysis mediated by natural killer cells. Am J Pathol 2005;166:443–53.
125. Sene D, Levasseur F, Abel M, et al. Hepatitis C virus (HCV) evades NKG2D-dependent NK cell responses through NS5A-mediated imbalance of inflammatory cytokines. PLoS Pathog 2010;6:e1001184.
126. Wen C, He X, Ma H, et al. Hepatitis C virus infection downregulates the ligands of the activating receptor NKG2D. Cell Mol Immunol 2008;5:475–8.
127. Nattermann J, Feldmann G, Ahlenstiel G, et al. Surface expression and cytolytic function of natural killer cell receptors is altered in chronic hepatitis C. Gut 2006; 55:869–77.
128. Oliviero B, Varchetta S, Paudice E, et al. Natural killer cell functional dichotomy in chronic hepatitis B and chronic hepatitis C virus infections. Gastroenterology 2009;137:1151–60, 1160.e1–7.
129. Bonorino P, Ramzan M, Camous X, et al. Fine characterization of intrahepatic NK cells expressing natural killer receptors in chronic hepatitis B and C. J Hepatol 2009;51:458–67.
130. Ahlenstiel G, Titerence RH, Koh C, et al. Natural killer cells are polarized toward cytotoxicity in chronic hepatitis C in an interferon-alfa-dependent manner. Gastroenterology 2010;138:325–35.e1-2.
131. Muhanna N, Abu Tair L, Doron S, et al. Amelioration of hepatic fibrosis by NK cell activation. Gut 2011;60:90–8.
132. Cheng YQ, Ren JP, Zhao J, et al. MicroRNA-155 regulates interferon-gamma production in natural killer cells via Tim-3 signalling in chronic hepatitis C virus infection. Immunology 2015;145(4):485–97.
133. Golden-Mason L, Bambha KM, Cheng L, et al. Natural killer inhibitory receptor expression associated with treatment failure and interleukin-28B genotype in patients with chronic hepatitis C. Hepatology 2011;54:1559–69.
134. Ahlenstiel G, Edlich B, Hogdal LJ, et al. Early changes in natural killer cell function indicate virologic response to interferon therapy for hepatitis C. Gastroenterology 2011;141:1231–9, 1239.e1–2.
135. Edlich B, Ahlenstiel G, Zabaleta Azpiroz A, et al. Early changes in interferon signaling define natural killer cell response and refractoriness to interferon-based therapy of hepatitis C patients. Hepatology 2012;55:39–48.
136. Exley MA, Koziel MJ. To be or not to be NKT: natural killer T cells in the liver. Hepatology 2004;40:1033–40.
137. Deignan T, Curry MP, Doherty DG, et al. Decrease in hepatic CD56(+) T cells and V alpha 24(+) natural killer T cells in chronic hepatitis C viral infection. J Hepatol 2002;37:101–8.
138. Lucas M, Gadola S, Meier U, et al. Frequency and phenotype of circulating Valpha24/Vbeta11 double-positive natural killer T cells during hepatitis C virus infection. J Virol 2003;77:2251–7.
139. Yamagiwa S, Matsuda Y, Ichida T, et al. Sustained response to interferon-alpha plus ribavirin therapy for chronic hepatitis C is closely associated with increased dynamism of intrahepatic natural killer and natural killer T cells. Hepatol Res 2008;38:664–72.
140. Inoue M, Kanto T, Miyatake H, et al. Enhanced ability of peripheral invariant natural killer T cells to produce IL-13 in chronic hepatitis C virus infection. J Hepatol 2006;45:190–6.

141. Golden-Mason L, Castelblanco N, O'Farrelly C, et al. Phenotypic and functional changes of cytotoxic CD56pos natural T cells determine outcome of acute hepatitis C virus infection. J Virol 2007;81:9292–8.

142. Wahl C, Bochtler P, Schirmbeck R, et al. Type I IFN-producing CD4 Valpha14i NKT cells facilitate priming of IL-10-producing CD8 T cells by hepatocytes. J Immunol 2007;178:2083–93.

143. Guidotti LG, Chisari FV. To kill or to cure: options in host defense against viral infection. Curr Opin Immunol 1996;8:478–83.

144. Diepolder HM, Zachoval R, Hoffmann RM, et al. Possible mechanism involving T-lymphocyte response to non-structural protein 3 in viral clearance in acute hepatitis C virus infection. Lancet 1995;346:1006–7.

145. Missale G, Bertoni R, Lamonaca V, et al. Different clinical behaviors of acute hepatitis C virus infection are associated with different vigor of the anti-viral cell-mediated immune response. J Clin Invest 1996;98:706–14.

146. Gerlach JT, Diepolder HM, Jung MC, et al. Recurrence of hepatitis C virus after loss of virus-specific CD4(+) T-cell response in acute hepatitis C. Gastroenterology 1999;117:933–41.

147. Ray SC, Wang YM, Laeyendecker O, et al. Acute hepatitis C virus structural gene sequences as predictors of persistent viremia: hypervariable region 1 as a decoy. J Virol 1999;73:2938–46.

148. Gruner NH, Gerlach TJ, Jung MC, et al. Association of hepatitis C virus-specific CD8+ T cells with viral clearance in acute hepatitis C. J Infect Dis 2000;181: 1528–36.

149. Lechner F, Gruener NH, Urbani S, et al. CD8+ T lymphocyte responses are induced during acute hepatitis C virus infection but are not sustained. Eur J Immunol 2000;30:2479–87.

150. Thimme R, Oldach D, Chang KM, et al. Determinants of viral clearance and persistence during acute hepatitis C virus infection. J Exp Med 2001;194:1395–406.

151. Chang KM. Immunopathogenesis of hepatitis C virus infection. Clin Liver Dis 2003;7:89–105.

152. Cooper S, Erickson AL, Adams EJ, et al. Analysis of a successful immune response against hepatitis C virus. Immunity 1999;10:439–49.

153. Thimme R, Bukh J, Spangenberg HC, et al. Viral and immunological determinants of hepatitis C virus clearance, persistence, and disease. Proc Natl Acad Sci U S A 2002;99:15661–8.

154. Zubkova I, Duan H, Wells F, et al. Hepatitis C virus clearance correlates with HLA-DR expression on proliferating CD8+ T cells in immune-primed chimpanzees. Hepatology 2014;59:803–13.

155. Grakoui A, Shoukry NH, Woollard DJ, et al. HCV persistence and immune evasion in the absence of memory T cell help. Science 2003;302:659–62.

156. Shoukry NH, Grakoui A, Houghton M, et al. Memory CD8+ T cells are required for protection from persistent hepatitis C virus infection. J Exp Med 2003;197:1645–55.

157. Thomson M, Nascimbeni M, Havert MB, et al. The clearance of hepatitis C virus infection in chimpanzees may not necessarily correlate with the appearance of acquired immunity. J Virol 2003;77:862–70.

158. Kaplan DE, Sugimoto K, Newton K, et al. Discordant role of CD4 T-cell response relative to neutralizing antibody and CD8 T-cell responses in acute hepatitis C. Gastroenterology 2007;132:654–66.

159. Folgori A, Spada E, Pezzanera M, et al. Early impairment of hepatitis C virus specific T cell proliferation during acute infection leads to failure of viral clearance. Gut 2006;55:1012–9.

160. Lechner F, Wong DK, Dunbar PR, et al. Analysis of successful immune responses in persons infected with hepatitis C virus. J Exp Med 2000;191: 1499–512.
161. Schulze zur Wiesch J, Lauer GM, Day CL, et al. Broad repertoire of the CD4+ Th cell response in spontaneously controlled hepatitis C virus infection includes dominant and highly promiscuous epitopes. J Immunol 2005;175:3603–13.
162. Smyk-Pearson S, Tester IA, Klarquist J, et al. Spontaneous recovery in acute human hepatitis C virus infection: functional T-cell thresholds and relative importance of CD4 help. J Virol 2008;82:1827–37.
163. Puig M, Mihalik K, Tilton JC, et al. CD4+ immune escape and subsequent T-cell failure following chimpanzee immunization against hepatitis C virus. Hepatology 2006;44:736–45.
164. Mondelli M, Alberti A, Tremolada F, et al. In-vitro cell-mediated cytotoxicity for autologous liver cells in chronic non-A, non-B hepatitis. Clin Exp Immunol 1986;63:147–55.
165. Kato T, Esumi M, Yamashita S, et al. Interferon-inducible gene expression in chimpanzee liver infected with hepatitis C virus. Virology 1992;190:856–60.
166. Hoffmann RM, Diepolder HM, Zachoval R, et al. Mapping of immunodominant CD4+ T lymphocyte epitopes of hepatitis C virus antigens and their relevance during the course of chronic infection. Hepatology 1995;21:632–8.
167. Chang KM, Thimme R, Melpolder JJ, et al. Differential CD4(+) and CD8(+) T-cell responsiveness in hepatitis C virus infection. Hepatology 2001;33:267–76.
168. Chang KM, Rehermann B, McHutchison JG, et al. Immunological significance of cytotoxic T lymphocyte epitope variants in patients chronically infected by the hepatitis C virus. J Clin Invest 1997;100:2376–85.
169. Kamal SM, Graham CS, He Q, et al. Kinetics of intrahepatic hepatitis C virus (HCV)-specific CD4+ T cell responses in HCV and Schistosoma mansoni coinfection: relation to progression of liver fibrosis. J Infect Dis 2004;189:1140–50.
170. Graham CS, Curry M, He Q, et al. Comparison of HCV-specific intrahepatic CD4+ T cells in HIV/HCV versus HCV. Hepatology 2004;40:125–32.
171. Weston SJ, Leistikow RL, Reddy KR, et al. Reconstitution of hepatitis C virus-specific T-cellmediated immunity after liver transplantation. Hepatology 2005; 41:72–81.
172. Berenguer M, Prieto M, Rayon JM, et al. Natural history of clinically compensated hepatitis C virus-related graft cirrhosis after liver transplantation. Hepatology 2000;32:852–8.
173. McCaughan GW, Zekry A. Effects of immunosuppression and organ transplantation on the natural history and immunopathogenesis of hepatitis C virus infection. Transpl Infect Dis 2000;2:166–85.
174. Nunez M, Soriano V. Hepatitis C virus (HCV) genotypes and disease progression in HIV/HCV-coinfected patients. J Infect Dis 2005;191:1–3.
175. Bertolino P, Trescol-Biemont MC, Thomas J, et al. Death by neglect as a deletional mechanism of peripheral tolerance. Int Immunol 1999;11:1225–38.
176. Wuensch SA, Pierce RH, Crispe IN. Local intrahepatic CD8+ T cell activation by a non-self-antigen results in full functional differentiation. J Immunol 2006;177: 1689–97.
177. Kruse N, Neumann K, Schrage A, et al. Priming of CD4(+) T cells by liver sinusoidal endothelial cells induces CD25(low) forkhead box protein 3- regulatory T cells suppressing autoimmune hepatitis. Hepatology 2009;50:1904–13.
178. Bull RA, Leung P, Gaudieri S, et al. Transmitted/founder viruses rapidly escape from CD8+ T cell responses in acute hepatitis C virus infection. J Virol 2015;89:5478–90.

179. Wang Y, Menne S, Jacob JR, et al. Role of type 1 versus type 2 immune responses in liver during the onset of chronic woodchuck hepatitis virus infection. Hepatology 2003;37:771–80.

180. Boettler T, Spangenberg HC, Neumann-Haefelin C, et al. T cells with a CD4+CD25+ regulatory phenotype suppress in vitro proliferation of virus-specific CD8+ T cells during chronic hepatitis C virus infection. J Virol 2005; 79:7860–7.

181. Rushbrook SM, Ward SM, Unitt E, et al. Regulatory T cells suppress in vitro proliferation of virus-specific CD8+ T cells during persistent hepatitis C virus infection. J Virol 2005;79:7852–9.

182. Sugimoto K, Stadanlick J, Ikeda F, et al. Influence of ethnicity in the outcome of hepatitis C virus infection and cellular immune response. Hepatology 2003;37: 590–9.

183. Ulsenheimer A, Gerlach JT, Gruener NH, et al. Detection of functionally altered hepatitis C virus-specific CD4 T cells in acute and chronic hepatitis C. Hepatology 2003;37:1189–98.

184. Wedemeyer H, He XS, Nascimbeni M, et al. Impaired effector function of hepatitis C virus-specific CD8+ T cells in chronic hepatitis C virus infection. J Immunol 2002;169:3447–58.

185. Ziegler S, Skibbe K, Walker A, et al. Impact of sequence variation in a dominant HLA-A*02-restricted epitope in hepatitis C virus on priming and cross-reactivity of CD8+ T cells. J Virol 2014;88:11080–90.

186. Azocar J, Clavijo OP, Yunis EJ. MHC class II genes in HCV viral clearance of hepatitis C infected Hispanic patients. Hum Immunol 2003;64:99–102.

187. Harris RA, Sugimoto K, Kaplan DE, et al. Human leukocyte antigen class II associations with hepatitis C virus clearance and virus-specific CD4 T cell response among Caucasians and African Americans. Hepatology 2008;48:70–9.

188. Erickson AL, Kimura Y, Igarashi S, et al. The outcome of hepatitis C virus infection is predicted by escape mutations in epitopes targeted by cytotoxic T lymphocytes. Immunity 2001;15:883–95.

189. Kittlesen DJ, Chianese-Bullock KA, Yao ZQ, et al. Interaction between complement receptor gC1qR and hepatitis C virus core protein inhibits T-lymphocyte proliferation. J Clin Invest 2000;106:1239–49.

190. Yao ZQ, Nguyen DT, Hiotellis AI, et al. Hepatitis C virus core protein inhibits human T lymphocyte responses by a complement-dependent regulatory pathway. J Immunol 2001;167:5264–72.

191. Li S, Floess S, Hamann A, et al. Analysis of FOXP3+ regulatory T cells that display apparent viral antigen specificity during chronic hepatitis C virus infection. PLoS Pathog 2009;5:e1000707.

192. Itose I, Kanto T, Kakita N, et al. Enhanced ability of regulatory T cells in chronic hepatitis C patients with persistently normal alanine aminotransferase levels than those with active hepatitis. J Viral Hepat 2009;16:844–52.

193. Sugimoto K, Ikeda F, Stadanlick J, et al. Suppression of HCV-specific T cells without differential hierarchy demonstrated ex-vivo in persistent HCV infection. Hepatology 2003;38(6):1437–48.

194. Cabrera R, Tu Z, Xu Y, et al. An immunomodulatory role for CD4(+)CD25(+) regulatory T lymphocytes in hepatitis C virus infection. Hepatology 2004;40: 1062–71.

195. Li S, Jones KL, Woollard DJ, et al. Defining target antigens for CD25+ FOXP3 + IFN-gamma- regulatory T cells in chronic hepatitis C virus infection. Immunol Cell Biol 2007;85:197–204.

196. Losikoff PT, Mishra S, Terry F, et al. HCV epitope, homologous to multiple human protein sequences, induces a regulatory T cell response in infected patients. J Hepatol 2015;62:48–55.
197. Hall CH, Kassel R, Tacke RS, et al. HCV+ hepatocytes induce human regulatory CD4+ T cells through the production of TGF-beta. PLoS One 2010;5:e12154.
198. Lapierre P, Janelle V, Langlois MP, et al. Expression of viral antigen by the liver leads to chronic infection through the generation of regulatory T cells. Cell Mol Gastroenterol Hepatol 2015;1(3):325–41.
199. Smyk-Pearson S, Golden-Mason L, Klarquist J, et al. Functional suppression by FoxP3+CD4+CD25(high) regulatory T cells during acute hepatitis C virus infection. J Infect Dis 2008;197:46–57.
200. Bolacchi F, Sinistro A, Ciaprini C, et al. Increased hepatitis C virus (HCV)-specific CD4+CD25+ regulatory T lymphocytes and reduced HCV-specific CD4+ T cell response in HCV-infected patients with normal versus abnormal alanine aminotransferase levels. Clin Exp Immunol 2006;144:188–96.
201. Ward SM, Fox BC, Brown PJ, et al. Quantification and localisation of FOXP3+ T lymphocytes and relation to hepatic inflammation during chronic HCV infection. J Hepatol 2007;47:316–24.
202. Sturm N, Thelu MA, Camous X, et al. Characterization and role of intra-hepatic regulatory T cells in chronic hepatitis C pathogenesis. J Hepatol 2010;53: 25–35.
203. Ju Y, Shang X, Liu Z, et al. The Tim-3/galectin-9 pathway involves in the homeostasis of hepatic Tregs in a mouse model of concanavalin A-induced hepatitis. Mol Immunol 2014;58:85–91.
204. Hara M, Kingsley CI, Niimi M, et al. IL-10 is required for regulatory T cells to mediate tolerance to alloantigens in vivo. J Immunol 2001;166:3789–96.
205. Levings MK, Sangregorio R, Galbiati F, et al. IFN-alpha and IL-10 induce the differentiation of human type 1 T regulatory cells. J Immunol 2001;166:5530–9.
206. Noel C, Florquin S, Goldman M, et al. Chronic exposure to superantigen induces regulatory CD4(+) T cells with IL-10-mediated suppressive activity. Int Immunol 2001;13:431–9.
207. Kingsley CI, Karim M, Bushell AR, et al. CD25+CD4+ regulatory T cells prevent graft rejection: CTLA-4- and IL-10-dependent immunoregulation of alloresponses. J Immunol 2002;168:1080–6.
208. Witsch EJ, Peiser M, Hutloff A, et al. ICOS and CD28 reversely regulate IL-10 on re-activation of human effector T cells with mature dendritic cells. Eur J Immunol 2002;32:2680–6.
209. Banz A, Peixoto A, Pontoux C, et al. A unique subpopulation of CD4+ regulatory T cells controls wasting disease, IL-10 secretion and T cell homeostasis. Eur J Immunol 2003;33:2419–28.
210. Sundstedt A, O'Neill EJ, Nicolson KS, et al. Role for IL-10 in suppression mediated by peptide-induced regulatory T cells in vivo. J Immunol 2003;170:1240–8.
211. Levings MK, Gregori S, Tresoldi E, et al. Differentiation of Tr1 cells by immature dendritic cells requires IL-10 but not CD25+CD4+ Treg cells. Blood 2004; 105(3):1162–9.
212. Vieira PL, Christensen JR, Minaee S, et al. IL-10-secreting regulatory T cells do not express Foxp3 but have comparable regulatory function to naturally occurring CD4+CD25+ regulatory T cells. J Immunol 2004;172:5986–93.
213. Zheng SG, Wang JH, Gray JD, et al. Natural and induced CD4+CD25+ cells educate CD4+CD25− cells to develop suppressive activity: the role of IL-2, TGF-beta, and IL-10. J Immunol 2004;172:5213–21.

214. Amaraa R, Mareckova H, Urbanek P, et al. Production of interleukins 10 and 12 by activated peripheral blood monocytes/macrophages in patients suffering from chronic hepatitis C virus infection with respect to the response to interferon and ribavirin treatment. Immunol Lett 2002;83:209–14.
215. Tsai SL, Liaw YF, Chen MH, et al. Detection of type 2-like T-helper cells in hepatitis C virus infection: implications for hepatitis C virus chronicity. Hepatology 1997;25:449–58.
216. Kimball P, Elswick RK, Shiffman M. Ethnicity and cytokine production gauge response of patients with hepatitis C to interferon-alpha therapy. J Med Virol 2001;65:510–6.
217. Godkin A, Jeanguet N, Thursz M, et al. Characterization of novel HLA-DR11-restricted HCV epitopes reveals both qualitative and quantitative differences in HCV-specific CD4+ T cell responses in chronically infected and non-viremic patients. Eur J Immunol 2001;31:1438–46.
218. Cramp ME, Rossol S, Chokshi S, et al. Hepatitis C virus-specific T-cell reactivity during interferon and ribavirin treatment in chronic hepatitis C. Gastroenterology 2000;118:346–55.
219. MacDonald AJ, Duffy M, Brady MT, et al. CD4 T helper type 1 and regulatory T cells induced against the same epitopes on the core protein in hepatitis C virus-infected persons. J Infect Dis 2002;185:720–7.
220. Koziel MJ, Dudley D, Wong JT, et al. Intrahepatic cytotoxic T lymphocytes specific for hepatitis C virus in persons with chronic hepatitis. J Immunol 1992;149: 3339–44 [Erratum appears in J Immunol 1993;150(6):2563].
221. Accapezzato D, Francavilla V, Paroli M, et al. Hepatic expansion of a virus-specific regulatory CD8(+) T cell population in chronic hepatitis C virus infection. J Clin Invest 2004;113:963–72.
222. Knapp S, Hennig BJ, Frodsham AJ, et al. Interleukin-10 promoter polymorphisms and the outcome of hepatitis C virus infection. Immunogenetics 2003; 55:362–9.
223. Mangia A, Santoro R, Piattelli M, et al. IL-10 haplotypes as possible predictors of spontaneous clearance of HCV infection. Cytokine 2004;25: 103–9.
224. Lio D, Caruso C, Di Stefano R, et al. IL-10 and TNF-alpha polymorphisms and the recovery from HCV infection. Hum Immunol 2003;64:674–80.
225. Edwards-Smith CJ, Jonsson JR, Purdie DM, et al. Interleukin-10 promoter polymorphism predicts initial response of chronic hepatitis C to interferon alfa. Hepatology 1999;30:526–30.
226. Yee LJ, Tang J, Gibson AW, et al. Interleukin 10 polymorphisms as predictors of sustained response in antiviral therapy for chronic hepatitis C infection. Hepatology 2001;33:708–12.
227. Kaplan DE, Ikeda F, Li Y, et al. Peripheral virus-specific T-cell interleukin-10 responses develop early in acute hepatitis C infection and become dominant in chronic hepatitis. J Hepatol 2008;48:903–13.
228. Kamal SM, Bianchi L, Al Tawil A, et al. Specific cellular immune response and cytokine patterns in patients coinfected with hepatitis C virus and Schistosoma mansoni. J Infect Dis 2001;184:972–82.
229. Nelson DR, Tu Z, Soldevila-Pico C, et al. Long-term interleukin 10 therapy in chronic hepatitis C patients has a proviral and anti-inflammatory effect. Hepatology 2003;38:859–68.
230. Barber DL, Wherry EJ, Masopust D, et al. Restoring function in exhausted CD8 T cells during chronic viral infection. Nature 2006;439:682–7.

231. Golden-Mason L, Palmer B, Klarquist J, et al. Upregulation of PD-1 expression on circulating and intrahepatic hepatitis C virus-specific CD8+ T cells associated with reversible immune dysfunction. J Virol 2007;81:9249–58.
232. Iwai Y, Terawaki S, Ikegawa M, et al. PD-1 inhibits antiviral immunity at the effector phase in the liver. J Exp Med 2003;198:39–50.
233. Urbani S, Amadei B, Tola D, et al. PD-1 expression in acute hepatitis C is associated with HCV-specific CD8 exhaustion. J Virol 2006;80(22):11398–403.
234. Kasprowicz V, Schulze Zur Wiesch J, Kuntzen T, et al. High level of PD-1 expression on hepatitis C virus (HCV)-specific CD8+ and CD4+ T cells during acute HCV infection, irrespective of clinical outcome. J Virol 2008;82:3154–60.
235. Raziorrouh B, Ulsenheimer A, Schraut W, et al. Inhibitory molecules that regulate expansion and restoration of HCV-specific CD4+ T cells in patients with chronic infection. Gastroenterology 2011;141:1422–31, 1431.e1–6.
236. Raghuraman S, Park H, Osburn WO, et al. Spontaneous clearance of chronic hepatitis C virus infection is associated with appearance of neutralizing antibodies and reversal of T-cell exhaustion. J Infect Dis 2012;205:763–71.
237. Radziewicz H, Ibegbu CC, Fernandez ML, et al. Liver-infiltrating lymphocytes in chronic human hepatitis C virus infection display an exhausted phenotype with high levels of PD-1 and low levels of CD127 expression. J Virol 2007;81: 2545–53.
238. Shen T, Zheng J, Xu C, et al. PD-1 expression on peripheral CD8+ TEM/TEMRA subsets closely correlated with HCV viral load in chronic hepatitis C patients. Virol J 2010;7:310.
239. Nakamoto N, Kaplan DE, Coleclough J, et al. Functional restoration of HCV-specific CD8 T cells by PD-1 blockade is defined by PD-1 expression and compartmentalization. Gastroenterology 2008;134:1927–37, 1937.e1–2.
240. Nakamoto N, Cho H, Shaked A, et al. Synergistic reversal of intrahepatic HCV-specific CD8 T cell exhaustion by combined PD-1/CTLA-4 blockade. PLoS Pathog 2009;5:e1000313.
241. Bengsch B, Seigel B, Ruhl M, et al. Coexpression of PD-1, 2B4, CD160 and KLRG1 on exhausted HCV-specific CD8+ T cells is linked to antigen recognition and T cell differentiation. PLoS Pathog 2010;6:e1000947.
242. McMahan RH, Golden-Mason L, Nishimura MI, et al. Tim-3 expression on PD-1+ HCV-specific human CTLs is associated with viral persistence, and its blockade restores hepatocyte-directed in vitro cytotoxicity. J Clin Invest 2010; 120:4546–57.
243. Schlaphoff V, Lunemann S, Suneetha PV, et al. Dual function of the NK cell receptor 2B4 (CD244) in the regulation of HCV-specific CD8+ T cells. PLoS Pathog 2011;7:e1002045.
244. Owusu Sekyere S, Suneetha PV, Kraft AR, et al. A heterogeneous hierarchy of co-regulatory receptors regulates exhaustion of HCV-specific CD8 T cells in patients with chronic hepatitis C. J Hepatol 2015;62:31–40.
245. Seigel B, Bengsch B, Lohmann V, et al. Factors that determine the antiviral efficacy of HCV-specific CD8(+) T cells ex vivo. Gastroenterology 2013;144: 426–36.
246. Nitschke K, Flecken T, Schmidt J, et al. Tetramer enrichment reveals the presence of phenotypically diverse hepatitis C virus-specific CD8+ T cells in chronic infection. J Virol 2015;89:25–34.
247. Fuller MJ, Callendret B, Zhu B, et al. Immunotherapy of chronic hepatitis C virus infection with antibodies against programmed cell death-1 (PD-1). Proc Natl Acad Sci U S A 2013;110:15001–6.

248. Gardiner D, Lalezari J, Lawitz E, et al. A randomized, double-blind, placebo-controlled assessment of BMS-936558, a fully human monoclonal antibody to programmed death-1 (PD-1), in patients with chronic hepatitis C virus infection. PLoS One 2013;8:e63818.
249. McHutchison JG, Kuo G, Houghton M, et al. Hepatitis C virus antibodies in acute icteric and chronic non-A, non-B hepatitis. Gastroenterology 1991;101:1117–9.
250. Peters T, Mohr L, Scheiffele F, et al. Antibodies and viremia in acute post-transfusion hepatitis C: a prospective study. J Med Virol 1994;42:420–7.
251. Netski DM, Mosbruger T, Depla E, et al. Humoral immune response in acute hepatitis C virus infection. Clin Infect Dis 2005;41:667–75.
252. Molina S, Castet V, Fournier-Wirth C, et al. The low-density lipoprotein receptor plays a role in the infection of primary human hepatocytes by hepatitis C virus. J Hepatol 2007;46:411–9.
253. Zeisel MB, Fofana I, Fafi-Kremer S, et al. Hepatitis C virus entry into hepato-cytes: molecular mechanisms and targets for antiviral therapies. J Hepatol 2011;54:566–76.
254. Pestka JM, Zeisel MB, Blaser E, et al. Rapid induction of virus-neutralizing antibodies and viral clearance in a single-source outbreak of hepatitis C. Proc Natl Acad Sci U S A 2007;104:6025–30.
255. Osburn WO, Snider AE, Wells BL, et al. Clearance of hepatitis C infection is associated with the early appearance of broad neutralizing antibody responses. Hepatology 2014;59:2140–51.
256. Bradley DW, Krawczynski K, Ebert JW, et al. Parenterally transmitted non-A, non-B hepatitis: virus-specific antibody response patterns in hepatitis C virus-infected chimpanzees. Gastroenterology 1990;99:1054–60.
257. Lanford RE, Notvall L, Barbosa LH, et al. Evaluation of a chimpanzee colony for antibodies to hepatitis C virus. J Med Virol 1991;34:148–53.
258. Beach MJ, Meeks EL, Mimms LT, et al. Temporal relationships of hepatitis C virus RNA and antibody responses following experimental infection of chimpanzees. J Med Virol 1992;36:226–37.
259. Hilfenhaus J, Krupka U, Nowak T, et al. Follow-up of hepatitis C virus infection in chimpanzees: determination of viraemia and specific humoral immune response. J Gen Virol 1992;73:1015–9.
260. Major ME, Mihalik K, Fernandez J, et al. Long-term follow-up of chimpanzees inoculated with the first infectious clone for hepatitis C virus. J Virol 1999;73: 3317–25.
261. Bassett SE, Thomas DL, Brasky KM, et al. Viral persistence, antibody to E1 and E2, and hypervariable region 1 sequence stability in hepatitis C virus-inoculated chimpanzees. J Virol 1999;73:1118–26.
262. Bassett SE, Guerra B, Brasky K, et al. Protective immune response to hepatitis C virus in chimpanzees rechallenged following clearance of primary infection. Hepatology 2001;33:1479–87.
263. Major ME, Mihalik K, Puig M, et al. Previously infected and recovered chimpanzees exhibit rapid responses that control hepatitis C virus replication upon re-challenge. J Virol 2002;76:6586–95.
264. Logvinoff C, Major ME, Oldach D, et al. Neutralizing antibody response during acute and chronic hepatitis C virus infection. Proc Natl Acad Sci U S A 2004; 101:10149–54.
265. Feray C, Gigou M, Samuel D, et al. Incidence of hepatitis C in patients receiving different preparations of hepatitis B immunoglobulins after liver transplantation. Ann Intern Med 1998;128:810–6.

266. Hjalmarsson S, Blomberg J, Grillner L, et al. Sequence evolution and cross-reactive antibody responses to hypervariable region 1 in acute hepatitis C virus infection. J Med Virol 2001;64:117–24.
267. Tarr AW, Urbanowicz RA, Hamed MR, et al. Hepatitis C patient-derived glycoproteins exhibit marked differences in susceptibility to serum neutralizing antibodies: genetic subtype defines antigenic but not neutralization serotype. J Virol 2011;85:4246–57.
268. Bailey JR, Wasilewski LN, Snider AE, et al. Naturally selected hepatitis C virus polymorphisms confer broad neutralizing antibody resistance. J Clin Invest 2015;125:437–47.
269. Meyer K, Banerjee A, Frey SE, et al. A weak neutralizing antibody response to hepatitis C virus envelope glycoprotein enhances virus infection. PLoS One 2011;6:e23699.
270. Takaki A, Wiese M, Maertens G, et al. Cellular immune responses persist and humoral responses decrease two decades after recovery from a single-source outbreak of hepatitis C. Nat Med 2000;6:578–82.
271. von Hahn T, Yoon JC, Alter H, et al. Hepatitis C virus continuously escapes from neutralizing antibody and T-cell responses during chronic infection in vivo. Gastroenterology 2007;132:667–78.
272. Dowd KA, Netski DM, Wang XH, et al. Selection pressure from neutralizing antibodies drives sequence evolution during acute infection with hepatitis C virus. Gastroenterology 2009;136:2377–86.
273. Osburn WO, Fisher BE, Dowd KA, et al. Spontaneous control of primary hepatitis C virus infection and immunity against persistent reinfection. Gastroenterology 2010;138:315–24.
274. Rosa D, Saletti G, De Gregorio E, et al. Activation of naive B lymphocytes via CD81, a pathogenetic mechanism for hepatitis C virus-associated B lymphocyte disorders. Proc Natl Acad Sci U S A 2005;102:18544–9.
275. Doi H, Iyer TK, Carpenter E, et al. Dysfunctional B-cell activation in cirrhosis resulting from hepatitis C infection associated with disappearance of CD27-positive B-cell population. Hepatology 2012;55:709–19.
276. Racanelli V, Frassanito MA, Leone P, et al. Antibody production and in vitro behavior of CD27-defined B-cell subsets: persistent hepatitis C virus infection changes the rules. J Virol 2006;80:3923–34.
277. Sugalski JM, Rodriguez B, Moir S, et al. Peripheral blood B cell subset skewing is associated with altered cell cycling and intrinsic resistance to apoptosis and reflects a state of immune activation in chronic hepatitis C virus infection. J Immunol 2010;185:3019–27.
278. Oliviero B, Cerino A, Varchetta S, et al. Enhanced B cell differentiation and reduced proliferative capacity in chronic hepatitis C and chronic hepatitis B virus infections. J Hepatol 2011;55:53–60.
279. Mizuochi T, Ito M, Takai K, et al. Peripheral blood memory B cells are resistant to apoptosis in chronic hepatitis C patients. Virus Res 2011;155:349–51.
280. Visentini M, Conti V, Cagliuso M, et al. Persistence of a large population of exhausted monoclonal B cells in mixed cryoglobuliemia after the eradication of hepatitis C virus infection. J Clin Immunol 2012;32:729–35.
281. Doi H, Tanoue S, Kaplan DE. Peripheral CD27-CD21- B-cells represent an exhausted lymphocyte population in hepatitis C cirrhosis. Clin Immunol 2014;150:184–91.
282. Oliviero B, Mantovani S, Ludovisi S, et al. Skewed B cells in chronic hepatitis C virus infection maintain their ability to respond to virus-induced activation. J Viral Hepat 2015;22:391–8.

283. Yan XB, Battaglia S, Boucreux D, et al. Mapping of the interacting domains of hepatitis C virus core protein and the double-stranded RNA-activated protein kinase PKR. Virus Res 2007;125:79–87.
284. Ryan EJ, Stevenson NJ, Hegarty JE, et al. Chronic hepatitis C infection blocks the ability of dendritic cells to secrete IFN-alpha and stimulate T-cell proliferation. J Viral Hepat 2011;18:840–51.
285. Kaukinen P, Sillanpaa M, Nousiainen L, et al. Hepatitis C virus NS2 protease inhibits host cell antiviral response by inhibiting IKKepsilon and TBK1 functions. J Med Virol 2013;85:71–82.
286. Sillanpaa M, Kaukinen P, Melen K, et al. Hepatitis C virus proteins interfere with the activation of chemokine gene promoters and downregulate chemokine gene expression. J Gen Virol 2008;89:432–43.
287. Saito T, Gale M Jr. Regulation of innate immunity against hepatitis C virus infection. Hepatol Res 2008;38:115–22.

Impact of Hepatitis C Virus Infection on Hepatocellular Carcinoma

Danielle M. Tholey, MD[a], Joseph Ahn, MD, MS[b],*

KEYWORDS

- Hepatocellular carcinoma • Hepatitis C virus • Direct-acting antivirals • Liver cancer

KEY POINTS

- Hepatitis C virus (HCV)–associated hepatocellular carcinoma (HCC) incidence is increasing in the United States.
- HCV core promoter protein and microRNA pathways play key roles in HCC carcinogenesis.
- Sustained virologic response decreases the risk of HCV-associated HCC.
- Individualized risk stratification in patients with HCV holds hope for further HCC risk reduction.

INTRODUCTION

Hepatocellular carcinoma (HCC) is a leading cause of liver-related death and the third most common cause of cancer death worldwide.[1] In the United States, the incidence of HCC is increasing, in part because of the growing impact of hepatitis C virus (HCV)–associated morbidity and mortality.[2,3] Without effective intervention, the number of patients with HCV-related cirrhosis or HCC is estimated to double by 2020.[3] This article reviews the latest efforts to discern the relationship of HCV with HCC, including virologic pathways to HCC, such as the role of the HCV core promoter protein and microRNA pathways. The impact of direct-acting antivirals (DAAs) on HCV-associated HCC and the persistent risk of HCC despite SVR are also reviewed with an emphasis on the need for individualized HCC risk stratification in patients with HCV.

Disclosures: No financial disclosures declared.
[a] Gastroenterology & Hepatology, Oregon Health & Sciences University, 3181 Southwest Sam Jackson Park Road, Portland, OR 97239, USA; [b] Division of Gastroenterology and Hepatology, Oregon Health & Sciences University, 3181 Southwest Sam Jackson Park Road, Mail Code L461, Portland, OR 97239, USA
* Corresponding author.
E-mail address: Ahnj@ohsu.edu

Gastroenterol Clin N Am 44 (2015) 761–773
http://dx.doi.org/10.1016/j.gtc.2015.07.005
0889-8553/15/$ – see front matter © 2015 Elsevier Inc. All rights reserved.

EPIDEMIOLOGY

HCV is associated with a 15-fold to 20-fold increased risk of HCC.[4] In patients with HCV, the annual incidence of HCC is estimated at 1% to 4% in cirrhotics compared with only 1% to 3% over a 30-year period in noncirrhotics.[4,5] The incidence of HCC in the United States has nearly doubled, from 3.1 per 100,000 to 5.1 per 100,000 people between 1992 and 2005. This trend of increasing HCC in the United States is postulated to be reflective of the progression of chronic HCV to cirrhosis in the aging baby boomer population.[2] As mortalities for HCC continue to increase, close monitoring of the state of HCC in the United States seems warranted.

RISK FACTORS FOR HEPATOCELLULAR CARCINOMA

HCC incidence is affected by many factors, including geographic location and ethnicity (**Table 1**). For example, East Asia and West Africa have a high prevalence of HCV and the highest global prevalence of HCC, with more than 80% of cases.[2,4,7] HCV prevalence in Japan is 1.9% to 3%[8] and 80% to 90% of patients with HCC are infected with HCV,[4] accounting for Japan's high HCC prevalence. In contrast, in the United States, which has a lower HCV prevalence of 1.8%, only 30% to 50% of patients with HCC are infected with HCV.[4,6] Japan's greater proportion of patients with HCC who are infected with HCV compared with the United States is attributed to an earlier onset of the HCV epidemic in Japan, suggesting that HCV-associated HCC incidence will continue to grow in the United States.[2,7]

Within the US population, HCC varies by ethnicity, with Hispanic patients at highest risk of HCC compared with white people and African Americans. A large cohort study of 150,000 US veterans showed that Hispanic patients had the highest annual HCC incidence at 7.8%.[9] The study postulated that a higher incidence of nonalcoholic fatty liver disease (NAFLD) in Hispanic patients could account for this higher HCC risk.

In addition to the impact of geographic region and ethnicity, many other risk factors affect the rates of HCC in patients with HCV. Major risk factors include concurrent liver disease, lifestyle, and viral factors.

Table 1
Geographic patterns of HCC prevalence and incidence

Prevalence of HCC	Region	Country	Incidence Rates (Cases per 100,000 Persons)
Very high prevalence	East Asia	Overall	20
		Mongolia	99
		Korea	49
		Japan	29
	West Africa	Mali	20
		Mozambique	
		Gambia	
Moderately high prevalence	Southern Europe	Italy	11–20
		Spain	11–20
	Latin America	—	10–20
Intermediate prevalence	Western Europe	France	5–10
		Germany	
Low prevalence	North America	United States	5.1[4,6]
		Canada	<5
	Northern Europe	Scandinavia	<5

Data from Refs.[2,4,6,7]

Concurrent Liver Disease

At present, the literature suggests that NAFLD, diabetes, and obesity contribute to an increased risk of HCC. Diabetes has reportedly been linked to a 2-fold to 37-fold increased risk of HCC.[10,11] Increased levels of homeostatic model assessment for Insulin resistance, which is an indicator for insulin resistance and a surrogate marker for the metabolic syndrome, have been measured in patients with HCC, suggesting that insulin resistance is associated with an increased risk of HCC.[11] Additional studies suggest that obesity may independently increase HCC risk or have a synergistic effect with diabetes via a central HCC pathway of increased steatosis.[12]

Similarly, coinfection with hepatitis B virus (HBV) increases the risk of HCC. In one small study, the cumulative lifetime incidence in coinfected men approached 38%, compared with 23% in monoinfected men.[5] HBV replication status is the crucial factor affecting the risk for HCC in patients with HCV. In another study, patients coinfected with HBV/HCV without detectable HBV DNA had HCC risk equal to that of mono-infected patients with HCV. However, patients with active HBV replication had twice the risk of HCC and a 21% increase in mortality risk.[13] The specific mechanism for this increased risk has not been fully elucidated, but has been attributed to the innate oncogenic potential of HBV covalently closed circular DNA during viral replication.[13] At present there is no shortened HCC screening interval recommended in patients coinfected with HCV/HBV.

Although HCV prevalence in the general US population is 1.8%, the prevalence is much higher in the HIV population, at 16%.[6,14] Improved survival of patients with HIV on antiretroviral therapy and the aggressiveness of HCV in patients with HIV has been associated with an increased risk of HCC. Between 1996 and 2009, there was a disproportionate 23-fold increase in HCC prevalence in coinfected patients compared with patients monoinfected with HIV.[14] This increase is attributed to decreased immune response in HIV, increased HCV replication, and an expedited evolution to cirrhosis, along with improved overall HIV-related survival. The aggressive nature of HCV/HIV coinfection and increased HCC risk mandates identifying HCV coinfection in patients with HIV and rigorous HCC surveillance in this population.

Lifestyle Factors

HCC risk is also linked to lifestyle factors such as coffee, smoking, and alcohol use. Coffee has been associated with both a decrease in the rate of progression to hepatic fibrosis and a decreased risk of HCC.[15,16] A large meta-analysis by Saab and colleagues[15] reviewed multiple studies supporting a dose-dependent decrease in HCC risk with at least 1 cup of coffee daily.[15,17] In addition, several studies support a significant decrease in HCC mortality with consumption of greater than or equal to 1 cup of coffee daily.[16] Specifically, a study by Kurozawa and colleagues[18] found a 69% reduction in HCC mortality in patients with HCV who drank 1 cup of coffee daily compared with non–coffee drinkers. At present, there are no randomized control trials on HCC and caffeine. Further, the previously mentioned cohort and case control studies have many potential confounders, including a higher incidence of alcohol use in coffee drinkers and lack of standardization regarding the volume and amount of caffeine in a cup of coffee.

In addition, it is well known that alcohol and smoking are associated with accelerated progression to HCC in HCV, likely via increased oxidative stress. There is a synergistic effect between alcohol and HCV on HCC, with a 2-fold increase in individuals who drink more than 60 g of alcohol daily.[19] Similarly, a recent meta-analysis has shown a significant increase in relative risk of HCC in smokers with HCV compared with nonsmokers with HCV, with relative risks of 23 and 7.9 respectively.[20] This increased risk with smoking may be confounded by alcohol because some patients tend to smoke while they drink.

Inherent Viral Factors

Genotype 3 was associated with an 80% higher risk of HCC than genotype 1 in a large Veterans' Affairs cohort of 100,000 patients controlled for age, body mass index, and viral therapy.[21] There was no consistent evidence that viral load affects HCC risk. In addition, although cirrhosis and stage 4 fibrosis are well-established risk factors for HCC, recent data suggest that stage 3 fibrosis also presents increased risk, with as many as 20% of patients progressing to HCC.[22] Additional data on these inherent viral factors are awaited.

VIROLOGY AND PATHOGENESIS

Both direct and indirect pathways of carcinogenesis are responsible for HCC development and understanding of these pathways will be key to devising new treatment strategies. Three major mechanisms of carcinogenesis have been proposed: direct pathways involving the HCV core protein, indirect injury from oxidative stress and steatosis leading to hepatocyte death, and microRNA (mi-RNA) instability.

HCV viral proteins can act directly on cell signaling pathways to promote HCC by inhibiting crucial cell cycle check points, inhibiting tumor suppressor genes and apoptosis regulators, or by causing activation of signaling pathways that upregulate growth and division[23–25] (**Table 2**). All these actions culminate in uncontrolled cell proliferation. The HCV core protein plays a key role in these deregulatory pathways by inhibiting the retinoblastoma protein (RB) and p53 tumor suppressor. Inhibition of RB causes dysfunction of important cell cycle check points involved in cell turnover and repair of faulty DNA sequences, resulting in uncontrolled proliferation of mutated HCV cells.[23,24] Also, HCV NS5B can inhibit other apoptosis regulators, such as BCL-2, and cause abnormal activation of signaling pathways that promote growth, such as Wnt/beta catenin and mammalian target of rapamycin (mTOR).[23,24,26] HCV core promoter protein also inhibits p53, which is the second most abundant tumor suppressor in the liver. It has been suggested that the loss of p53 and retinoblastoma could be synergistic, leading to a greater degree of carcinogenesis.[23] HCV core protein may also indirectly facilitate HCC by increasing oxidative damage via increased steatosis, lipogenesis, and promotion of protein misfolding in the endoplasmic reticulum.[23,27]

Other indirect pathways to HCC have been proposed, including the bystander effect.[23,28] In the bystander effect, the immune system produces proapoptotic signals to fight the replicating HCV virus, causing death of HCV-infected hepatocytes. As a result of this widespread hepatocyte death, hepatocyte proliferation is enhanced to maintain hepatic synthetic function. In the midst of this rapid proliferation, uninfected bystander cells can accumulate mutations, which in an environment of oxidative stress can promote carcinogenesis. This theory has been partially shown in mouse studies, which show that stimulation of rapid hepatocyte turnover and apoptosis can serve as a driver for HCC.[28]

In addition, HCC carcinogenesis is affected by mi-RNAs, a group of complex gene regulators that control expression of apoptosis, proliferation, and differentiation of cells.[23,29] Alterations in the expression of various mi-RNAs are associated with HCC. For example, silencing miR-122, which is crucial for HCV replication, has been associated with an antiviral effect in monkeys. In addition, inhibiting miR-21 in

Table 2
Summary of HCC carcinogenic pathways

Theory	Pathway	Direct or Indirect Effect	Basic Mechanism of Action	Deficiency of Function or Abnormal Activation	Specific Pathways or Molecules Involved
1	HCV core protein	Direct	Upregulates proliferation pathways	Activation	mTOR Wnt/Beta
1	HCV core protein	Direct	Inhibition of tumor suppressor genes (p53 and RB)	Deficiency	P53 Retinoblastoma
1	HCV core protein	Direct	Disables cell cycle checkpoints to allow continued division	Deficiency	G1-S
1	HCV core protein	Direct	Interferes with DNA repair via inhibiting retinoblastoma at G2-M cell cycle check point	Deficiency	G2-M
1	HCV core protein	Direct	Inhibits apoptosis regulators	Deficiency	BCL-2
1	HCV core protein	Indirect	Increases stress and oxidative damage	Neither	—
2	Bystander effect	Indirect	Death of HCV-infected cells by immune system leads to rapid proliferation of new hepatocytes and increased risk for mutations to accumulate	Deficiency	No specific markers
3	MicroRNAs	unclear	Regulators of gene expression	Activating in some cases and deficiency in others	miR-22 miR-122

Abbreviations: mTOR, mammalian target of rapamycin; RB, retinoblastoma protein.
Data from Lemon SM, McGivern DR. Is hepatitis C virus carcinogenic? Gastroenterology 2012;142(6):1274–78.

cultured HCC cells leads to decreased tumor proliferation and invasion.[29] Elucidating the relationship of these various mi-RNAs may offer promising therapeutic targets.

Although progress has been made in understanding these pathways, significant obstacles remain in identifying potential viral targets for treatment and HCC risk reduction.

IMPACT OF ANTIVIRAL THERAPY ON HEPATOCELLULAR CARCINOMA
Impact of Interferon Therapy

Interferon (IFN) is successful in reducing the risk of HCC as long as SVR is achieved.[30–32] SVR decreases the risk of HCC because of improvement in fibrosis and reduction in inflammation.[33] Compared with nonresponders, achievement of SVR resulted in an 11% risk reduction and 4.6% absolute risk reduction.[31] Even without SVR, patients with HCV relapse are 2 times less likely to develop HCC than nonresponders.[31] Five-year HCC incidence rates were significantly lower in patients with transient virologic response (3%) compared with nonresponders (7.9%; $P = .03$)[34] Although SVR is the optimal outcome, these findings suggested that even a temporary period of decreased inflammation by HCV treatment may be beneficial.

Although SVR reduces the risk of HCC, the risk of HCC persists, especially in patients with advanced fibrosis. Ikeda and colleagues[35] observed that HCC risk gradually increased over a 9-year period despite achieving SVR. Specifically, 5-year and 10-year incidence rates after SVR in chronic HCV were 1.2% and 4.3%, respectively[36] compared with a 5-year incidence of 20% in patients with HCV cirrhosis.[34] Morgan and colleagues[30] compared the risk of HCC in cirrhotics to that in patients with all stages of fibrosis and discovered that, despite achieving SVR, 4.2% of cirrhotics developed HCC as opposed to 1.5% of those with all stages of fibrosis.

In addition, HCV treatment after ablation or resection of HCC is effective in reducing new HCC foci and mortality in patients who achieve SVR. Improved survival is seen, with a 5-year survival of 76% compared with 60% in those not treated with IFN.[31] However, even with SVR, there is still a 35% risk of HCC recurrence in these patients.[31]

There are studies that reported that IFN therapy was unsuccessful in decreasing HCC risk. However, patients in these studies did not achieve SVR, had a short follow-up period, or had confounding variables that could increase the risk of HCC, such as a high proportion of subjects with diabetes or decompensated cirrhosis.[37] On the whole, it seems that, with achievement of SVR, IFN is successful in decreasing the risk of HCC.

Impact of Direct-acting Antivirals

Given the recent approval of DAAs such as NS3/4A protease inhibitors, NS5B polymerase inhibitors, and NS5A complex inhibitors, there are limited data on their impact on HCC risk reduction. Based on the data from the IFN era, it is intuitive that achievement of SVR by IFN or DAA treatment would lead to similar HCC risk reduction. Significantly higher SVR rates of greater than 90% in DAAs, reported even in challenging HCV populations at increased risk of HCC, should result in reduced HCC risk that will be evident with time as these treatments are widely adopted into clinical practice.[38,39] Specific data are awaited to confirm these strong hypotheses.

Predictors of Hepatocellular Carcinoma After Sustained Virologic Response

Because a reduced but durable risk of HCC persists despite SVR, there has been interest in identifying risk factors for HCC development after SVR. These risk factors are identical to initial HCC risk factors such as cirrhosis, duration of HCV infection, and comorbid conditions such as diabetes mellitus and HBV. Other factors include male gender, exposure to multiple IFN treatments, age, and surrogate markers for advanced fibrosis, such as albumin level, platelet count, and increased aspartate aminotransferase level.[35,40] At this point, there are insufficient data to guide HCC risk stratification and surveillance intervals in patients with HCV who have achieved SVR. Ongoing HCC surveillance should continue for those with advanced fibrosis despite achieving SVR.

SURVEILLANCE

The goal of HCC screening is to detect early HCCs to decrease overall mortality secondary to HCC. Screening for HCC has been shown to be cost-effective once the risk of HCC is greater than 1.5% per year and current American Association for the Study of Liver Diseases (AASLD) guidelines suggest dynamic imaging once patients develop cirrhosis.[41] However, there are subpopulations that may be considered for screening despite the absence of overt cirrhosis, because up to 20% of HCCs develop in the absence of cirrhosis.[22] Patients with advanced fibrosis such as METAVIR stage F3, can develop HCC and have recently been identified as an at-risk group for HCC.[42] Subsequently, the European Association For the Study of the Liver (EASL) HCC guidelines recommended surveillance every 6 months in at-risk patients, including those with advanced fibrosis.[43] A recent study noted that patients with HCV with advanced fibrosis have significantly reduced decompensation-free survival and HCC-free survival after 7 years compared with those with only mild fibrosis (FO–F2).[42] At 18 years of follow-up, HCC-free survival was only 78% in those with advanced fibrosis as opposed to approximately 98% to 100% at 15 years in those with F0 to F2 fibrosis.[42] The investigators of this study surmised that this increase in liver-related complications after 7 years represented the time required for progression to cirrhosis. Thus, they recommended screening patients with advanced fibrosis for HCC after 7 years from the F3 identification.

Patients with mild fibrosis, defined as METAVIR stage F0-to F2, are at very low risk for HCC. As such, EASL and AASLD guidelines do not recommend HCC screening in these patients.[41,43] Although the risk of HCC in patients with mild fibrosis is very low, elderly patients with mild fibrosis, older than 75 years, manifested a higher risk of HCC compared with patients less than 75 years old.[44] A study by Lewis and colleagues[44] showed an HCC prevalence of 10.6% in these elderly patients without cirrhosis, a prevalence rate that would surpass the greater than 1.5% annual risk required for screening to be effective. However, the sample size in this study was small and various confounders were present.

Despite these guidelines and the recognition of the fatality of HCC, adherence rates for HCC surveillance remain poor.[45,46] Annual surveillance with alpha-fetoprotein and ultrasonography occurred in only 2% of patients in a large cohort of 1480 patients with HCV.[46] Other studies have shown that surveillance of any form occurs annually in less than 13% to 20% of patients,[45] whereas screening practices meeting guidelines recommendations occurs in less than 5% of patients.[45] Potential causes of limited adherence include inadequate recall practices, patient noncompliance, and a lack of patient education or awareness of their diagnosis. Suboptimal outcomes in HCC are attributed to inadequate surveillance, leading to a reduction in timely access to potentially curative therapy in patients at treatable stages of HCC.

Transient elastography or FibroScan may have a role in improved detection of HCC in HCV by increasing identification of patients who are offered HCC surveillance via facilitating detection of advanced fibrosis.[47,48] The cost-effectiveness and impact of elastography on HCC detection was assessed using a Markov model based on incidence and disease progression rates using national database information from the United Kingdom. This study showed the potential to detect 40% more HCCs occurring in noncirrhotics or 30 extra cases per 10,000 patients,[48] assuming at least 20% compliance rates for HCC surveillance.[48] However, based on the current limited compliance rates, elastography may not be an effective strategy because it does not address the more basic issue of appropriate surveillance of patients already at increased risk for HCC. However, it remains a promising tool that requires further research to determine its potential role in improving HCV-associated HCC outcomes.

PROGNOSIS/OUTCOMES

As HCC incidence increases, outcomes continue to be poor, with high mortalities. Between 2002 and 2008, 5-year survival rates for HCC were a dismal 15% in the United States.[1] Compared with HCV cirrhotics, 5-year survival rates are slightly higher in those with chronic HCV at 35%, but still poor overall.[6,32] Death from HCC was more frequent in patients with HCV[32] (**Table 3**).

Patients coinfected with HCV/HIV have even poorer outcomes, with a younger age of onset, more advanced tumors at diagnosis, and aggressive clinical course with lower survival rates.[49] Survival at 2 years is only 11% in coinfected patients, as opposed to 41% in patients monoinfected with HCV.[50]

Trends in Mortality

Mortality from HCC continues to increase in the United States, from 2.5 per 100,000 persons in 2007 to 4.3 per 100,000 persons between 2006 and 2010.[1,6] Between 2006 and 2010, HCC mortality increased with increasing age.[6] However, for the first time, a significant decrease was seen in HCC mortality in patients between the ages of 35 and 49 years.[6] This may be reflective of decreased exposure to HCV risk factors, surveillance measures, and more effective antiviral therapy. Because this is the first decade in which a downward trend in mortality has been appreciated in the younger generations, further follow-up is awaited to assess whether this trend will continue. If sustained, this trend would provide hope that HCC mortality may have peaked and will decrease over the coming years, especially with advances in treatment.

Effect of Hepatocellular Carcinoma on Posttransplant Survival

Although liver transplant offers the potential for cure, posttransplant survival in patients with HCC with HCV is decreased compared with those without HCV. In patients

Table 3	
HCC survival rates by HCV subpopulation	
Patient Group	**5-y Survival Rates (%)**
Chronic HCV[6,32]	35
HCV cirrhosis[1]	15
HIV/HCV[50]	11[a]
Posttransplant[51,52]	69–76
Postresection[54]	70

Survival is measured as percentage of total patients still living.
[a] Represents 2-year survival.

Table 4
Posttransplant survival and HCC recurrence–free survival rates by HCV status

		Survival Rate Posttransplant (%)		
	HCV Status	**1 y**	**3 y**	**5 y**
Posttransplant survival	HCV positive	81–87	57–71	69–76
	HCV negative	89–94	77–82	49–59
HCC recurrence–free survival	HCV positive	70	43	37
	HCV negative	88	73	61

Data from Hu Z, Li Z, Xiang J, et al. Intent-to-treat analysis of liver transplant for hepatocellular carcinoma in the MELD era: impact of hepatitis C and advanced status. Dig Dis Sci 2014;59(12):3062–72; and Bozorgzadeh A, Orloff M, Abt P, et al. Survival outcomes in liver transplantation for hepatocellular carcinoma, comparing impact of hepatitis C versus other etiology of cirrhosis. Liver Transpl 2007;13(6):807–13.

with HCC with HCV compared with patients with HCC without HCV, a statistically significant decrease in survival was appreciated: at 1 year, 81% to 87% versus 89% to 94%; at 3 years, 57% to 71% versus 77% to 82%; and at 5 years, 49% to 59% versus 69% to 76% (P<.001 and P<.049)[51,52] (**Table 4**). In addition, long-term posttransplant survival is worse in patients with HCV, manifesting twice the mortality risk at 10 years, with rates of 35%.[53] Although overall survival rates in transplanted patients with HCV and HCC are lower than in those without HCV, intervention with transplant or resection greatly increases survival. Transplant or resection of early HCCs has 5-year survival rates of approximately 70% compared with rates of 15% in patients with late-stage HCCs.[54]

Tumor-free survival was decreased in posttransplant patients with HCV compared with those without HCV, with average survival of 17 months versus 32 months (P = .016).[52] Poor survival and HCC recurrence posttransplant in patients with HCV is related to accelerated replication of HCV and progression to cirrhosis in the setting of immunosuppression. Although HCV cirrhosis typically occurs after 20 to 30 years of infection, recurrent cirrhosis occurs much faster posttransplant, with cirrhosis risk increasing within 5 years.[55] This background of inflammation and rapid progression to cirrhosis likely further contributes to recurrence of HCC. Thus recurrence of advanced fibrosis and cirrhosis after liver transplant denotes recurrent risk for HCC, and mandates careful surveillance of these patients for HCC recurrence. This finding also provides impetus for aggressive monitoring of posttransplant HCV and HCV treatment.[52,54]

SUMMARY

As the baby boomer population ages in the United States, rates of HCV cirrhosis and HCC are projected to increase, making prevention and early identification of HCC crucial. This article identifies many special populations that are at higher risk for HCV-associated HCC, including patients with NAFLD, HIV coinfection, Hispanic descent, and patients without SVR.

Individualized risk stratification for HCC and personalized management in patients with HCV will be an important field for future study. In addition to studies focusing on the incorporation of new screening tools, such as transient elastography, methods for increasing surveillance adherence rates will remain an important priority. In addition, the impact of DAA therapies on potential HCC risk reduction coupled with analysis of their cost-effectiveness is yet to be reported. In addition, pursuing the mechanism of carcinogenesis of HCC in HCV and unraveling the mysteries of hepatic fibrosis will be a burgeoning topic to answer why patients with SVR have persistent risk of HCC. The impact of the ever-improving arsenal of DAA therapies against HCV with their increased rates of SVR on HCC incidence reduction is eagerly awaited.

REFERENCES

1. Bosetti C, Turati F, La Vecchia C. Hepatocellular carcinoma epidemiology. Best Pract Res Clin Gastroenterol 2014;28(5):753–70.
2. Gomaa AI, Khan SA, Toledano MB, et al. Hepatocellular carcinoma: epidemiology, risk factors and pathogenesis. World J Gastroenterol 2008;14(27):4300–8.
3. Davis GL, Alter MJ, El-Serag H, et al. Aging of hepatitis C virus (HCV)-infected persons in the United States: a multiple cohort model of HCV prevalence and disease progression. Gastroenterology 2010;138(2):513–21, 521.e1–6.
4. El-Serag HB. Epidemiology of viral hepatitis and hepatocellular carcinoma. Gastroenterology 2012;142(6):1264–73.e1.
5. Huang YT, Jen CL, Yang HI, et al. Lifetime risk and sex difference of hepatocellular carcinoma among patients with chronic hepatitis B and C. J Clin Oncol 2011; 29(27):3643–50.
6. Altekruse SF, Henley SJ, Cucinelli JE, et al. Changing hepatocellular carcinoma incidence and liver cancer mortality rates in the United States. Am J Gastroenterol 2014;109(4):542–53.
7. Ferlay J, Shin HR, Bray F, et al. Estimates of worldwide burden of cancer in 2008: GLOBOCAN 2008. Int J Cancer 2010;127(12):2893–917.
8. Sievert W, Altraif I, Razavi HA, et al. A systematic review of hepatitis C virus epidemiology in Asia, Australia and Egypt. Liver Int 2011;31(Suppl 2):61–80.
9. El-Serag HB, Kramer J, Duan Z, et al. Racial differences in the progression to cirrhosis and hepatocellular carcinoma in HCV-infected veterans. Am J Gastroenterol 2014;109(9):1427–35.
10. Davila JA, Morgan RO, Shaib Y, et al. Diabetes increases the risk of hepatocellular carcinoma in the United States: a population based case control study. Gut 2005;54(4):533–9.
11. Khattab MA, Eslam M, Mousa YI, et al. Association between metabolic abnormalities and hepatitis C-related hepatocellular carcinoma. Ann Hepatol 2012;11(4): 487–94.
12. N'Kontchou G, Paries J, Htar MT, et al. Risk factors for hepatocellular carcinoma in patients with alcoholic or viral C cirrhosis. Clin Gastroenterol Hepatol 2006;4(8): 1062–8.
13. Kruse RL, Kramer JR, Tyson GL, et al. Clinical outcomes of hepatitis B virus coinfection in a United States cohort of hepatitis C virus-infected patients. Hepatology 2014;60(6):1871–8.
14. Ioannou GN, Bryson CL, Weiss NS, et al. The prevalence of cirrhosis and hepatocellular carcinoma in patients with human immunodeficiency virus infection. Hepatology 2013;57(1):249–57.
15. Saab S, Mallam D, Cox GA 2nd, et al. Impact of coffee on liver diseases: a systematic review. Liver Int 2014;34(4):495–504.
16. Wakai K, Kurozawa Y, Shibata A, et al. Liver cancer risk, coffee, and hepatitis C virus infection: a nested case-control study in Japan. Br J Cancer 2007;97(3): 426–8.
17. Bravi F, Bosetti C, Tavani A, et al. Coffee reduces risk for hepatocellular carcinoma: an updated meta-analysis. Clin Gastroenterol Hepatol 2013;11(11):1413–21.e1.

18. Kurozawa Y, Ogimoto I, Shibata A, et al. Coffee and risk of death from hepatocellular carcinoma in a large cohort study in Japan. Br J Cancer 2005;93(5):607–10.

19. Donato F, Boffetta P, Puoti M. A meta-analysis of epidemiological studies on the combined effect of hepatitis B and C virus infections in causing hepatocellular carcinoma. Int J Cancer 1998;75(3):347–54.

20. Chuang SC, Lee YC, Hashibe M, et al. Interaction between cigarette smoking and hepatitis B and C virus infection on the risk of liver cancer: a meta-analysis. Cancer Epidemiol Biomarkers Prev 2010;19(5):1261–8.

21. Kanwal F, Kramer JR, Ilyas J, et al. HCV genotype 3 is associated with an increased risk of cirrhosis and hepatocellular cancer in a national sample of U.S. veterans with HCV. Hepatology 2014;60(1):98–105.

22. Alkofer B, Lepennec V, Chiche L. Hepatocellular cancer in the non-cirrhotic liver. J Visc Surg 2011;148(1):3–11.

23. Lemon SM, McGivern DR. Is hepatitis C virus carcinogenic? Gastroenterology 2012;142(6):1274–8.

24. Kannan RP, Hensley LL, Evers LE, et al. Hepatitis C virus infection causes cell cycle arrest at the level of initiation of mitosis. J Virol 2011;85(16):7989–8001.

25. Walters KA, Syder AJ, Lederer SL, et al. Genomic analysis reveals a potential role for cell cycle perturbation in HCV-mediated apoptosis of cultured hepatocytes. PLoS Pathog 2009;5(1):e1000269.

26. Park CY, Choi SH, Kang SM, et al. Nonstructural 5A protein activates beta-catenin signaling cascades: implication of hepatitis C virus-induced liver pathogenesis. J Hepatol 2009;51(5):853–64.

27. Li Y, Boehning DF, Qian T, et al. Hepatitis C virus core protein increases mitochondrial ROS production by stimulation of Ca2+ uniporter activity. FASEB J 2007; 21(10):2474–85.

28. Qiu W, Wang X, Leibowitz B, et al. PUMA-mediated apoptosis drives chemical hepatocarcinogenesis in mice. Hepatology 2011;54(4):1249–58.

29. Meng F, Henson R, Wehbe-Janek H, et al. MicroRNA-21 regulates expression of the PTEN tumor suppressor gene in human hepatocellular cancer. Gastroenterology 2007;133(2):647–58.

30. Morgan RL, Baack B, Smith BD, et al. Eradication of hepatitis C virus infection and the development of hepatocellular carcinoma: a meta-analysis of observational studies. Ann Intern Med 2013;158(5 Pt 1):329–37.

31. Singal AG, Volk ML, Jensen D, et al. A sustained viral response is associated with reduced liver-related morbidity and mortality in patients with hepatitis C virus. Clin Gastroenterol Hepatol 2010;8(3):280–8, 288.e1.

32. Omland LH, Krarup H, Jepsen P, et al. Mortality in patients with chronic and cleared hepatitis C viral infection: a nationwide cohort study. J Hepatol 2010;53(1):36–42.

33. George SL, Bacon BR, Brunt EM, et al. Clinical, virologic, histologic, and biochemical outcomes after successful HCV therapy: a 5-year follow-up of 150 patients. Hepatology 2009;49(3):729–38.

34. Hikmet A, Macit S, Ersin A, et al. Efficacy of pegylated interferon alpha and ribavirin treatment on risk of hepatocellular carcinoma in patients with chronic hepatitis C a prospective study. Hepatol Int 2015;9(Supp 1):S75 [APSAL abstract: 2183].

35. Ikeda M, Fujiyama S, Tanaka M, et al. Risk factors for development of hepatocellular carcinoma in patients with chronic hepatitis C after sustained response to interferon. J Gastroenterol 2005;40(2):148–56.

36. Toyoda H, Kumada T, Tada T, et al. Risk factors of HCC development in non-cirrhotic patients with sustained virologic response for chronic HCV infection. J Gastroenterol Hepatol 2015;30(7):1183–9.

37. Veldt BJ, Heathcote EJ, Wedemeyer H, et al. Sustained virologic response and clinical outcomes in patients with chronic hepatitis C and advanced fibrosis. Ann Intern Med 2007;147(10):677–84.

38. Manns M, Pol S, Jacobson IM, et al. All-oral daclatasvir plus asunaprevir for hepatitis C virus genotype 1b: a multinational, phase 3, multicohort study. Lancet 2014;384(9954):1597–605.

39. Lawitz E, Sulkowski MS, Ghalib R, et al. Simeprevir plus sofosbuvir, with or without ribavirin, to treat chronic infection with hepatitis C virus genotype 1 in non-responders to pegylated interferon and ribavirin and treatment-naive patients: the COSMOS randomised study. Lancet 2014;384(9956):1756–65.

40. Makiyama A, Itoh Y, Kasahara A, et al. Characteristics of patients with chronic hepatitis C who develop hepatocellular carcinoma after a sustained response to interferon therapy. Cancer 2004;101(7):1616–22.

41. Bruix J, Sherman M, American Association for the Study of Liver Diseases. Management of hepatocellular carcinoma: an update. Hepatology 2011;53(3):1020–2.

42. Huang Y, de Boer WB, Adams LA, et al. Clinical outcomes of chronic hepatitis C patients related to baseline liver fibrosis stage: a hospital-based linkage study. Intern Med J 2015;45(1):48–54.

43. European Association For the Study of the Liver, European Organisation for Research and Treatment of Cancer. EASL-EORTC clinical practice guidelines: management of hepatocellular carcinoma. J Hepatol 2012;56(4):908–43.

44. Lewis S, Roayaie S, Ward SC, et al. Hepatocellular carcinoma in chronic hepatitis C in the absence of advanced fibrosis or cirrhosis. AJR Am J Roentgenol 2013; 200(6):W610–6.

45. Singal AG, Li X, Tiro J, et al. Racial, social, and clinical determinants of hepatocellular carcinoma surveillance. Am J Med 2015;128(1):90.e1–7.

46. El-Serag HB, Kramer JR, Chen GJ, et al. Effectiveness of AFP and ultrasound tests on hepatocellular carcinoma mortality in HCV-infected patients in the USA. Gut 2011;60(7):992–7.

47. Masuzaki R, Tateishi R, Yoshida H, et al. Prospective risk assessment for hepatocellular carcinoma development in patients with chronic hepatitis C by transient elastography. Hepatology 2009;49(6):1954–61.

48. Canavan C, Eisenburg J, Meng L, et al. Ultrasound elastography for fibrosis surveillance is cost effective in patients with chronic hepatitis C virus in the UK. Dig Dis Sci 2013;58(9):2691–704.

49. Bourcier V, Winnock M, Ait Ahmed M, et al. Primary liver cancer is more aggressive in HIV-HCV coinfection than in HCV infection. A prospective study (ANRS CO13 Hepavih and CO12 Cirvir). Clin Res Hepatol Gastroenterol 2012;36(3): 214–21.

50. Puoti M, Bruno R, Soriano V, et al. Hepatocellular carcinoma in HIV-infected patients: epidemiological features, clinical presentation and outcome. AIDS 2004; 18(17):2285–93.

51. Hu Z, Li Z, Xiang J, et al. Intent-to-treat analysis of liver transplant for hepatocellular carcinoma in the MELD era: impact of hepatitis C and advanced status. Dig Dis Sci 2014;59(12):3062–72.

52. Bozorgzadeh A, Orloff M, Abt P, et al. Survival outcomes in liver transplantation for hepatocellular carcinoma, comparing impact of hepatitis C versus other etiology of cirrhosis. Liver Transpl 2007;13(6):807–13.

53. Dumitra S, Alabbad SI, Barkun JS, et al. Hepatitis C infection and hepatocellular carcinoma in liver transplantation: a 20-year experience. HPB (Oxford) 2013; 15(9):724–31.

54. Mazzaferro V, Regalia E, Doci R, et al. Liver transplantation for the treatment of small hepatocellular carcinomas in patients with cirrhosis. N Engl J Med 1996; 334(11):693–9.
55. Crosbie OM, Alexander GJ. Liver transplantation for hepatitis C virus related cirrhosis. Baillieres Best Pract Res Clin Gastroenterol 2000;14(2):307–25.

Extrahepatic Manifestations of Hepatitis C Virus

Mauro Viganò, MD, PhD[a], Massimo Colombo, MD[b],*

KEYWORDS

- Extrahepatic manifestations • HCV • Cryoglobulins • B-cell non–Hodgkin lymphoma
- Interferon

KEY POINTS

- Hepatitis C virus (HCV) infection is associated with injury of organs other than the liver, which is thought to contribute to increased rates of morbidity and all-cause mortality.
- Extrahepatic manifestations (EHMs) of HCV infection are variegate because they include mixed cryoglobulinemia (MC), lymphomas, membranous glomerulonephritis, porphyria cutanea tarda (PCT), lichen planus, thyroiditis, sicca syndrome, polyarthritis, diabetes mellitus (DM), cardiovascular diseases, and neurocognitive impairment.
- MC is the dominant EHM because it can be detected in half of all HCV-infected patients, yet less than 5% of the affected subjects develop a cryoglobulinemic syndrome.
- HCV eradication through antiviral therapy protects against the clinical consequences of such EHMs as cryoglobulinemic vasculitis, glomerulonephritis and polyneuropathy, lymphoma, and diabetes. Deferral of HCV infection treatment favors the onset of irreversible organ injury.

INTRODUCTION

HCV infection is a multifaceted disease, associated with chronic and typically slowly developing injury of the liver and a potential to affect other organs including the kidney, skin, thyroid, eyes, joints, nervous system, and immune system.[1,2] In the past decades, a variety of symptoms occurring in HCV-infected patients such as fatigue,

Conflict of Interest: M. Viganò: speaking and teaching: Roche, Gilead Sciences, BMS; Massimo Colombo: grant and research support: Merck, Roche, BMS, Gilead Sciences; advisory committees: Merck, Roche, Novartis, Bayer, BMS, Gilead Sciences, Tibotec, Vertex, Janssen Cilag, Achillion, Lundbeck, Abbott, Boehringer Ingelheim,Wasserman; speaking and teaching: Tibotec, Roche, Novarti-s, Bayer, BMS, Gilead Sciences, Vertex, Glaxo, Janssen Cilag, Merck, Abbott.
[a] Hepatology Division, Ospedale San Giuseppe, Università degli Studi di Milano, Via San Vittore 12, Milan 20122, Italy; [b] Division of Gastroenterology and Hepatology, "A. M. and A. Migliavacca" Center for Liver Disease, Fondazione IRCCS Ca' Granda Ospedale Maggiore Policlinico, Università degli Studi di Milano, Via F. Sforza 35, Milan 20122, Italy
* Corresponding author.
E-mail address: massimo.colombo@unimi.it

Gastroenterol Clin N Am 44 (2015) 775–791
http://dx.doi.org/10.1016/j.gtc.2015.07.006
0889-8553/15/$ – see front matter © 2015 Elsevier Inc. All rights reserved.

gastro.theclinics.com

musculoskeletal pain, depression, and irritability have been recognized and attributed to EHMs of HCV infection. More recently, both in the West and in the East, the role of HCV in all-cause mortality has also emerged through studies comparing the outcome of untreated patients with patients treated with antiviral therapy.[3–5] Although cirrhosis-related death invariably is the dominant cause of mortality in all studies, significant rates of deaths caused by extrahepatic events have also been identified. As a matter of fact, HCV has been recognized as the major viral cause of MC, which in turn affects half of all chronically infected patients and may be implicated in multiorgan damage. Some cases of MC have been associated with other viral infections, including human immunodeficiency virus, Epstein Barr virus, and parvoviruses.[6] Evidence has also accumulated supporting an association between HCV infection and an increased risk of lymphoproliferative disorders in the domain of B-cell non–Hodgkin lymphoma (NHL), type 2 diabetes, cerebrovascular and cardiovascular events, PCT, and lichen planus.[7] It is not surprising, therefore, that the lifetime cumulative risk for an HCV-infected patient to develop at least one EHM is thought to largely exceed 50%, likely being a consequence of either the ability of the virus to target and infect lymphocytes or the virus expressing reactive proteins, which boost tissue deposition of immune complexes and initiation of immune-mediated cytotoxic reactions.[2,7] While EHMs such as MC have strongly been associated with HCV both clinically and pathologically, the link between the virus and other clinical complications is difficult to explain, being mostly supported by prevalence studies and, in a few reports, by additional response to antiviral treatment (**Box 1**).[7] The latter is the case for the basis of an association between chronic HCV infection and B-cell NHL, which relies on robust

---

Box 1
EHMs of HCV infection

Established association

MC/cryoglobulinemic vasculitis

B-cell NHL

Significant association

PCT

Lichen planus

Monoclonal gammophaties

Possible association

Sicca syndrome

Corneal ulcers (Mooren ulcers)

Thyroid disease

Noncryoglobulin nephropathies

Neuropathy

Pulmonary fibrosis

Type 2 diabetes

Arthralgias, myalgias, inflammatory polyarthritis

Autoimmune thrombocytopenia

epidemiologic data coupled with reports of prevention and reversal of the tumor after HCV eradication with antiviral therapy.[8,9] More recently, the central nervous system (CNS) involvement of HCV infection resulting in impairment of several neurocognitive functions has been substantiated by clinical studies coupled with brain imaging investigations, leading to the demonstration that such a dysfunction was reversible on treatment-related clearance of HCV.[10]

MIXED CRYOGLOBULINEMIA

MC is an autoimmune, lymphoproliferative disorder characterized by circulating immune complexes named cryoglobulins (CGs) that reversibly precipitate at low temperatures.[7] MC is the dominant and most thoroughly documented EHM of HCV infection, which in some patients results in systemic vasculitis after the deposition of CGs in small- and medium-sized blood vessels. The relationship between HCV and CGs is substantiated by the exceedingly high rates (up to 90%) of patients with CGs who have circulating anti-HCV antibodies and the finding that about half of all HCV-infected patients have circulating CGs, although less than 5% of these subjects will ultimately develop an overt MC syndrome (MCS).[7,11–13] As the prevalence of MC increases with the duration of the infection, not surprisingly, liver abnormalities were found to persist almost twice as long in patients with MC as in those without it.[12] Although clinically benign, MC is classified as a lymphoproliferative disorder that predisposes to NHL in about 5% to 10% of the patients at a risk threshold that is about 35 times higher than that in the general population.[14] CGs consist of polyclonal IgGs and monoclonal or polyclonal IgM with rheumatoid factor activity sustained by the clonal expansion of B cells and are categorized on the basis of the clonality of the responsible immunoglobulin. In type I CGs, the cryoprecipitate contains an isolated monoclonal immunoglobulin IgG or IgM, whereas type II CGs are mixed, with a cryoprecipitate consisting of polyclonal immunoglobulins (mainly IgG) mixed with monoclonal immunoglobulins IgM, IgG, or IgA. Type III CGs are mixed, the cryoprecipitate containing both polyclonal IgG and IgM.[15] HCV infection is strongly associated with the latter 2 types of MC.[16]

As the clinical manifestations of MC are the consequence of a systemic vasculitis involving mainly the skin, joints, peripheral nervous system, and kidneys,[7] the disease expression (MCS) of CGs is heterogeneous, ranging from the classic triad of mild palpable purpura, weakness, and arthralgia to such life-threatening organ damage as type I membranoproliferative glomerulonephritis (MPGN) and widespread vasculitis with pulmonary hemorrhage, gastrointestinal ischemia, as well as cardiac and CNS involvement. Skin is commonly involved in up to 95% of cases of MCS in the form of cutaneous vasculitis ranging from a palpable purpura and petechiae in the lower extremities to chronic cutaneous ulcers, Raynaud phenomenon, and acrocyanosis.[17] Biopsy of the skin lesions reveals small vessels that are affected by immune complex vasculitis, whereas mononuclear cells heavily infiltrate the vessel walls.[18] Arthralgia without arthritis is common, typically affecting the proximal interphalangeal joints of the hands, metacarpophalangeal joints, knees, and hips.[19] The most frequently reported neurologic manifestation of MCS is a peripheral neuropathy with distal sensory or mixed, sensorimotor polyneuropathy, usually presenting with painful asymmetric paresthesia, numbness, burning, needles-and-pins sensation, skin crawling, and itching that mostly involve hands and feet. At biopsy, axonal damage with epineuronal vasculitic infiltration and endoneuronal microangiopathy has often been demonstrated. Less frequently, multiple mononeuropathies and, even more anecdotally, CNS involvement have been reported.[20–23] In 30% to 60% of patients with MCS, the kidneys are involved, mostly as an MPGN with subendothelial deposits of proteins. The most frequent clinical presentation of renal involvement during MCS is proteinuria with microscopic hematuria and a variable degree of renal insufficiency.[24–26] The most characteristic histologic findings are capillary thrombi consisting of precipitated CGs that can be visualized with light microscopy.[25]

The universally accepted pathogenesis of HCV-related MC is a chronic antigenic stimulation of the immune system, which facilitates clonal B-lymphocyte expansion.[27] A possible culprit is an increase of B-cell survival because of the inhibition of apoptosis by Bcl2 activation or by the interaction of HCV E2 envelope protein with the glycoprotein CD81 on the surface of B cells, which ultimately downregulates the activation threshold leading to persistent cell stimulation.[28,29] The recognition of a molecular mimicry between HCV-specific proteins and certain autoantigens and of NS5A and core proteins of HCV being able to stimulate autoantigen production by the immune system may also account for both B-lymphocyte activation and autoimmune reactions in MCS.[30] All these abnormalities could be the consequence of an altered expression of regulatory microRNAs (miRNAs), as recently suggested by the finding of an overexpression of miRNA 17-92 in the circulating lymphocytes of patients with MC that was reverted by interferon therapy.[31]

TREATMENT OF MIXED CRYOGLOBULINEMIA SYNDROME

Antiviral therapy with interferon is the mainstay for the long-term control of MCS because HCV RNA suppression leads to interruption of lymphocyte stimulation by HCV and results in an improvement or disappearance of most clinical and laboratory manifestations of virus-related MCS (**Table 1**). While cumulatively the achievement of a sustained virological response (SVR) to interferon-based therapy has resulted in the recovery from signs and symptoms of MCS in up to 90% of patients, access to interferon therapy was restricted in most patients with advanced hepatitis owing to an increased risk of life-threatening adverse reactions to interferons or myelosuppression.[32–38] Regrettably, for interferon-ineligible patients, symptomatic treatment of the clinical manifestations of MC without suppressing HCV leads to a transient control of the clinical syndrome only. Thus, virus eradication should be attempted as a first-line therapeutic option in patients with HCV infection with MCS, although either onset or worsening of vasculitic manifestations such as peripheral neuropathy, nephropathy, and skin ulcers have occasionally been reported after administration of interferon.[39] The expected clinical benefit of an SVR is the resolution of polyarthropathy, vasculitis, dermatologic lesions, glomerulonephritis, and proteinuria, whereas most patients with significant renal impairment from HCV-induced glomerulonephritis and those with a peripheral neuropathy with significant neural injury may not fully recover after viral eradication.[32,39] In a study of pegylated interferon (Peg-IFN)/ribavirin (Rbv) therapy of 253 patients with HCV-associated MC (121 symptomatic), all patients with SVR experienced either a complete or a partial clinical response, and in most responders, MCS disappeared, contrary to all virological nonresponders who were also clinical nonresponders, despite a transient improvement in some cases.[38] Triple therapy with first-generation protease inhibitors has resulted in high rates of virus clearance, yet with substantial toxicity rates. In an open-label prospective single-center cohort study, the safety and efficacy of 48 weeks' combination therapy with Peg-IFN/Rbv plus an NS3/4A protease inhibitor boceprevir (n = 13) or telaprevir (n = 17) was evaluated in 30 genotype-1-infected patients with severe and/or refractory MC.[37] At week 72, 20 patients (67%) achieved an SVR combined with a complete clinical response, whereas 14 (47%) experienced serious adverse events, all patients being mostly those

Table 1
Selected studies with interferon-based treatment of symptomatic patients with HCV-related MC

Author, Reference, yr	Treated Patients	Cirrhosis (%)	Genotype 1 (%)	Antiviral Regimen	Duration of Treatment (mo)	Sustained Virological Response (%)	Complete Clinical Response (%)	Adverse Events (%)
Saadoun et al,[33] 2010	55	Na	63	Peg-IFNa2b or 2a/Rbv	12	60	73	54
Mazzaro et al,[34] 2011	86	5	49	Peg-IFNa2b/Rbv	6/12	50	88	9
El Khayat et al,[35] 2012	46	Na	0	Peg-IFNa2a/Rbv	12	48	48	22
Gragnani et al,[36] 2014	5	100	100	Peg-IFNa2b/Rbv/BOC	12	0	0	55
Saadoun et al,[37] 2015	30	40	100	Peg-IFNa2b or 2a/Rbv/PI	12	67	67	47
Gragnani et al,[38] 2015	121	29	45	Peg-IFNa2b or 2a/Rbv	12	52	50	29

Abbreviations: BOC, boceprevir; Na, not available; Peg-IFN, pegylated interferon; PI, protease inhibitor; Rbv, ribavirin.

with advanced liver fibrosis and a low platelet count.[37] In another prospective study, 35 genotype-1-infected patients with MC who received a 48 weeks' course of Peg-IFN/Rbv plus boceprevir experienced a significant reduction of cryocrit values and an improvement in symptoms; however, they achieved lower SVR rates compared with matched MC-free controls (24% vs 70%; P = .01).[36] Although neither efficacy nor safety data are available for the treatment of HCV-related MC with all oral regimens based on new direct-acting antiviral agents (DAA), high SVR rates and excellent safety and tolerability records can be anticipated with those regimens.[1] However, the demonstration that HCV suppression following direct antiviral therapy restores NK cell function related innate immunity should alert against the clinical risks of immune reconstitution that might also ensue in patients with MCS following exposure to all oral DAA.[40]

Targeting the effector arm of MCS with rituximab (RTX), a monoclonal chimeric antibody against B-cell-specific surface antigen CD20, which inhibits B-cell function, has been reported to induce clinical benefits such as a reduction of both CG levels and clinical manifestations. Nevertheless, suppression of B cells by RTX treatment may favor HCV RNA replication, even though this apparently does not significantly harm the liver.[41–45] After a weekly dosing of 375 mg/m^2 of RTX for 4 consecutive weeks, the vast majority of patients with an MCS could achieve a complete response in the skin, joint, and neuromuscular domain, whereas most patients were able to discontinue corticosteroids.[41] In a randomized controlled trial of 57 patients with MC vasculitis not responding to or unfit for antiviral treatment, RTX showed a better efficacy than such conventional treatments as glucocorticoids, azathioprine, cyclophosphamide, or plasmapheresis.[44] In another study, the administration of RTX was also shown to be safe and associated with clinical improvement in patients with advanced liver disease.[46] When the association of RTX with Peg-IFN/Rbv was evaluated against Peg-IFN/Rbv alone, the former regimen led to more clinical remissions and higher rates of renal response and CG clearance than the RTX-free regimen, but both regimens had comparable rates of safety and clinical and virological adverse events.[33,47]

Other options to treat MCS included short-term steroid administration that may help control minor intermittent inflammatory events, yet it is unsuccessful in patients with major disorders such as neuropathy or nephropathy, while it may boost viral replication. Measures such as plasma exchange or administration of antigen-free diets (low-antigen-content [LAC] diet) aimed to stimulate immunocomplex clearance proved to be safe, whereas the administration of such immunosuppressive regimens as cyclophosphamide or azathioprine carry the potential risk of toxicity related to virus reactivation. While an LAC diet has led to improvement of minor manifestations of MC in some patients and therefore is considered the standard of care for the early stages of the syndrome,[48] immunosuppressive regimens are indicated to treat patients with acute, life-threatening manifestations of organ involvement who do not respond to steroids, although these drugs may occasionally cause severe adverse reactions and liver disease progression.[48–50] Although patients with mild to moderate HCV-related MCS should be prioritized to receive antiviral treatment, RTX is the standard of care for patients with worsening of renal function, neuropathy, skin disease, and intestinal ischemia and needs be initiated before or in parallel with antiviral therapy. Patients with life-threatening organ involvement and those with refractory HCV-related MCS or underlying B-cell NHL need to be prioritized to lifesaving options based on steroids, plasma exchange, cyclophosphamide, and/or RTX. In this latter group of patients, antiviral therapy should therefore be deferred (**Fig. 1**).

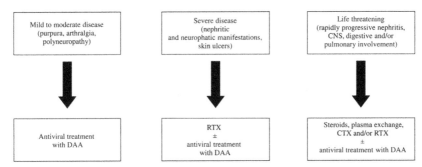

Fig. 1. Therapy for HCV-related MC. CTX, cyclophosphamide.

LYMPHOPROLIFERATIVE DISORDERS

The well-documented, strong association between HCV and B-cell NHL follows a geographic gradient whereby the incidence rates are higher in northern countries than in the southern ones.[51–58] A most convincing pathogenetic link between HCV and lymphoma was the finding of lower cumulative incidence rates of lymphoma in patients in whom HCV was successfully eradicated following interferon therapy based on a large population study in Japan.[8] In this study, a lymphoma developed in 2.6% of patients with HCV infection over 15 years of observation compared with none among patients who achieved an SVR following interferon-based therapy. The causal role of HCV in the lymphoproliferative disorders is further highlighted by the report of episodes of viral relapse occurring in parallel with lymphoma recurrence.[9,59] Despite scanty data on HCV replication within B lymphocytes, chronic antigenic stimulation by the virus is thought to trigger B-cell proliferation, resulting in a wide spectrum of injuries ranging from minor expansion of B-cell populations to an aggressive high-grade lymphoma.[7] The most common types of B-cell NHL associated with HCV are lymphoplasmacytic lymphoma; marginal zone lymphoma (MZL), in particular splenic marginal zone lymphomas (SMZLs); and diffuse large B-cell NHL. Approximately two-thirds of the HCV-related NHLs are low-grade tumors with predominantly extranodal involvement of organs such as liver, spleen, salivary glands, and stomach compared with 19% of non-HCV-related lymphomas.[60,61] Other hematologic disorders in the course of HCV infection include gammopathies of uncertain significance mainly composed of IgM kappa, present in up to 11% of CG-free patients with HCV infection.[62] Clinical surveillance of patients with monoclonal gammopathies is deemed necessary owing to the fact that these patients carry a risk of progressing to multiple myeloma. It should be recognized that MC may be a bridge disorder between HCV infection and several hematological malignancies, a clinical switch that can take place in up to 10% of patients with circulating CGs.[63] B-cell neoplasia more often affects patients with longstanding infections and diagnosis of MC, keeping in mind that HCV infection has been reported in up to 35% of patients with B-cell NHL and in almost 90% of patients with NHL with circulating CGs.[64] The pathogenic mechanism of lymphoproliferative disorders is likely a long-standing infection with HCV resulting in clonal B-cell expansion of CG-secreting lymphocytes and ultimately in a combination of genetic and environmental factors causing a mutational event including activation of oncogenes leading to neoplastic transformation of B cells. Another possible mechanism underlying B-cell transformation during hepatitis C is the inhibition of apoptosis of HCV-infected lymphocytes by (18-14) translocation, which results in an overexpression of the bcl2 oncogene, coupled with a second mutation (myc oncogene) that leads to the development of a lymphoma.[65,66]

TREATMENT OF LYMPHOPROLIFERATIVE DISORDERS

Remission of a low-grade NHL after HCV eradication is well documented.[67–76] In the late 1990s, regression of a splenic lymphoma with villous lymphocytes (SLVL) was documented in HCV-seropositive patients who responded to interferon-based therapy,[68] whereas the oncologic benefits provided by a virological response to interferon were documented in patients with other indolent lymphoma subtypes, such as mucosa-associated lymphoid tissue lymphomas, SMZLs, and disseminated MZLs.[69] Antiviral therapy for HCV-seropositive patients with a lymphoma is a double-faceted one aiming to eradicate the etiologic factor and to revert genetic alterations of lymphoma cells together with regression of expanded B-cell clones.[32,69–72] This notwithstanding, B-cell clonality may persist in patients with SVR despite achievement of a clinical remission, as it was shown to be the case for patients with SLVL, suggesting the existence of "no-return points" in the HCV-driven lymphoma, which render the neoplastic cell process less and less dependent on the etiologic agent.[69,73] At variance with mild indolent NHL that may go onto remission following HCV eradication, patients with either a diffuse or a high-grade lymphoma typically require chemotherapy to gain oncological remission independent of an SVR.[67,69] In patients with aggressive lymphomas, the therapeutic efficacy of antiviral regimens is counteracted by the long time required to deliver antineoplastic effects and, most importantly, by the risk of treatment refractoriness that may be acquired through additional oncogenic mutations that are no more antigen driven.[69] In patients with HCV infection with an aggressive NHL, anthracycline-based chemotherapy coupled with RTX is the standard of care, whereas in patients with HCV-associated MC, RTX-based chemotherapy has a less-beneficial safety profile because of increased risk of hematological toxicity, viral breakthrough, hepatitis flares, and drug toxicity from altered drug metabolism.[77,78] Interferon-based treatment following chemotherapy-induced remission of NHL may provide additional clinical benefits, including prolonged disease-free survival.[79,80]

In summary, available data suggest that low-grade lymphomas may be cured by antiviral therapy, whereas intermediate- and high-grade NHL benefit from chemotherapy only. However, the outcome of interferon-based therapy is jeopardized by the risk of hematological toxicity (**Fig. 2**). Therapy with interferon is an option to consolidate the response to chemotherapy owing to the combined antiviral and immunomodulatory activity of this cytokine.

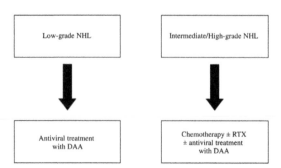

Fig. 2. Therapy for HCV-related NHL.

PORPHYRIA CUTANEA TARDA

PCT is caused by the inhibition of hepatic uroporphyrinogen decarboxylase activity resulting in overproduction of uroporphyrinogen in blood and urine. Clinical features of PCT include photosensitivity, skin fragility, bruising, vesicles and bullae that may become hemorrhagic, hypopigmentation or hyperpigmentation, alopecia, hirsutism, and skin thickening. The prevalence of HCV infection in patients with PCT is high, that is, about 50%, and likely accounts for hepatic iron overload in genetically predisposed individuals.[81–84] This interpretation matches anecdotal reports of PCT features disappearing following interferon therapy, yet randomized clinical trials to prove this are lacking.[85] Phlebotomy was successful in reducing the characteristic iron overload encountered in this disorder.

LICHEN PLANUS

Lichen planus is a recurrent pruritic eruption characterized by flat-topped scarlet papules that can develop on any skin site of arms, trunk, genital, nails and scalp, and mucosal membranes.[86] The prevalence of serum HCV in patients with oral lichen planus is around 27%, and HCV RNA has been detected in oral mucous membranes of the affected patients.[87,88] Unfortunately, remission of lichen planus following antiviral therapy is not the rule.[89,90]

THYROID DISORDERS

Hypothyroidism is the most common thyroid disorder encountered in patients chronically infected by HCV. In this population, up to 13% have clinical hypothyroidism and up to 25% have circulating thyroid antibodies.[91–93] These antibodies can help in identifying patients with HCV infection who are at an increased risk of thyroid dysfunction following interferon therapy.[94]

ARTHRALGIAS AND ARTHRITIS

Arthralgias and/or arthritis affect the vast majority of patients with MC and may manifest as bilateral joint pain and symmetric, nondeforming inflammation, mainly of knees and hands, and more rarely elbows and ankles. Characteristically, HCV-related arthritis does not lead to joint destruction and may be present in less than 10% of all MC-free HCV-infected patients.[95] In patients with clinical signs and symptoms or rheumatologic involvement, attention should be paid to define whether arthralgias, myalgias, and arthritis are primarily related to the HCV infection rather than to a newly developing rheumatologic disease.

SICCA SYNDROME AND SJÖGREN SYNDROME

Chronic lymphocytic sialoadenitis similar to the salivary and ocular disorders seen in the idiopathic Sjögren syndrome may approximately affect 50% of patients with HCV infection. Sjögren syndrome is defined by the presence of xerostomia, xerophthalmia, anti-Sjögren's syndrome A (SSA) or anti-Sjögren's syndrome B (SSB) antibodies, and typical salivary gland histology; yet less than 5% of these patients are infected by HCV.[96] In the transgenic mice, expression of envelope proteins of HCV is associated with development of sicca syndrome.[97]

DIABETES MELLITUS AND VASCULAR DISORDERS

DM arises from a complex interaction between HCV and the low inflammation status generated by insulin resistance. DM is more commonly diagnosed in patients with chronic hepatitis C than in the general population and is particularly strongly associated with advanced liver fibrosis or cirrhosis.[98,99] The association of DM and HCV is also suggested by the remarkable reduction of DM risk seen in patients with HCV infection responding to interferon-based therapy, and, even more convincingly, by the observation that in the diabetic population, interferon therapy led to a reduction of mortality from renal failure, stroke, and cardiovascular events.[100–102] The causal role of HCV in cardiovascular diseases is well grounded, mimicking in fact the pathologic activity of several other types of chronic infection. Working in this direction is the association of HCV with an increased risk of carotid artery plaques and carotid intima-media thickening, including a possible local direct role of the virus in initiating the plaque independent of classic risk factors for atherosclerosis.[103–105] While the risk of atherosclerosis in patients with HCV infection is likely driven by active viral replication, which leads to the release of proatherogenic cytokines,[106–108] HCV infection was clearly associated with an increased risk of coronary artery disease after adjustment for classic cardiovascular risk factors.[109] In the end, the best piece of evidence linking HCV infection to EHMs is the increased rates of mortality from diabetes, cardiovascular diseases, and renal failure that were shown to revert in patients with HCV infection responding to interferon therapy.[3–5,101,110] This is the observation of a large study in Taiwan based on the Risk Evaluation of Viral Load Elevation and Associated Liver Disease/Cancer-Hepatitis B Virus (REVEAL) cohort and the scrutiny of the nationwide registry for disease diagnosis and mortality, which demonstrated mortality from diabetes, cardiac events, and renal failure to be increased by 49%, 50%, and 17%, respectively, among viremic patients compared with HCV-RNA-seronegative patients.[5] These findings were replicated by surveys in the East and West documenting a clear-cut protective effect of interferon-related clearance of HCV on patient survival.[3,4,111,112] What remains to be clarified is whether the survival benefits provided by interferon will also be seen in DAA-treated cohorts that have abundant interferon-ineligible patients with advanced liver impairment and severe comorbidities.

NEUROCOGNITIVE IMPAIRMENT

The reversal of the typical symptoms of neurocognitive impairment such as depression, fatigue, and reduced quality of life on achieving HCV clearance with the potent and well-tolerated DAA regimens has conclusively validated the association between HCV and several CNS dysfunctions.[113] Approximately one-third of patients with advanced HCV infection have symptoms related to neurocognitive impairment,[114] which may be a direct consequence of HCV affecting the CNS through serotonergic and dopaminergic mechanisms.[115] The eradication of HCV is associated with improvement not only of CNS symptoms but also of brain metabolism, as demonstrated by MRI.[10]

SUMMARY

The pathogenicity of HCV is not limited to the liver, owing to the fact that the virus may cause significant morbidity related to EHM that in some patients overrides that related to the liver in terms of clinical severity. The pathogenic role of HCV in EHM is clearly explained by the declining rates of all-cause mortality that have been documented in patients with chronic HCV infection who successfully responded to interferon therapy. Although this may have several practical implications on the current strategies of hepatitis C therapy, it should be emphasized that antiviral therapy for HCV infection has clearly been shown to be effective against a wide spectrum of EHMs including CG-associated vasculitis, membranous glomerulonephritis, B-cell lymphoma, and diabetes. The fact that not all patients with a severe injury to extrahepatic sites clinically benefited by an SVR suggests that there are risks in deferring antiviral therapy until patients become symptomatic and further argues against the policy of only treating symptomatic patients, one that has gained popularity in Europe given the high cost of all oral DAA regimens.

REFERENCES

1. Webster DP, Klenerman P, Dusheiko GM. Hepatitis C. Lancet 2015;385(9973):1124–35.
2. Cacoub P, Poynard T, Ghillani P, et al. Extrahepatic manifestations of chronic hepatitis C. MULTIVIRC Group Multidepartment virus C. Arthritis Rheum 1999;42:2204–12.
3. van der Meer AJ, Veldt BJ, Feld JJ, et al. Association between sustained virological response and all-cause mortality among patients with chronic hepatitis C and advanced hepatic fibrosis. JAMA 2012;308:2584–93.
4. Hsu YC, Ho HJ, Huang YT, et al. Association between antiviral treatment and extrahepatic outcomes in patients with hepatitis C virus infection. Gut 2015;64:495–503.
5. Lee MH, Yang HI, Lu SN, et al. Chronic hepatitis C virus infection increases mortality from hepatic and extrahepatic diseases: a community-based long-term prospective study. J Infect Dis 2012;206:469–77.
6. Guillevin L. Infections in vasculitis. Best Pract Res Clin Rheumatol 2013;27:19–31.
7. Cacoub P, Gragnani L, Comarmond C, et al. Extrahepatic manifestations of chronic hepatitis C virus infection. Dig Liver Dis 2014;46(Suppl 5):S165–73.
8. Kawamura Y, Ikeda K, Arase Y, et al. Viral elimination reduces incidence of malignant lymphoma in patients with hepatitis C. Am J Med 2007;120:1034–41.
9. Casato M, Mecucci C, Agnello V, et al. Regression of lymphoproliferative disorder after treatment for hepatitis C virus infection in a patient with partial trisomy 3 Bcl-2 overexpression, and type II cryoglobulinemia. Blood 2002;99:2259–61.
10. Byrnes V, Miller A, Lowry D, et al. Effects of anti-viral therapy and HCV clearance on cerebral metabolism and cognition. J Hepatol 2012;56:549–56.
11. Viganò M, Lampertico P, Rumi MG, et al. Natural history and clinical impact of cryoglobulins in chronic hepatitis C: 10-year prospective study of 343 patients. Gastroenterology 2007;133:835–42.
12. Lunel M, Musset L, Cacoub P, et al. Cryoglobulinemia in chronic liver diseases: role of hepatitis C virus and liver damage. Gastroenterology 1994;106:1291–300.
13. Wong VS, Egner W, Elsey T, et al. Incidence, character and clinical relevance of mixed cryoglobulinemia in patients with chronic hepatitis C virus infection. Clin Exp Immunol 1996;104:25–31.
14. Zignego AL, Giannini C, Gragnani L. HCV and lymphoproliferation. Clin Dev Immunol 2012;2012:980942.
15. Brouet JC, Clauvel JP, Danon F, et al. Biologic and clinical significance of cryoglobulins. A report of 86 cases. Am J Med 1974;57:775–88.

16. Agnello V, Chung RT, Kaplan LM. A role for hepatitis C virus in type II cryoglobulinemia. N Engl J Med 1992;327:1490–5.
17. Dammacco F, Sansonno D, Piccoli C, et al. The cryoglobulins: an overview. Eur J Clin Invest 2001;31:628–38.
18. Sansonno D, Cornacchiuolo V, Iacobelli AR, et al. Localization of hepatitis C virus antigens in liver and skin tissues of chronic hepatitis C virus infected patients with mixed cryoglobulinemia. Hepatology 1995;21:305–12.
19. Ramos-Casals M, Trejo O, Garcia-Carrasco M, et al. Therapeutic management of extrahepatic manifestations in patients with chronic hepatitis C virus infection. Rheumatology (Oxford) 2003;42:818–28.
20. Ferri C, La Civita L, Cirafisi C, et al. Peripheral neuropathy in mixed cryoglobulinemia: clinical and electrophysiologic investigations. J Rheumatol 1992;19:889–95.
21. Tembl JI, Ferrer JM, Sevilla MT, et al. Neurological complications associated with hepatitis C virus infection. Neurology 1999;53:861–4.
22. Lidove O, Cacoub P, Hausfater P, et al. Cryoglobulinemia and hepatitis C: worsening of pheripheral neuropathy after interferon á treatment. Gastroenterol Clin Biol 1999;23:403–6.
23. Casato M, Saadun D, Marchetti A, et al. Central nervous system involvement in hepatitis C virus cryoglobulinemia vasculitis: a multicenter case control study using magnetic resonance imaging and neuropsychological tests. J Rheumatol 2005;32:484–8.
24. Johnson RJ, Gretch DR, Yamabe H, et al. Membranoproliferative glomerulonephritis associated with hepatitis C virus infection. N Engl J Med 1993;328:465–70.
25. Daghestani L, Pomeroy C. Renal manifestations of hepatitis C infection. Am J Med 1999;106:347–54.
26. Tarantino A, Campise M, Banfi G, et al. Long-term predictors of survival in essential mixed cryoglobulinemic glomerulonephritis. Kidney Int 1995;47:618–23.
27. Ferri C, Zignego A, Pileri S. Cryoglobulins. J Clin Pathol 2002;55:4–13.
28. Zignego A, Ferri C, Giannelli F, et al. Prevalence of bcl-2 rearrangement in patients with hepatitis C virus related mixed cryoglobulinemia with or without B-cell lymphomas. Ann Intern Med 2002;137:571–80.
29. Flint M, McKeating JA. The role of the hepatic C virus glycoproteins in infection. Rev Med Virol 2000;10:101–17.
30. De Re V, Sansonno D, Simula M, et al. HCV-NS3 and IgG-Fc cross reactive IgM in patients with type II mixed cryoglobulinemia and B-cell clonal proliferations. Leukemia 2006;20:1145–54.
31. Piluso A, Gragnani L, Genovesi A, et al. MIR-17/92 expression pattern: a molecular signature of HCV-related mixed cryoglobulinemia. J Hepatol 2015;62:S221.
32. Cacoub P, Terrier B, Saadoun D. Hepatitis C virus-induced vasculitis: therapeutic options. Ann Rheum Dis 2014;73:24–30.
33. Saadoun D, Resche Rigon M, Sene D, et al. Rituximab plus Peg-interferon-alpha/ribavirin compared with Peg-interferon-alpha/ribavirin in hepatitis C-related mixed cryoglobulinemia. Blood 2010;116:326–34.
34. Mazzaro C, Monti G, Saccardo F, et al. Efficacy and safety of peginterferon alfa-2b plus ribavirin for HCV-positive mixed cryoglobulinemia: a multicentre open-label study. Clin Exp Rheumatol 2011;29:933–41.
35. El Khayat HR, Fouad YM, Ahmad EA, et al. Hepatitis C virus (genotype 4)-associated mixed cryoglobulinemia vasculitis: effects of antiviral treatment. Hepatol Int 2012;6:606–12.

36. Gragnani L, Fabbrizzi A, Triboli E, et al. Triple antiviral therapy in hepatitis C virus infection with or without mixed cryoglobulinaemia: a prospective, controlled pilot study. Dig Liver Dis 2014;46:833–7.
37. Saadoun D, Resche Rigon M, Pol S, et al. Peg-IFN-ribavirin/protease inhibitor combination in severe hepatitis C virus associated mixed cryoglobulinemia vasculitis. J Hepatol 2015;62:24–30.
38. Gragnani L, Fognani E, Piluso A, et al. Long-term effect of HCV eradication in patients with mixed cryoglobulinemia: a prospective, controlled, open-label, cohort study. Hepatology 2015;61:1145–53.
39. Alric L, Plaisier E, Thebault S, et al. Influence of antiviral therapy in hepatitis C virus-associated cryoglobulinemic MPGN. Am J Kidney Dis 2004;43:617–23.
40. Serti E, Chepa-Lotrea X, Kim YJ, et al. Successful Interferon-Free Therapy of Chronic Hepatitis C Virus Infection Normalizes Natural Killer Cell Function. Gastroenterology 2015;149:190–200.
41. Sansonno D, De Re V, Lauletta G, et al. Monoclonal antibody treatment of mixed cryoglobulinemia resistant to interferon alpha with an anti-CD20. Blood 2003; 101:3818–26.
42. Zaja F, De Vita S, Mazzaro C, et al. Efficacy and safety of rituximab in type II mixed cryoglobulinemia. Blood 2003;101:3827–34.
43. Cacoub P, Delluc A, Saadoun D, et al. Anti-CD20 monoclonal antibody (rituximab) treatment for cryoglobulinemic vasculitis: where do we stand? Ann Rheum Dis 2008;67:283–7.
44. De Vita S, Quartuccio L, Isola M, et al. A randomized controlled trial of rituximab for the treatment of severe cryoglobulinemic vasculitis. Arthritis Rheum 2012;64: 843–53.
45. Sneller MC, Hu Z, Langford CA. A randomized controlled trial of rituximab following failure of antiviral therapy for hepatitis C virus-associated cryoglobulinemic vasculitis. Arthritis Rheum 2012;64:835–42.
46. Petrarca A, Rigacci L, Caini P, et al. Safety and efficacy of rituximab in patients with hepatitis C virus-related mixed cryoglobulinemia and severe liver disease. Blood 2010;116:335–42.
47. Dammacco F, Tucci FA, Lauletta G, et al. Pegylated interferon-alpha, ribavirin and rituximab combined therapy of hepatitis C virus-related mixed cryoglobulinemia: a long-term study. Blood 2010;116:343–53.
48. Zignego AL, Ferri C, Pileri SA, et al. Extrahepatic manifestations of Hepatitis C Virus infection: a general overview and guidelines for a clinical approach. Dig Liver Dis 2007;39:2–17.
49. Ferri C, Giuggioli D, Cazzato M, et al. HCV-related cryoglobulinemic vasculitis: an up date on its etiopathogenesis and therapeutic strategies. Clin Exp Rheumatol 2003;21(Suppl.):S78–84.
50. Ballare M, Bobbio F, Poggi S, et al. A pilot study on the effectiveness of cyclosporine in type II mixed cryoglobulinemia. Clin Exp Rheumatol 1995;13(Suppl 13):S201–3.
51. Matsuo K, Kusano A, Sugumar A, et al. Effect of hepatitis C virus infection on the risk of non-Hodgkin's lymphoma: a meta-analysis of epidemiological studies. Cancer Sci 2004;95:745–52.
52. De Sanjose S, Benavente Y, Vajdic CM, et al. Hepatitis C and non-Hodgkins lymphoma among 4784 cases and 6269 controls from the International Lymphoma Epidemiology Consortium. Clin Gastroenterol Hepatol 2008;6:451–8.
53. Zuckerman E, Zuckerman T, Levine AM, et al. Hepatitis C virus infection in patients with B-cell non-Hodgkin lymphoma. Ann Intern Med 1997;127:423–8.

54. Gisbert JP, García-Buey L, Pajares JM, et al. Prevalence of hepatitis C virus infection in B-cell non-Hodgkin's lymphoma: systematic review and meta-analysis. Gastroenterology 2003;125:1723–32.

55. Dal Maso L, Franceschi S. Hepatitis C virus and risk of lymphoma and other lymphoid neoplasms: a meta-analysis of epidemiologic studies. Cancer Epidemiol Biomarkers Prev 2006;15:2078–85.

56. Dammacco F, Gatti P, Sansonno D. Hepatitis C virus infection, mixed cryoglobulinemia, and non-Hodgkin's lymphoma: an emerging picture. Leuk Lymphoma 1998;31:463–76.

57. Mele A, Pulsoni A, Bianco E, et al. Hepatitis C virus and B-cell non-Hodgkin lymphomas: an Italian multicenter case-control study. Blood 2003;102:996–9.

58. Negri E, Little D, Boiocchi M, et al. B-cell non-Hodgkin's lymphoma and hepatitis C virus infection: a systematic review. Int J Cancer 2004;111:1–8.

59. Kayali Z, Buckwold VE, Zimmerman B, et al. Hepatitis C, cryoglobulinemia, and cirrhosis: a meta-analysis. Hepatology 2002;36:978–85.

60. Monti G, Galli M, Invernizzi F, et al. Cryoglobulinaemias: a multi-centre study of the early clinical and laboratory manifestations of primary and secondary disease. GISC. Italian Group for the Study of Cryoglobulinaemias. QJM 1995;88: 115–26.

61. De Vita S, Sacco C, Sansonno D, et al. Characterization of overt B-cell lymphomas in patients with hepatitis C virus infection. Blood 1997;90:776–82.

62. Andreone P, Zignego AL, Cursaro C, et al. Prevalence of monoclonal gammopathies in patients with hepatitis C virus infection. Ann Intern Med 1998;129:294–8.

63. Rasul I, Shepherd FA, Kamel-Reid S, et al. Detection of occult low-grade B-cell non-Hodgkin's lymphoma in patients with chronic hepatitis C virus infection and mixed cryoglobulinemia. Hepatology 1999;29:543–7.

64. Dammacco F, Sansonno D, Piccoli C, et al. The lymphoid system in hepatitis C virus infection: autoimmunity, mixed cryoglobulinemia, and overt B-cell malignancy. Semin Liver Dis 2000;20:143–57.

65. Zignego A, Giannelli F, Marocchi ME, et al. T(14;18) trans-location in chronic hepatitis C virus infection. Hepatology 2000;31:474–9.

66. Ellis M, Rathaus M, Amiel A, et al. Monoclonal lymphocyte proliferation and bcl-2 rearrangement in essential mixed cryoglobulinemia. Eur J Clin Invest 1995;25: 833–7.

67. Gisbert JP, Garcia-Buey L, Pajares JM, et al. Systematic review: regression of lymphoproliferative disorders after treatment for hepatitis C infection. Aliment Pharmacol Ther 2005;21:653–62.

68. Hermine O, Lefrère F, Bronowicki J-P, et al. Regression of splenic lymphoma with villous lymphocytes after treatment of hepatitis C virus infection. N Engl J Med 2002;347:89–94.

69. Peveling-Oberhag J, Arcaini L, Hansmann ML, et al. Hepatitis C-associated B-cell non-Hodgkin lymphomas. Epidemiology, molecular signature and clinical management. J Hepatol 2013;59:169–77.

70. Paulli M, Arcaini L, Lucioni M, et al. Subcutaneous 'lipoma-like' B-cell lymphoma associated with HCV infection: a new presentation of primary extranodal marginal zone B-cell lymphoma of MALT. Ann Oncol 2010;21:1189–95.

71. Giannelli F, Moscarella S, Giannini C, et al. Effect of antiviral treatment in patients with chronic HCV infection and t(14;18) translocation. Blood 2003;102: 1196–201.

72. Kelaidi C, Rollot F, Park S, et al. Response to antiviral treatment in hepatitis C virus-associated marginal zone lymphomas. Leukemia 2004;18:1711–6.

73. Saadoun D, Suarez F, Lefrere F, et al. Splenic lymphoma with villous lympho-cytes, associated with type II cryoglobulinemia and HCV infection: a new entity? Blood 2005;105:74–6.

74. Vallisa D, Bernuzzi P, Arcaini L, et al. Role of anti-hepatitis C virus (HCV) treat-ment in HCV-related, low-grade, B-cell, non-Hodgkin's lymphoma: a multicenter Italian experience. J Clin Oncol 2005;23:468–73.

75. Mazzaro C, De Re V, Spina M, et al. Pegylated-interferon plus ribavirin for HCV-positive indolent non-Hodgkin lymphomas. Br J Haematol 2009;145:255–7.

76. Arcaini L, Vallisa D, Rattotti S, et al. Antiviral treatment in patients with indolent B-cell lymphomas associated with HCV infection: a study of the Fondazione Ital-iana Linfomi. Ann Oncol 2014;25:1404–10.

77. Arcaini L, Merli M, Passamonti F, et al. Impact of treatment-related liver toxicity on the outcome of HCV positive non-Hodgkin's lymphomas. Am J Hematol 2010; 85:46–50.

78. Viganò M, Degasperi E, Aghemo A, et al. Anti-TNF drugs in patients with hep-atitis B or C virus infection: safety and clinical management. Expert Opin Biol Ther 2012;12:193–207.

79. Musto P, Dell'Olio M, Carotenuto M, et al. Hepatitis C virus infection: a new bridge between hematologists and gastroenterologists? Blood 1996;88: 752–4.

80. La Mura V, De Renzo A, Perna F, et al. Antiviral therapy after complete response to chemotherapy could be efficacious in HCV-positive non-Hodgkin's lym-phoma. J Hepatol 2008;49:557–63.

81. Fargion S, Piperno A, Cappellini MD, et al. Hepatitis C virus and porphyria cu-tanea tarda: evidence of a strong association. Hepatology 1992;16:1322–6.

82. DeCastro M, Sanchez J, Herrera JF, et al. Hepatitis C virus antibodies and liver disease in patients with porphyria cutanea tarda. Hepatology 1993;17:551–7.

83. O'Reilly FM, Darby C, Fogarty J, et al. Porphyrin metabolism in hepatitis C infec-tion. Photodermatol Photoimmunol Photomed 1996;12:31–3.

84. Bonkovsky HL, Poh-Fitzpatrick M, Pimstone N, et al. Porphyria cutanea tarda, hepatitis C, and HFE gene mutations in North America. Hepatology 1998;27: 1661–9.

85. Okano J, Horie Y, Kawasaki H, et al. Interferon treatment of porphyria cutanea tarda associated with chronic hepatitis type C. Hepatogastroenterology 1997; 44:525–8.

86. Thornhill MH. Immune mechanisms in oral lichen planus. Acta Odontol Scand 2001;59:174–7.

87. Carrozzo M, Gandolfo S, Carbone M, et al. Hepatitis C virus infection in Italian patients with oral lichen planus: a prospective case-control study. J Oral Pathol Med 1996;25:527–33.

88. Nagao Y, Kameyama T, Sata M. Hepatitis C virus RNA detection in oral lichen planus tissue. Am J Gastroenterol 1998;93:850.

89. Doutre MS, Beylot C, Couzigou P, et al. Lichen planus and hepatitis C virus: disappearance of lichen under interferon alpha therapy. Dermatology 1992; 184:229.

90. Areias J, Velho GC, Cerqueira R, et al. Lichen planus and chronic hepatitis C: exacerbation of the lichen under interferon-alpha-2a therapy. Eur J Gastroen-terol Hepatol 1996;8:825–8.

91. Huang MJ, Tsai SL, Huang BY, et al. Prevalence and significance of thyroid au-toantibodies in patients with chronic hepatitis C virus infection: a prospective controlled study. Clin Endocrinol 1999;50:503–9.

92. Antonelli A, Ferri C, Fallahi P. Thyroid cancer in patients with hepatitis C infection. JAMA 1999;281:1588.

93. Antonelli A, Ferri C, Pampana A, et al. Thyroid disorders in chronic hepatitis C. Am J Med 2004;117:10–3.

94. Prummel MF, Laurberg P. Interferon-alpha and autoimmune thyroid disease. Thyroid 2003;13:547–51.

95. Lee YH, Ji JD, Yeon JE, et al. Cryoglobulinaemia and rheumatic manifestations in patients with hepatitis C virus infection. Ann Rheum Dis 1998;57:728–31.

96. Haddad J, Deny P, Munz-Gotheil C, et al. Lymphocytic sialadenitis of Sjogren's syndrome associated with chronic hepatitis C virus liver disease. Lancet 1992; 339:321–3.

97. Koike K, Moriya K, Ishibashi K, et al. Sialadenitis histologically resembling Sjogren syndrome in mice transgenic for hepatitis C virus envelope genes. Proc Natl Acad Sci U S A 1997;94:233–6.

98. Fallahi P, Ferrari SM, Colaci M, et al. Hepatitis C virus infection and type 2 diabetes. Clin Ter 2013;164:e393–404.

99. Zein NN, Abdulkarim AS, Weisner RH, et al. Prevalence of diabetes mellitus in patients with end-stage liver cirrhosis due to hepatitis C, alcohol or cholestatic disease. J Hepatol 2000;32:209–17.

100. Arase Y, Suzuki F, Suzuki Y, et al. Sustained virological response reduces incidence of onset of type 2 diabetes in chronic hepatitis C. Hepatology 2009;49: 739–44.

101. Aghemo A, Prati GM, Rumi MG, et al. Sustained virological response prevents the development of insulin resistance in patients with chronic hepatitis C. Hepatology 2012;56:1681–7.

102. Hsu YC, Lin JT, Ho HJ, et al. Antiviral treatment for hepatitis C virus infection is associated with improved renal and cardiovascular outcomes in diabetic patients. Hepatology 2014;59:1293–302.

103. Ishizaka N, Ishizaka Y, Takahashi E, et al. Association between hepatitis C virus seropositivity, carotid-artery plaque, and intima-media thickening. Lancet 2002; 359:133–5.

104. Lindsberg PJ, Grau AJ. Inflammation and infections as risk factors for ischemic stroke. Stroke 2003;34:2518–32.

105. Palm F, Urbanek C, Grau A. Infection, its treatment and the risk for stroke. Curr Vasc Pharmacol 2009;7:146–52.

106. Boddi M, Abbate R, Chellini B, et al. HCV infection facilitates asymptomatic carotid atherosclerosis: preliminary report of HCV RNA localization in human carotid plaques. Dig Liver Dis 2007;39(Suppl. 1):S55–60.

107. Boddi M, Abbate R, Chellini B, et al. Hepatitis C virus RNA localization in human carotid plaques. J Clin Virol 2010;47:72–5.

108. Adinolfi LE, Zampino R, Restivo L, et al. Chronic hepatitis C virus infection and atherosclerosis: clinical impact and mechanisms. World J Gastroenterol 2014; 20:3410–7.

109. He H, Kang R, Zhao Z. Hepatitis C virus infection and risk of stroke: a systematic review and meta-analysis. PLos One 2013;8:e58130.

110. Hsu CS, Kao JH, Chao YC, et al. Interferon-based therapy reduces risk of stroke in chronic hepatitis C patients: a population-based cohort study in Taiwan. Aliment Pharmacol Ther 2013;38:415–23.

111. Backus LI, Boothroyd DB, Phillips BR, et al. A sustained virologic response reduces risk of all-cause mortality in patients with hepatitis C. Clin Gastroenterol Hepatol 2011;9:509–16.

112. Innes HA, McDonald SA, Dillon JF, et al. Toward a more complete understanding of the association between a hepatitis C sustained viral response and cause-specific outcomes. Hepatology 2015. http://dx.doi.org/10.1002/hep.27766.

113. Younossi ZM, Singer ME, Mir HM, et al. Impact of interferon free regimens on clinical and cost outcomes for chronic hepatitis C genotype 1 patients. J Hepatol 2014;60:530–7.

114. McAndrews MP, Farcnik K, Carlen P, et al. Prevalence and significance of neuro-cognitive dysfunction in hepatitis C in the absence of correlated risk factors. Hepatology 2005;41:801–8.

115. Cozzi A, Zignego AL, Carpendo R, et al. Low serum tryptophan levels, reduced macrophage IDO activity and high frequency of psychopathology in HCV patients. J Viral Hepat 2006;13:402–8.

Hepatitis C: An Eastern Perspective

Yock Young Dan, MBBS, PhD, MRCP, MMed[a,b,c],
Seng Gee Lim, MBBS, FRACP, FRCP, MD, Cert Immunology[a,b,c,d,e,*]

KEYWORDS

- Hepatitis C • Asia • Cost-effectiveness • Roadmap strategy

KEY POINTS

- More than 50% of Hepatitis C carriers worldwide reside in Asia but prevalence is heterogenous with pockets of high and low prevalence, and variable genotype - in East Asia, genotype 1b predominates, while in South and South East Asia, genotype 3 is a dominant genotype, while in Indochina genotype 6 is dominant.
- Asians have a much higher prevalence of favourable IL28CC interferon good responder genotype which leads to a high sustained virological response (SVR) rate of over 70%.
- The registration approvals of new DAAs lag behind that of Western countries, and with some Asian countries requiring a registration trial, leading to delays of 3–4 years, however, generic licensing and access programs in low income countries will make these drugs more accessible.
- Due to the diversity in the epidemiology and genotype distribution, healthcare systems, economic status, reimbursement policies, and access to the new DAAs, a one size fits all strategy is unlikely with the current treatment strategies.
- A roadmap for HCV management based on available therapies and their SVR rates provides guidance for treatment selection.

INTRODUCTION

More than 170 million persons globally may be infected with HCV,[1] with over 60% living in Asia and an estimated burden of 124 million.[2] In the recent Global Burden of Disease Survey,[3] viral hepatitis accounted for more than 1 million deaths in Asia, of which about 20% are due to chronic hepatitis C. This large burden of disease is

[a] Department of Medicine, Yong Loo Lin School of Medicine, National University of Singapore, 1E, Kent Ridge Road, NUHS Tower Block Level 10, Singapore 119228, Singapore; [b] Division of Gastroenterology and Hepatology, National University Health System, Singapore, Singapore; [c] Cancer Science Institute, National University of Singapore, Singapore, Singapore; [d] Institute of Molecular and Cell Biology, Agency for Science and Technology, 61 Biopolis Drive, Singapore 138673, Singapore; [e] Department of Gastroenterology and Hepatology, National University Hospital, 1E Lower Kent Ridge Road, Singapore 119228, Singapore
* Corresponding author. Department of Gastroenterology and Hepatology, National University Hospital, 1E Lower Kent Ridge Road, Singapore 119228, Singapore.
E-mail address: mdclimsg@nus.edu.sg

Gastroenterol Clin N Am 44 (2015) 793–805
http://dx.doi.org/10.1016/j.gtc.2015.07.007
0889-8553/15/$ – see front matter © 2015 Elsevier Inc. All rights reserved.

compounded by several issues such as inadequate data on disease prevalence, poor screening programs, lack of infrastructure, insufficient number of trained health care personnel, policy inaction, delayed access, and lower priority with regards to health care budgets. Unlike the United States, which is a country, and the European Union, which is a politico-economic union of nations, Asia is made up of a wide variety of nations with a variety of health care systems and gross domestic product (GDP) from the very lowest (Bangladesh GDP per capita $2853) to the highest (Macau $138,025). Hepatitis C disease, like many infectious diseases, is closely linked to the socioeconomic status of the country. In many Asian countries, including some of the most populous ones, which were lower in the list of countries ranked by GDP until recently,[4] not only are health care budgets under duress but priority for viral hepatitis is also low. Consequently, the HCV problem in Asia is a complex one, and each country has specific issues that need to be addressed.

THE EAST AS CLUSTERS OF SIMILAR COUNTRIES

Given the vastness and the variability of the multitude of countries in the East, the Global Burden of Disease Study[5] has grouped countries based on epidemiologic homogeneity so as to allow meaningful health care conclusions to be drawn for countries that are clustered in the same group (**Table 1**). However, one can also view countries based on their health care reimbursement patterns: full or almost full reimbursement, partial reimbursement, or no reimbursement.[6] Health care reimbursement leads to a single payer and hence a stronger negotiating position with regards to drug costs from pharmaceutical companies. Where there is no single payer, the cost of drugs is set by the pharmaceutical company based on market forces.

Table 1
Estimated prevalence of HCV in Asia Pacific countries using global burden of disease grouping

	Countries	Health Care Affordability (GDP)	Prevalence (%)
Group 1: High-income Asia Pacific	Singapore, Japan, South Korea	+++	0.5–1.4
Group 2: Central Asia	Armenia, Uzbekistan, Mongolia, Kazakhstan	+ to ++	3.8 (3.0–4.5)
Group 3: East Asia	China, Special Administrative Regions, Taiwan	++ to +++	3.7 (3.4–4.5)
Group 4: South Asia	Bangladesh, India, Pakistan	+	3.4 (2.6–4.4)
Group 5: Southeast Asia	Malaysia, Myanmar, Vietnam, Cambodia, Thailand	+ to ++	2.0 (1.7–2.3)
Group 6: Australasia	Australia, New Zealand	+++	2.7 (2.2–3.22)

Prevalence *Data from* Mohd Hanafiah K, Groeger J, Flaxman AD, et al. Global epidemiology of hepatitis C virus infection: new estimates of age-specific antibody to HCV seroprevalence. Hepatology 2013;57(4):1333–42; Sievert W, Altraif I, Razavi HA, et al. A systematic review of hepatitis C virus epidemiology in Asia, Australia and Egypt. Liver Int 2011;31 Suppl 2:61–80; and Relative GDP (per capita) *Data from* International Monetary Fund. World Economy Outlook Database. 2015. Available at: https://www.imf.org/external/pubs/ft/weo/2015/01/weodata/index.aspx. Accessed April 22, 2015.

VARIED EPIDEMIOLOGY

The true prevalence rate of HCV infection in the East remains less well defined because of the lack of good-quality community studies in many countries. A systematic review of the epidemiology of HCV infection in the East was performed recently.[7] Even within the same country, there may be high discordance in HCV prevalence rates between studies because of the multiethnicity and socioeconomic heterogeneity within the same country. A typical case is Taiwan where a nationwide seroepidemiology survey of 7 townships showed variation of 1.6% in the lowest to 19.6% in the highest.[8] The difference was thought to be related to differences in risk factors, the most common being blood transfusion and unsafe injection practices, acupuncture, and tattooing. In China, studies have reported an estimated prevalence of 1% to 1.9%[7]; however, a recent seroepidemiology update indicated a much lower prevalence of 0.43%, which was consistent across the different regions in China.[9] One of the reasons for this decrease was the use of newer-generation anti-HCV enzyme-linked immunosorbent assay, which had fewer false-positive results than the previous studies. However, there may be pockets of high prevalence in high-risk groups, such as rural Henan, where paid blood donation is commonly practiced and prevalence rates of up to 9.6% have been reported.[10] In most countries, epidemiologic data are from older serology studies or from blood donor groups, which underestimate the actual prevalence.[2]

Attempts have been made to mathematically predict the actual prevalence in various countries.[2] Using these predictions, the countries with the highest prevalence are those in Central, South, and East Asia (Mongolia, China, Taiwan, and Pakistan), with prevalence rates exceeding 3%. The 2 countries with the highest recorded prevalence are Pakistan (4.7%)[11] and Taiwan (4.4%).[12] Australia, New Zealand, and the Southeast Asian countries are moderate in prevalence (2%–3%). The high-income Asian countries such as Japan, South Korea, and Singapore, having the highest community hygiene standards, have the lowest HCV serology prevalence.[2] Without good prevalence data, prioritization for action is difficult to mobilize from both policy makers and the public. Estimates of disease burden are also misleading.

COMPLEX GENOTYPE DISTRIBUTION

The diversity of HCV genotypes in the East[7] is related to the highly heterogeneous ethnicity and routes of transmission in Asia Pacific countries. Genotype 1b is the predominant genotype (45%–64%) in countries in East Asia such as China, Taiwan, South Korea, and Japan, followed by genotype 2. Australia has a fairly equal mix of genotypes 1 and 3 (54% and 37%, respectively). In South Asia and southeastern parts of Asia, the predominant genotype was genotype 3 (45%–79%), in Thailand, India, and Pakistan. Vietnam has a high predominance of genotypes 1 and 6 (30% and 54%, respectively), a pattern that is not shared by other Asian countries. The differences in genotype distribution have significant implications for Asian countries. In particular, genotype 3, the predominant genotype in South Asia and Southeast Asia, now recognized to be associated with worse prognosis, is also a difficult-to-treat genotype.[13] There are more limited therapeutic options for genotype 3 because most of the new all-oral DAAs are active against genotype 1 and they have more limited activity against genotype 3.[13] For Indochina, where genotype 6 is the dominant genotype, there are few studies on antiviral efficacy. These scenarios make recommendations and guidelines of limited value in these countries.

DIFFERING HEPATITIS C VIRUS TREATMENTS

In many Asian countries, the standard of care (SOC) still remains a combination of pegylated interferon and ribavirin (PR), which achieves an SVR in approximately 74% of patients in the largest Asian randomized control study. This situation is attributed to the high prevalence of the IL28B good-responder (CC) genotype in 80% of the patients,[14] the most common genotype in Asians.[15] In contrast, only 50% of Caucasian HCV genotype 1–infected subjects achieve SVR with PR.[16] Unfortunately, most Asians present with advanced disease and many have also failed PR therapy; consequently, there is a large unmet need for new treatments. With the approval of boceprevir, the efficacy of boceprevir triple therapy was evaluated in an early access program of the most difficult-to-treat patient category in Asians, those who had failed therapy and had advanced fibrosis or cirrhosis.[17] The overall sustained virological response at week 12 post treatment (SVR12) was 61% and was similar in both Asian and Caucasian patients, and although there was no mortality in this study, there were significant serious adverse events and adverse events that led to many treatment discontinuations. Consequently, more effective anti-HCV treatments are needed in patients who may otherwise progress to liver cirrhosis and hepatocellular carcinoma (HCC). Although the first-wave DAAs, telaprevir and boceprevir, were approved in the United States and the European Union in 2011, telaprevir was approved only in Japan in Asia. Boceprevir was subsequently approved in many Asian countries, but its use has declined considerably recently. Production of telaprevir has been discontinued, and boceprevir is likely to be discontinued in the near future.

The second-wave DAAs still used an interferon backbone. Simeprevir, peginterferon, and ribavirin as well as sofosbuvir, peginterferon, and ribavirin were approved for treatment of genotype 1 in the United States and European Union. The phase 3 studies were performed in the United States and European Union and had few Asian patients, with the exception of Japan. Although the efficacy of these drugs was superior to that of the first-wave DAAs, the responses were still less than ideal and came with adverse events because of the use of peginterferon and ribavirin. In Asia, simeprevir has been approved only in Japan at a reduced dose of 100 mg/d with PR for 24 weeks. This regimen led to SVR rates of 88.6% in treatment-naive genotype 1–infected patients,[18] similar to Western studies in which simeprevir 150 mg/d with PR achieves SVR rates of 80%. Studies on sofosbuvir and PR for 12 weeks achieved high rates of SVR in Western studies in treatment-naive patients,[19] but there are no randomized control trials on treatment-experienced patients, particularly in the more difficult-to-treat group of treatment-experienced patients with cirrhosis. Real-world data from HCV TRIO suggest that this is a suboptimal regimen in such patients.[20] In Asia, approval has lagged behind Western countries; although registration has been filed in multiple counties, approval has been limited to a few Asian countries (**Table 2**), but is expected to be complete in Asia by 2018–2019. A roadmap to guide clinicians on the efficacy of various available therapies can be viewed in **Fig. 1**.

There have been limited studies with the all-oral DAAs in Asia. One of the few DAA combinations to be tested in Asia was the all-oral combination of asunaprevir and daclatasvir, which has been approved in Japan but can only be used for genotype 1b, a strain that is by far the most common genotype 1 subtype in Asia. In a phase 3 international study (HALLMARK-DUAL),[21] 307 treatment-naïve nonresponders to PR or PR intolerant genotype 1b–infected patients were treated with asuneprevir and daclatasvir for 12 or 24 weeks. SVR12 was 90% in patients in the treatment-naive cohort, 82% in the nonresponder cohort, and 82% in the ineligible, intolerant, or ineligible and intolerant cohort, 168 (82%; 95% CI, 77–87) in the nonresponder cohort,

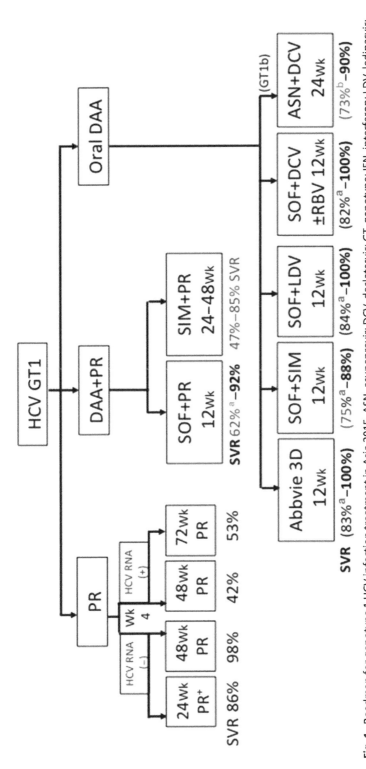

Fig. 1. Roadmap for genotype 1 HCV infection treatment in Asia 2015. ASN, asuneprevir; DCV, daclatasvir; GT, genotype; IFN, interferon; LDV, ledipasvir; P, peginterferon; R, ribavirin; SIM, simeprevir; SOF, sofosbuvir. [a]For treatment-experienced cirrhosis, [b]for cirrhosis, [c]advanced cirrhosis with low platelet count. (*Data from* Refs.[21,24,39])

and 192 (82%; 95% CI, 77–87) in the ineligible, intolerant, or ineligible and intolerant cohort. An open-label study of genotype 1b–infected patients (interferon-ineligible/intolerant patients and nonresponders) was performed in Japan.[22] Sustained virological response at week 24 post treatment was achieved by 87.4% of interferon-ineligible/intolerant patients and 80.5% of nonresponder (null and partial) patients; rates were similar in patients with cirrhosis (90.9%) and without cirrhosis (84.0%). The combination of asuneprevir and daclatasvir was approved for treatment of genotype 1b chronic hepatitis C in Japan in July 2014, being the first DAA all-oral combination to achieve initial global registration in Asia[23]; this was largely because of the high efficacy of the combination in genotype 1b infection, which is by far the predominant genotype 1 subtype in Japan. The combination has substantially lower efficacy in genotype 1a infection and is prone to develop drug-resistant mutations. Other recently approved DAAs, such as sofosbuvir, sofosbuvir and ledipasvir (Harvoni), and Abbvie 3D combination ± ribavirin (Viekira Pak), have not been tested in the East, and most studies of these DAAs have few Asian patients. However, there is no reason to suspect that the efficacy of these DAAs are likely to be different from that of the Western phase 3 studies. The efficacy of these drugs in different HCV-infected populations has been updated in the most recent European Association for Study of Liver (EASL) clinical practice guidelines.[24]

Genotype 3 poses a major problem in South Asia and Southeast Asia, where it is the dominant genotype in some countries such as Pakistan. Treatment with PR for 24 weeks is the SOC in most Asian countries, although treatment extension to 48 weeks is common for those with cirrhosis. Unfortunately, there are not much clinical trial data to support this strategy, and if patients are positive for HCV RNA at week 4, SVR rates seem suboptimal.[25] Sofosbuvir and daclatasvir for 12 weeks is also an option but as daclatasvir is not readily available in Asia, this may not be a suitable option; sofosbuvir and ribavirin for 24 weeks can be used in treatment-experienced patients with cirrhosis (**Fig. 2**), but this has poor efficacy (60% SVR).[26] However, this strategy may still be useful in Asia for treatment-naive patients even with cirrhosis despite the lack of recommendation from EASL guidelines.[24]

IMPLICATIONS OF FAVORABLE INTERFERON-RESPONSIVE GENES

Meta-analyses have shown that the strongest single nucleotide polymorphism upstream of the IL28B gene that is favorable for achieving an SVR is the rs12979860 CC in Caucasians, whereas in Asians, the rs8099917TT genotype is more predictive of SVR with PR. The pooled prevalence of the favorable IL28B genotype is more common in Asians (73%) than in Caucasians (41%) and African Americans (13%).[27] The higher prevalence of a favorable genotype results in a high SVR using PR in genotype 1–infected patients in Asians making this still acceptable as a treatment option. The potential for shortened duration of PR treatment and favorable cost-effectiveness may make this classic regimen still relevant especially if affordability and access to new drugs limit their use.

DIVERSE BARRIERS IN ACCESS TO CARE
Registration Trials Are Needed in Some Asian Countries

There are numerous barriers to access of the new DAA interferon-free agents in Asia. As Asia comprises many different countries, each with its own regulatory requirements, new drug applications need to be filed for each country. In addition, the specific requirements for registration differ widely.[28] In some countries (China, Taiwan, South Korea, and Vietnam), local clinical trials need to be conducted as a registration

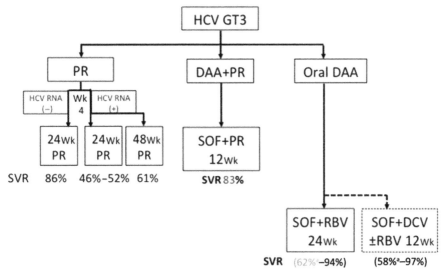

Fig. 2. Roadmap for genotype 3 HCV infection treatment in Asia 2015. DCV, daclatasvir; GT, genotype; P, peginterferon; R, ribavirin; SOF, sofosbuvir. [a]Treatment-experienced cirrhosis. (*Data from* Refs.[24,25,43])

requirement, which consequently leads to a considerable delay, as the trials need to be completed and data analyzed before the registration documents can be submitted, reviewed, and subsequently approved.

Registration Time Lines

Owing to the diverse health care systems in Asia, the time lines for registration are highly variable, but the minimum period is 12 months with some registrations taking as long as 4 years mainly because of administrative and bureaucratic processes.[29] A fast-track process may be available in some countries. In high-income Asia Pacific countries (group 1), Australasia (group 6), and East Asia (group 3), the processes are more established, and the time lines for drug approval are usually clearer. The estimated approval dates for different all-oral DAAs are listed in **Table 2**.

Health Care Systems in the East

Owing to the high variability in economic spending power in health care among Asian countries, the health systems are highly heterogeneous and 70% of the countries in Asia have GDP per capita lower than $20,000.[4] Health expenditure as a percentage of GDP in 2010 was 4.5% in the Asian region. This indicator varied from 2% in Myanmar to up to 10.1% in New Zealand, but almost all countries fall short of the Organisation for Economic Cooperation and Development average of 9.5%.[30] Unlike in the West where universal health care is available either through single payer or through comprehensive insurance, most health care systems in Asia are based on a hybrid system whereby government subsidies are limited, and patient is the direct payer for expensive or new drugs.[30] Subvention policies are thus arbitrary and vary significantly. Although PR is funded by many governments, access is not universal and is virtually absent in the lower-income countries where competition for the health dollar is high and universal health care is not available. Even in developed countries, the high cost of the DAAs would overwhelm the health budgets of most countries.[31]

Table 2
Expected approval dates for DAAs (pharmaceutical sources)

Country	Sofosbuvir	Harvoni	Viekira Pak	Asuneprevir & Daclatasvir
Australia	Approved	Second half 2015	Second half 2016	Second half 2015
Bangladesh	No filing	No filing	No filing	NA
China	Q2 2018	Q2 2019	Second half 2018	Registration trial completing 2017
Hong Kong	Approved	Q3 2016	Second half 2015	Second half 2015
India	Approved	Second half 2016	No filing	NA
Indonesia	Q3 2016	Q4 2016/1Q 2017	No filing	NA
Japan	Approved	Second half 2015	Second half 2016	2014 approved
Macau	Approved	Approved	Available since 2015	Second half 2015
Malaysia	Q2 2016	Q1 2017	Second half 2015	2016/2017
Myanmar	Q2 2018	Q2 2018	No filing	NA
New Zealand	Approved	Approved	Second half 2016	Second half 2015
Pakistan	Approved	Second half 2016	No filing	NA
Philippines	Q3 2015	Q2 2018	No filing	2016/2017
Singapore	Approved	Q3 2016	First half 2016	July 2015
South Korea	Q4 2015	Q4 2015	Second half 2016	May 2015 Approved
Taiwan	Q3 2015	Q3 2016	Second half 2016	Second half 2015
Thailand	Second half 2015	Second half 2016	No filing	2016
Vietnam	2017	NA	No filing	NA
Mongolia	Approved	Second half 2015	NA	NA

Abbreviations: NA, not available; Q1, quarter 1; Q2, quarter 2; Q3, quarter 3; Q4, quarter 4.

Public Health Policies

In the East, with the lack of screening programs and universal health care, the majority of HCV-infected patients do not know they are infected. Patient advocacy group, health care workers, and policy makers need to put in place more comprehensive screening strategies now that all-oral therapy with high SVR rates can lead ultimately to eradication of HCV. Such a program would include the following aims:

- Conducting local epidemiology studies to identify the at-risk group for screening
- Educating the public to create awareness for screening
- Using demonstration programs to evaluate the best methods for screening and treatment uptake

- Establishing screening outreach programs integrated with community health care with trained personnel to provide counseling and evaluation
- Making available screening test (serology of HCV antigen) and mechanism for follow-up for confirmatory test, including HCV RNA, genotype testing, and evaluation of liver fibrosis
- Creating access to affordable medication
- Monitoring of compliance, outcomes of treatment, and resistance
- Creating public health policies to reduce further transmission by targeting the at-risk sources, for example, screening at blood banks, avoiding reuse needles, and reworking dialysis protocols

These strategies can be challenging in countries where affordability and infrastructure for rural access remain limited.

Cost-Effectiveness Analysis in the East

PR, PR/DAA, and all-oral DAA regimens have been shown to be cost-effective in the United States and Europe. In Asia, the authors' analysis showed that all 3 regimens are cost-effective in Singapore with incremental cost effective ratio (ICER) ranging from $14,000 to $18,000.[32] These figures would be lower than the GDP per capita of about half the countries in Asia. Using the World Health Organization guidelines of using the GDP per capita as the threshold for cost-effectiveness, this suggests that HCV treatment is potentially cost-effective in half the countries in Asia.

In the high-income countries where liver transplant is used to treat patients with liver complications, treatment of HCV infection becomes even more cost-effective as SVR results in savings by avoiding liver complications such as liver failure and HCC.[32] In fact, it has been shown that targeted population screening of high-risk groups in Japan can be cost-effective.[33]

Cost-Effectiveness Versus Affordability: Competition for the Health Dollar

Cost-effectiveness does not equate affordability, and the limited health care budget in many of the Asian countries means that there is tremendous competition for every health dollar. The life expectancy in Asia is 71 years compared with 79 years in the West,[34] but in parts of central Asia, this can be as low as 65 years because of diarrheal disease, violence, and metabolic disease.[32] Consequently, prioritization for hepatitis C treatment may not be high in the health care agenda.

Access and Other Programs

Under the HCV treatment expansion program, Gilead (Gilead Sciences, Foster City, CA, USA) has licensed generic pharmaceutical manufacturers to produce sofosbuvir for low-income countries based on GDP.[35] Countries in Asia that would benefit from this program include Afghanistan, Bangladesh, Bhutan, Cambodia, Indonesia, India, Mongolia, Myanmar, Central Asian countries, Pakistan, Sri Lanka, and Vietnam. This program would open up access to many of the low-income countries in Asia, but several challenges still exist. These include the final cost of these generic versions in relation to patients' affordability, the need for an infrastructure to identify patients and for them to obtain access to these drugs, and the need to ensure that noncompliance does not result in emergence of widespread resistance in the community.[36,37] However, the commitment to and scale of HCV programs by governments in the East is still lacking compared with the tremendous strides made in Egypt. National liver associations and nongovernmental organizations such as the Coalition for Eradication of Viral Hepatitis in the Asia Pacific and WHO are mapping out strategies, but the impact of these are likely to be limited without the infrastructure and resources of each nation.

MANAGEMENT OF HEPATITIS C VIRUS INFECTION IN THE EAST

Because of the differences in HCV prevalence, genotype, health care systems, economic priorities, and infrastructure, it would be challenging indeed to propose a one-size-fits-all therapy for HCV infection, especially at this time when therapeutic strategies are still in a state of flux and there is no pangenotypic therapy. In general, treatment of HCV infection can be divided into 2 groups: where there is public reimbursement and where there is none. In the former, government policy dictates first-line and rescue therapy, whereas in the latter, affordability and market forces dictate treatment uptake. For instance, in Australia, although sofosbuvir has been approved for treatment of HCV infection, reimbursement has not been approved; hence, those who wish to have sofosbuvir-based therapy have to pay out of pocket for the therapy. First-line therapy still remains simeprevir triple therapy. In Asia, only in Japan has an all-oral therapy, asuneprevir and daclatasvir, been approved for treatment of genotype 1b infection. Consequently, Japanese HCV guidelines are different from those of the rest of Asia, as they would be in Australia. However, in the remainder of Asia, where these new DAAs are not as yet approved, PR remains the SOC. With the impending approval of sofosbuvir, the prospect of short-term (12 weeks) treatment with sofosbuvir and PR with high SVR rates for genotype 1 infection in treatment-naive patients has led many to defer therapy until it is approved. In high-income countries, such as Singapore, Hong Kong, and Macau, there is no reimbursement; hence, treatment is based on affordability. In low-income countries such as Pakistan, sofosbuvir and PR can be obtained at low cost through the Gilead Access Program through government-approved schemes. For genotype 3, the possibility of either sofosbuvir and PR for 12 weeks or interferon-free therapy with sofosbuvir and ribavirin for 24 weeks leads to reasonable SVR rates, although the latter is not recommended in the most recent EASL guidelines; this may be a good option in countries that have access to the generic version of sofosbuvir. The alternative option of sofosbuvir and daclatasvir is less likely because of the lack of availability and cost of daclatasvir in Asia. Sofosbuvir and PR is also a suitable alternative. A new roadmap for management is proposed (see **Figs. 1** and **2**), which may be useful since the last Asian Pacific Association for the Study of the Liver guidelines were published in 2012,[38] and provides updated information subsequent to the approval of boceprevir[39] and the most recent EASL clinical practice guidelines.[24] Using the roadmap, choices can be made depending on the availability and cost of the treatment available. Ultimately, the choice is whether PR should be used as the initial therapy. As rescue therapy for treatment-experienced patients, the results are suboptimal. A clear idea of risk benefit is needed. With the new DAAs, SVR rates more than 90% are now the SOC. Consequently, expectations of therapy fall into this range, but the cost of failure is high both in financial terms and in the lack of rescue options. Although PR is the only treatment option available in many countries such as China, it has many well-known limitations in those considered difficult-to-treat patients, such as those with advanced or decompensated cirrhosis, those who underwent liver or renal transplant, those with human immunodeficiency virus coinfection, and those with autoimmune disease. Such patients certainly need access to all-oral DAAs.

LOOKING AHEAD TO THE FUTURE

The East lags behind the West with regards to availability of therapy for HCV infection, but eventually availability will be widespread. However, therapy for HCV infection is evolving rapidly, and new treatment regimens that offer high SVR rates and are better options for therapy are becoming available. Consequently, the East may be able to benefit by avoiding the experience of using therapies as they become available and leapfrog to the most optimal therapies. The previously hard-to-treat subpopulations may no longer be considered hard to treat with the new DAAs. Treatment of treatment-naive patients with genotype 1 infection with 8 weeks of therapy with high SVR rates is now possible, and studies show that 6 weeks of all-oral therapy is possible. As we push the boundaries of shortening therapy, we are also exploring the prospect of pangenotypic therapy, although no regimen currently meets that ideal. However, the huge burden of undiscovered and undiagnosed disease remains the biggest challenge.[40] In the United States, birth cohort screening has been advocated by the Centers for Disease Control and Prevention to screen those with the highest risk.[41] Demonstration studies have indicated the successful approaches to this. However, strategies that work in the East have not been tested and are likely to be different because of cultural, infrastructure, and access to care reasons. Another impediment is the necessity of HCV RNA testing, which is expensive and may take up to 4 weeks to obtain a result. Point-of-care testing[42] is now actively being pursued to resolve this bottleneck. Other challenges include the lack of trained health care workers needed to manage the anticipated epidemic of cases needing therapy. With simple treatment strategies, treatment may be initiated by general practitioners and even practice nurses.

SUMMARY

The rapid advances in treatment of HCV infection have led to a paradigm change that HCV is curable and can potentially be eradicated. The majority of the HCV burden is in Asia where significant challenges exist in the attempts to eradicate this disease. There is a need to engage policy makers to increase awareness in community, provide public education and influence change of practices to reduce HCV transmission, and develop public health care infrastructure to reach out and identify patients in the community and make drugs accessible to these patients. We are in a dynamic transition period where competition will likely drive prices down, but a comprehensive understanding of the social targets will be needed to allow one to tailor and optimize an effective multipronged approach to counter HCV in Asia. Eradication of HCV, although still a dream, is now technically possible and must remain our working aim.

REFERENCES

1. Lavanchy D. Evolving epidemiology of hepatitis C virus. Clin Microbiol Infect 2011;17(2):107–15.
2. Mohd Hanafiah K, Groeger J, Flaxman AD, et al. Global epidemiology of hepatitis C virus infection: new estimates of age-specific antibody to HCV seroprevalence. Hepatology 2013;57(4):1333–42.
3. Lozano R, Naghavi M, Foreman K, et al. Global and regional mortality from 235 causes of death for 20 age groups in 1990 and 2010: a systematic analysis for the Global Burden of Disease Study 2010. Lancet 2012;380(9859):2095–128.

4. International Monetary Fund. World Economy Outlook Database. 2015. Available at: https://www.imf.org/external/pubs/ft/weo/2015/01/weodata/index.aspx. Accessed April 22, 2015.

5. Global Burden of Diseases Study. Global burden of diseases, injuries and risk factors study operations manual. 2009. Available at: http://www.healthdata.org/GBD. Accessed April 23, 2015.

6. Lim SG, Amarapurkar DN, Chan HL, et al. Reimbursement policies in the Asia-Pacific for chronic hepatitis B. Hepatol Int 2015;9(1):43–51.

7. Sievert W, Altraif I, Razavi HA, et al. A systematic review of hepatitis C virus epidemiology in Asia, Australia and Egypt. Liver Int 2011;31(Suppl 2):61–80.

8. Sun CA, Chen HC, Lu CF, et al. Transmission of hepatitis C virus in Taiwan: prevalence and risk factors based on a nationwide survey. J Med Virol 1999;59(3):290–6.

9. Cui Y, Jia J. Update on epidemiology of hepatitis B and C in China. J Gastroenterol Hepatol 2013;28(Suppl 1):7–10.

10. Zhang M, Sun XD, Mark SD, et al. Hepatitis C virus infection, Linxian, China. Emerg Infect Dis 2005;11(1):17–21.

11. Umar M, Bushra HT, Ahmad M, et al. Hepatitis C in Pakistan: a review of available data. Hepat Mon 2010;10(3):205–14.

12. Chen CH, Yang PM, Huang GT, et al. Estimation of seroprevalence of hepatitis B virus and hepatitis C virus in Taiwan from a large-scale survey of free hepatitis screening participants. J Formos Med Assoc 2007;106(2):148–55.

13. Ampuero J, Romero-Gomez M, Reddy KR. Review article: HCV genotype 3 - the new treatment challenge. Aliment Pharmacol Ther 2014;39(7):686–98.

14. Liu CH, Liang CC, Liu CJ, et al. Interleukin 28B genetic polymorphisms and viral factors help identify HCV genotype-1 patients who benefit from 24-week pegylated interferon plus ribavirin therapy. Antivir Ther 2012;17(3):477–84.

15. Thomas DL, Thio CL, Martin MP, et al. Genetic variation in IL28B and spontaneous clearance of hepatitis C virus. Nature 2009;461(7265):798–801.

16. Fried MW, Shiffman ML, Reddy KR, et al. Peginterferon alfa-2a plus ribavirin for chronic hepatitis C virus infection. N Engl J Med 2002;347(13):975–82.

17. Sukeepaisarnjaroen W, Pham T, Tanwandee T, et al. Boceprevir early-access for advanced-fibrosis/cirrhosis in Asia-Pacific hepatitis C virus genotype 1 non-responders/relapsers. World J Gastroenterol 2015;21(28):8660–9.

18. Dieterich D, Bacon BR, Flamm SL, et al. Evaluation of sofosbuvir and simeprevir-based regimens in the TRIO network: academic and community treatment of a real-world, heterogeneous population. Washington, DC: American Association of the Study of Liver Disease; 2014.

19. Hayashi N, Izumi N, Kumada H, et al. Simeprevir with peginterferon/ribavirin for treatment-naive hepatitis C genotype 1 patients in Japan: CONCERTO-1, a phase III trial. J Hepatol 2014;61(2):219–27.

20. Lawitz E, Gane EJ. Sofosbuvir for previously untreated chronic hepatitis C infection. N Engl J Med 2013;369(7):678–9.

21. Manns M, Pol S, Jacobson IM, et al. All-oral daclatasvir plus asunaprevir for hepatitis C virus genotype 1b: a multinational, phase 3, multicohort study. Lancet 2014;384(9954):1597–605.

22. Kumada H, Suzuki Y, Ikeda K, et al. Daclatasvir plus asunaprevir for chronic HCV genotype 1b infection. Hepatology 2014;59(6):2083–91.

23. Poole RM. Daclatasvir + asunaprevir: first global approval. Drugs 2014;74(13):1559–71.

24. European Association for Study of Liver. EASL recommendations on treatment of hepatitis C 2015. J Hepatol 2015;63(1):199–236.

25. Shiffman ML, Cheinquer H, Berg CP, et al. Extended treatment with pegylated interferon alfa/ribavirin in patients with genotype 2/3 chronic hepatitis C who do not achieve a rapid virological response: final analysis of the randomised N-CORE trial. Hepatol Int 2014;8(4):517–26.

26. Zeuzem S, Dusheiko GM, Salupere R, et al. Sofosbuvir and ribavirin in HCV genotypes 2 and 3. N Engl J Med 2014;370(21):1993–2001.

27. Rangnekar AS, Fontana RJ. Meta-analysis: IL-28B genotype and sustained viral clearance in HCV genotype 1 patients. Aliment Pharmacol Ther 2012;36(2):104–14.

28. Kudrin A. Challenges in the clinical development requirements for the marketing authorization of new medicines in Southeast Asia. J Clin Pharmacol 2009;49(3): 268–80.

29. Duggal E, Singh R, Kakar S. Fast track approaches for drug approval across the globe. Asian Pacific Journal of Health Sciences 2014;1(1):2–12.

30. Tarn YH, Hu S, Kamae I, et al. Health-care systems and pharmacoeconomic research in Asia-Pacific region. Value Health 2008;11(Suppl 1):S137–55.

31. Hoofnagle JH, Sherker AH. Therapy for hepatitis C–the costs of success. N Engl J Med 2014;370(16):1552–3.

32. Dan YY, Ferrante SA, Elbasha EH, et al. Cost-effectiveness of boceprevir co-administration versus pegylated interferon-alpha2b and ribavirin only for patients with hepatitis C genotype 1 in Singapore. Antivir Ther 2015;20(2): 209–16.

33. Nakamura J, Terajima K, Aoyagi Y, et al. Cost-effectiveness of the national screening program for hepatitis C virus in the general population and the high-risk groups. Tohoku J Exp Med 2008;215(1):33–42.

34. OECD/WHO. Life expectancy at birth, in Health at a Glance: Asia/Pacific 2012. 2012. Available at: http://www.oecd-ilibrary.org/social-issues-migration-health/health-at-a-glance-asia-pacific-2012_9789264183902-en. Accessed May 22, 2014.

35. Gilead Sciences media files: Chronic hepatitis C treatment expansion. Generic manufacturing for developing countries. Available at: http://www.gilead.com/~/media/files/pdfs/other/hcvgenericagreementfactsheet.pdf?la=en. Accessed April 2014.

36. Suthar AB, Harries AD. A public health approach to hepatitis C control in low- and middle-income countries. PLoS Med 2015;12(3):e1001795.

37. Wei L, Lok AS. Impact of new hepatitis C treatments in different regions of the world. Gastroenterology 2014;146(5):1145–50.e1–4.

38. Omata M, Kanda T, Yu ML, et al. APASL consensus statements and management algorithms for hepatitis C virus infection. Hepatol Int 2012;6:409–35.

39. Lim SG. Chronic hepatitis C genotype 1 treatment roadmap for resource constrained settings. World J Gastroenterol 2015;21(6):1972–81.

40. Goldberg D, Anderson E. Hepatitis C: who is at risk and how do we identify them? J Viral Hepat 2004;11(Suppl 1):12–8.

41. Smith BD, Morgan RL, Beckett GA, et al. Hepatitis C virus testing of persons born during 1945–1965: recommendations from the Centers for Disease Control and Prevention. Ann Intern Med 2012;157(11):817–22.

42. Parisi MR, Soldini L, Vidoni G, et al. Point-of-care testing for HCV infection: recent advances and implications for alternative screening. New Microbiol 2014;37(4): 449–57.

43. Andriulli A, Mangia A, Iacobellis A, et al. Meta-analysis: the outcome of anti-viral therapy in HCV genotype 2 and genotype 3 infected patients with chronic hepatitis. Aliment Pharmacol Ther 2008;28(4):397–404.

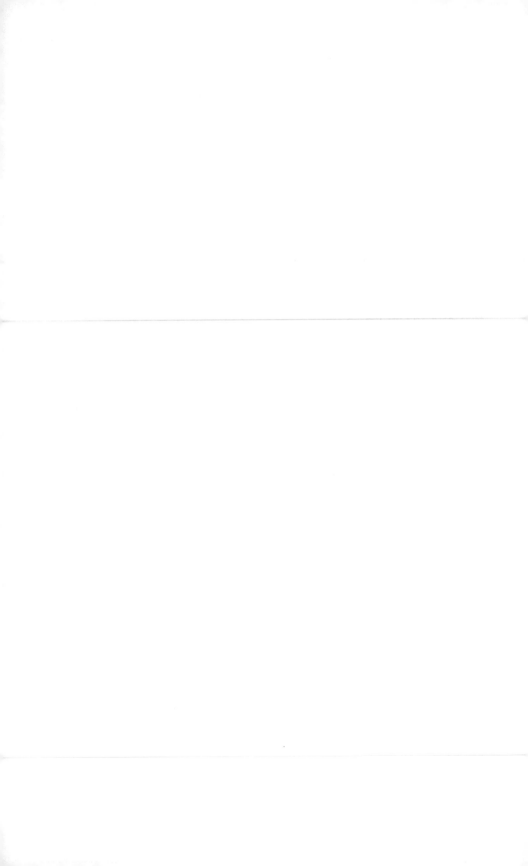

Hepatitis C Virus
A European Perspective

 CrossMark

Georg Dultz, MD, Stefan Zeuzem, MD, PhD*

KEYWORDS

- Hepatitis C virus (HCV) • Cirrhosis • European guidelines
- Direct-acting antiviral agents (DAA) • Interferon-free

KEY POINTS

- Properties of the hepatitis C virus (HCV) disease burden are heterogeneous across Europe with differences in incidence, prevalence, diagnosis and treatment rates, transmission routes, and genotype distribution.
- Injective drug use has replaced medical procedures as the major transmission risk factor for HCV in Europe.
- Recent estimates expect an increase in HCV-related morbidity and mortality in most European countries until 2030 even when current treatment options are taken into account.
- Highly efficient interferon-free treatment regimens are available for all HCV genotypes. Interferon-containing treatment regimens have limited relevance in some European countries with less developed health care systems and for selected difficult-to-cure patients.
- Accessible and affordable treatment options with high efficacy have to be complemented by improved prevention and screening strategies for a sustained reduction of HCV-related morbidity and mortality on the European continent.

INTRODUCTION

Chronic HCV infection is a major public health burden in Europe, being one of the leading causes of chronic liver disease, liver cirrhosis, and hepatocellular carcinoma (HCC). As a consequence, chronic HCV infection is a common cause for liver transplants across the continent.[1,2] The prevalence of HCV infection in the geographic area of Europe ranges from 0.4% to 1.5% in Western Europe and 0.7% to 3.2% in Central Europe to 0.9% to 1.7% in Eastern Europe.[3] The limited availability of reliable data from some regions, especially Eastern Europe, and the fact that some patient

Disclosures: No disclosures (G. Dultz); Consultancy for Abbvie, BMS, Gilead, Janssen, and Merck (S. Zeuzem).
Department of Medicine 1, Goethe University Hospital, Theodor-Stern-Kai 7, Frankfurt 60590, Germany
* Corresponding author.
E-mail address: zeuzem@em.uni-frankfurt.de

populations such as prison inmates or socially excluded groups with a higher HCV prevalence are not reached by surveys lead to an underestimation of the total number of infected individuals.[2,4–6] Owing to the diverse historical developments and backgrounds in different European countries and regions, the characteristics of the HCV-infected population and risk factors for transmission are highly variable across European countries. To date, injective drug use is the leading cause for chronic HCV infection in most parts of Europe, whereas contaminated syringes in medical procedures were a major cause of infection in rural areas with limited medical care in Eastern European countries such as Greece, Turkey, and Romania.[7] A substantial proportion of the HCV-infected population in most Western European countries, such as Belgium, France, and Germany, acquired the infection in the 1970s and 1980s similar to the high proportion of baby boomers among HCV-infected patients in North America, whereas the increase in injective drug use (IDU) in many Eastern European countries during the last 2 decades led to more recent HCV infection and a younger HCV-infected cohort in countries such as the Czech Republic.[8–12] That is why epidemiologic models predict the peak prevalence of HCV-related complications (transplant, cirrhosis, and HCC) by 2030 for Western Europe and much later for parts of Eastern Europe.[10]

HCV treatment is still changing rapidly as the first approved direct antiviral agents (DAAs) telaprevir and boceprevir were outpaced by new highly effective and interferon-free treatment regimens within the last 2 years. In Europe, NS5B polymerase inhibitor sofosbuvir, NS3/4A protease inhibitor simeprevir, and NS5A inhibitor daclatasvir in interferon-based and interferon-free treatment and combination regimens, as well as the ritonavir-boosted combination of NS3/4A protease inhibitor paritaprevir and NS5A inhibitor ombitasvir with NS5B-polymerase inhibitor dasabuvir, are approved by the European Medicines Agency for the treatment of chronic HCV infection according to genotype, prior treatment, and stage of liver disease. Nevertheless, interferon-containing treatment regimens with or without the first-generation NS3/4A protease inhibitors telaprevir and boceprevir are still in use in some Eastern European countries with less developed health care systems owing to the lower treatment costs.[13,14]

The European perspective on HCV infection regarding epidemiologic features of disease burden in European countries, consequences of chronic HCV-related liver disease, and future challenges, as well as the currently available treatment options, are reviewed herein.

THE EPIDEMIOLOGY OF HEPATITIS C VIRUS INFECTION IN EUROPE

Epidemiologic data on HCV prevalence, diagnosis rate, genotype distribution, and major risk factors for HCV transmission for several representative European countries are illustrated in **Fig. 1**.

Hepatitis C Virus Prevalence, Diagnosis Rate, and Screening Strategies

For interpretation of the HCV prevalence in Europe, it is worth knowing that the epidemiologic data are based mostly on reports from national HCV surveillance systems, which leads to a heterogeneity in data quality and completeness between countries. Especially in some Eastern European countries where no HCV surveillance system exists, the data were extrapolated from local studies.[15] Furthermore, selected groups with a naturally high HCV prevalence, such as prison inmates or socially excluded groups, are not represented sufficiently in the reports, leading to an underestimation of the total number of infected individuals.[16]

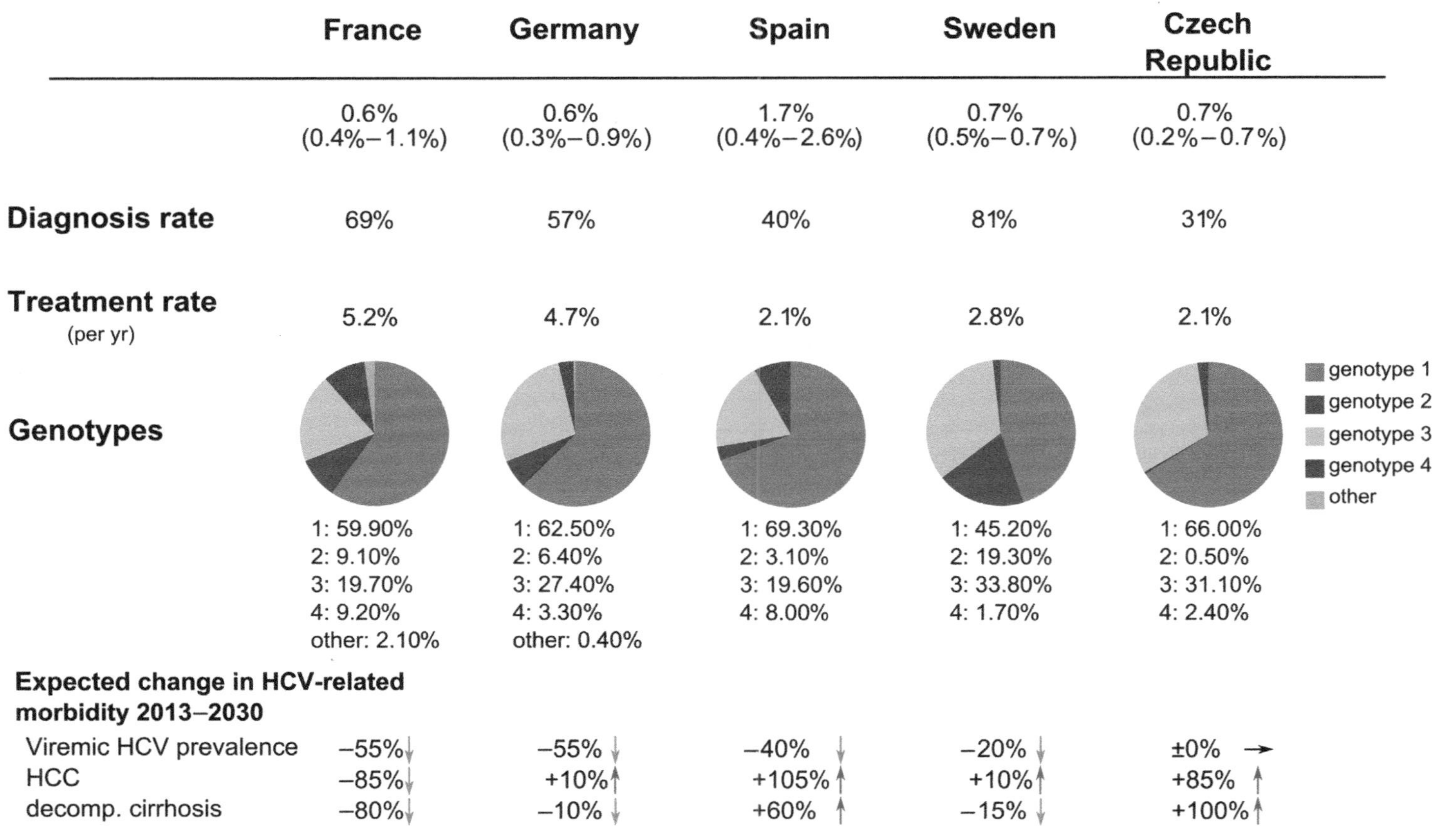

	France	Germany	Spain	Sweden	Czech Republic
Diagnosis rate	0.6% (0.4%–1.1%)	0.6% (0.3%–0.9%)	1.7% (0.4%–2.6%)	0.7% (0.5%–0.7%)	0.7% (0.2%–0.7%)
Treatment rate (per yr)	69%	57%	40%	81%	31%
	5.2%	4.7%	2.1%	2.8%	2.1%
Genotypes	1: 59.90% 2: 9.10% 3: 19.70% 4: 9.20% other: 2.10%	1: 62.50% 2: 6.40% 3: 27.40% 4: 3.30% other: 0.40%	1: 69.30% 2: 3.10% 3: 19.60% 4: 8.00%	1: 45.20% 2: 19.30% 3: 33.80% 4: 1.70%	1: 66.00% 2: 0.50% 3: 31.10% 4: 2.40%
Expected change in HCV-related morbidity 2013–2030					
Viremic HCV prevalence	−55%	−55%	−40%	−20%	±0%
HCC	−85%	+10%	+105%	+10%	+85%
decomp. cirrhosis	−80%	−10%	+60%	−15%	+100%

Legend: genotype 1, genotype 2, genotype 3, genotype 4, other

Fig. 1. Properties of HCV-related disease burden in representative European countries. The figure illustrates that countries with high treatment and diagnosis rates are expected to reduce HCV-related morbidity in the next 15 years. (Data from Razavi H, Waked I, Sarrazin C, et al. The present and future disease burden of hepatitis C virus (HCV) infection with today's treatment paradigm. J Viral Hepat 2014;21 Suppl 1:34–59; and Gower E, Estes C, Blach S, et al. Global epidemiology and genotype distribution of the hepatitis C virus infection. J Hepatol 2014;61(1 Suppl):S45–57.)

The prevalence of HCV infection in the geographic area of Europe ranges from 0.4% to 1.5% in Western Europe and 0.7% to 3.2% in Central Europe to 0.9% to 1.7% in Eastern Europe.[3] HCV hotspots with a prevalence of 3% or more are found in Romania and some rural areas in Greece and Italy.[2,4] Thus, estimations for the total number of HCV-infected persons in Europe range from 11,500,000 to 19,000,000.[2,4] As highly efficient treatment options become available, the new diagnosis of to date unknown HCV infections is a key factor and a prerequisite for the efficient reduction of the European HCV disease burden. The diagnosis rate varies between European countries and is high in Denmark (59%), France (69%), Germany (57%), and Sweden (81%). Low diagnosis rates are found in the Czech Republic (31%), Portugal (33%), and Turkey (16%).[6,10] HCV screening programs are implemented in almost all European countries for organ and blood donors as well as for patients undergoing hemodialysis, but up to now risk groups such as injecting drug users, prison inmates, or health care workers are not included in routine HCV screenings in some parts of Europe. In 2012, an HCV screening program for all baby boomers born between 1945 and 1965 was implemented in the United States because more than 75% of HCV-infected patients belong to that age group. In Europe, similar programs were considered but not yet implemented as the age distribution is not as narrow as in the United States. The growing challenge of HCV infections in migrants is not yet addressed by screening programs, although this sensitive subject deserves attention as, for example, approximately one-quarter of HCV-infected patients in Germany are not of German origin.[17]

Effective screening programs for risk groups proved to be successful and cost-effective.[18–20] The access to HCV screening and subsequent treatment of injecting drug users, who form the new major HCV cohort in Europe for upcoming decades, is an elementary task on the European continent.[21]

Routes of Hepatitis C Virus Transmission

Iatrogenic transmission

Before screening assays were available, blood transfusions or invasive medical procedures were the leading cause for HCV transmission in the 1970s and 1980s across Europe. After the implementation of routine screening assays in 1990, the infection rates by blood transfusion were reduced tremendously from 0.45% to less than 0.001% per blood unit.[22] Simultaneously, the high rate of HCV transmission in hemophiliacs by contaminated clotting factors was eliminated by the use of recombinant products.[23,24] According to a French cross-sectional survey, HCV transmission in hemodialysis units was reduced to 0.45% per year and the prevalence of anti-HCV antibodies in patients undergoing dialysis has decreased in most European countries.[25,26] Although the transmission of HCV by invasive medical procedures was reduced significantly in most Central and Western European countries over the last decades, hospital admissions and invasive medical procedures were still among the major risk factors in 2 studies among patients with acute hepatitis C infection in the 1990s and 2000s in Spain and Germany.[27,28] The extraordinary high prevalence in some areas of southern Italy is due to the frequent use of glass multiuse syringes for intravenous therapies in the past.[29,30] A continued high iatrogenic transmission rate in Europe is observed in rural areas with limited medical care, such as in parts of Romania, Crete, or Turkey.[31–33] Nevertheless, IDU has outpaced other risk factors of HCV transmission in most European countries, and individuals with IDU will form the future major HCV cohort on the continent.[2,34–36]

Injective drug use

Most newly acquired HCV infections in Europe are related to injective drug use.[10] Up to 1 million active injective drug users live in the European Union with a prevalence of anti-HCV antibodies ranging between 45% and 90%.[37–43] The incidence of HCV infection was highest in the 1980s and early 1990s before the implementation of HIV prevention programs.[44] Prevention strategies against IDU-transmitted infections by enhanced access to sterile injection equipment, self-injection facilities, professional counseling, and substitution programs have lowered transmission rates among illicit drug users in Western Europe during the last decades.[44–47] According to the Swiss HIV cohort study, the HCV incidence in individuals with IDU decreased from 13.89 per 100 person-years in 1998 to 2.24 in 2011.[45] Similar progress was reported for other Western European countries.[47–49] However, the infection rates among injective drug users even in Western Europe remain high, and further measurements to improve prevention, diagnosis rates, and treatment access are necessary. Prevention programs are implemented insufficiently or lacking in most Eastern European countries, including Russia leading to an increase in HCV incidence during the last years parallel to the increase in IDU.[2,12,50]

Hepatitis C virus in the migrant population

An increasing proportion of the HCV-infected cohort in Western Europe consists of immigrants coming from countries with high HCV prevalence. Approximately a quarter of HCV-infected patients in Germany and The Netherlands are migrants mostly from Poland, Russia, and Turkey.[17,51] In all European countries (with reliable data) except Italy, the anti-HCV prevalence was shown to be higher in the migrant population than in the general population of the same country. Hence, the implementation of screening strategies for migrants from high-prevalence countries might help to reduce HCV disease burden and long-term complications in the future.[51]

Genotype Distribution

HCV genotype 1 accounts for most HCV infections across the European continent (Western Europe, 59%; Eastern Europe, 65%; Central Europe, 89%) followed by genotype 3 (25%, 30%, 9%), genotype 2 (10.8%, 4.4%, 0.1%), and genotype 4 (4.9%, 0.1%, 1.3%). The genotype distribution is influenced considerably by routes of HCV transmission. Transmission by contaminated blood products was traditionally related to infections with genotype 1b, whereas genotypes 1a and 3 are associated with IDU-related infections.[52] Accordingly, in countries with IDU as the major transmission route in the prevalent HCV cohort (eg, United Kingdom, Sweden), genotypes 1a and 3 account for most cases. Countries where most infections are associated with iatrogenic transmission (eg, Spain, Turkey), genotype 1b is most common. As IDU outpaced transmission by blood products or medical procedures as the main risk factor across the European continent, genotypes 1a and 3 are on the increase, especially in countries with an increasing number of illicit drug users, mostly in Eastern Europe.[2,6] Genotype 4 is more common in Central and Southern Europe (Spain 8%, France 9.2%, Switzerland 10.3%, Greece 13.9%) in contrast to North America, where it accounts for less than 2% of HCV infections.[3] That is why pharmaceutical companies promoted the approval of their therapeutic regimens with genotype 4 activity for the treatment of genotype 4 in the European Union, whereas approval by the US Food and Drug Administration (FDA) for genotype 4 is lacking.

Hepatitis C Virus–Related Mortality, Transplant, and Future Perspectives

Hepatitis C virus and mortality

HCV infection is one of the leading causes of chronic liver disease in Europe. After 20 to 30 years of chronic HCV infection, 20% to 30% of the patients have developed liver cirrhosis with a risk to develop HCC of 1% to 4% per year.[53,54] The World Health

Organization (WHO) mortality reports include data on deaths associated with acute HCV infection, liver cirrhosis, and HCC. It is estimated that about 35% of deaths related to cirrhosis and 32% related to HCC are associated with HCV infection in the WHO region of Europe.[1,55] Based on those numbers, in 2012, about 96,000 deaths in Europe can be attributed to HCV infection leading to an HCV-related mortality of 10.61 per 100,000, which is higher than the mortality related to human immunodeficiency virus infection/AIDS (92,700; 10.2 per 100,000).[56] The mortality associated with HCV-related HCC follows an East-West gradient with a higher mortality observed in Western Europe. The opposite effect applies for the mortality of HCV-related cirrhosis, which is higher in Eastern Europe. These findings might be related to a higher prevalence of coexisting risk factors in HCV-infected patients in Eastern Europe, such as excessive alcohol intake or coinfection with hepatitis B, leading to an increase in mortality in patients with cirrhosis before they develop HCC.[1,57] Furthermore, the diagnosis and reporting of HCCs might be less reliable in parts of Eastern Europe with less developed health care systems.[55]

Hepatitis C virus and transplant

HCV is one of the leading causes for liver transplant in Europe. Prospective data on all liver transplants in Europe are collected by the European Liver Transplant Registry (ELTR). About 11,454 of 48,218 (24%) liver transplants between 1999 and 2009 were HCV related (assuming that 32% of HCC-associated transplants were HCV related as no HCV-specific data for HCC is published) (**Fig. 2**). In the same period, HCV infection accounted for 60% of transplants with viral hepatitis-related cirrhosis as the primary diagnosis.[58] Given the high proportion of patients with HCV infection on the liver transplant waiting list and the mismatch of needed and available organs, it is obvious that a substantial amount of waiting list mortality concerns patients with

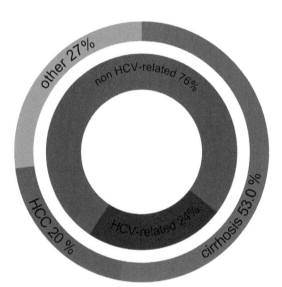

Fig. 2. Distribution of indications for liver transplant (outer circle) and HCV-related transplants (inner circle) in Europe, 1999 to 2009. One-quarter of liver transplants in Europe between 1999 and 2009 were HCV related. The quarter was formed by patients with cirrhosis and HCC. (*Data from* Adam R, Karam V, Delvart V, et al. Evolution of indications and results of liver transplantation in Europe. A report from the European Liver Transplant Registry (ELTR). J Hepatol 2012;57(3):675–88.)

HCV. The disparity of the number of waiting list patients and organ transplants in the Eurotransplant region (Austria, Belgium, Croatia, Germany, Hungary, Luxembourg, The Netherlands, and Slovenia) emerging for more than a decade is illustrated in **Fig. 3**. Recent estimates expect the number of liver transplants for HCV-related liver disease to increase until the year 2030 in almost all European countries even when current treatment options are taken into account. Accordingly, future efforts have to focus on HCV prevention to further reduce HCV incidence as well as on the improvement of diagnosis and treatment rates to reduce the HCV disease burden in Europe for the upcoming decades.[10]

Future perspectives of hepatitis C virus disease burden in Europe
The incidence of HCV infection is decreasing across Europe because of the decrease in iatrogenic HCV transmissions and the implementation of prevention programs against IDU-transmitted infections. In addition, with the beginning of the current millennium and the introduction of pegylated interferon, effective treatment possibilities that helped to decrease the existing HCV disease burden became available. This development will be boosted enormously by the currently available treatment options with DAAs. Nevertheless, although a study that modeled the future developments of HCV disease burden in Europe predicted a decrease in viremic HCV infections in most European countries (Belgium, Denmark, England, France, Germany, Portugal, Spain, Sweden, Switzerland, and Turkey) except the Czech Republic until 2030, an increase in the number of HCCs, in compensated and decompensated cirrhosis, and in liver-related mortality is expected in the same period.[10] This development is associated with the aging of the large number of patients who acquired the infection more than 20 years ago, forming a cohort with a peak prevalence of HCV-related complications to be expected in the next 15 years. As diagnosis and treatment rates are historically high in Austria, France, Germany, and Sweden, it is estimated that the prevalence of HCV-related sequelae will peak in those countries before 2030. In countries such as

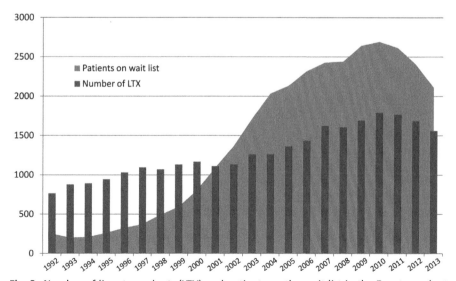

Fig. 3. Number of liver transplants (LTX) and patients on the wait list in the Eurotransplant region, 1992–2013. The figure illustrates the evolving mismatch of transplants and patients on the wait list after the millennium change in the Eurotransplant region. (*Data from* Eurotransplant annual reports. Available at: www.eurotransplant.org.)

the Czech republic, with a young HCV cohort that acquired the infection more recently, mostly by IDU, complications of chronic HCV infection are estimated to peak even after 2030.[10] The change in the HCV-related morbidity in representative European countries is illustrated in **Fig. 1**. These data emphasize that efficient treatment options alone are insufficient in the struggle for a reduction of HCV-related complications in the European population. Rather, a team play of improved prevention and screening strategies with accessible and affordable treatment options is essential for a sustained reduction of HCV-related morbidity and mortality.

APPROVED HEPATITIS C VIRUS TREATMENT OPTIONS IN THE EUROPEAN UNION

Since the approval of the first DAAs telaprevir and boceprevir in 2011, the portfolio of highly effective HCV treatment options has increased tremendously. In the last 2 years, 7 new DAAs have been approved in the European Union, which are NS5B polymerase inhibitor sofosbuvir, NS3/4A protease inhibitor simeprevir, and NS5A inhibitor dacla-tasvir, as well as the ritonavir-boosted combination of NS3/4A protease inhibitor pari-taprevir and NS5A inhibitor ombitasvir with NS5B polymerase inhibitor dasabuvir. **Fig. 4** illustrates the timeline for DAA approvals in the United States and Europe, showing the dense order of approvals within the last year. Most therapeutic regimens were approved in close succession in the United States and Europe; only for daclatasvir FDA approval is still pending. With the availability of highly effective and short interferon-free treatment protocols even for former difficult-to-cure patients with cirrhosis or therapy experience, interferon-based therapies can no longer be recom-mended as first-line treatments. Nevertheless, interferon keeps its relevance in coun-tries with less developed health care systems and limited access to the new DAAs as well as for selected difficult-to-cure cases. The following paragraphs summarize the available interferon-free treatment options for the different genotypes and their imple-mentation in European treatment protocols. Owing to the density of new DAA approvals in the last year, some treatment options are not yet implemented into guidelines.

Genotypes 1 and 4

Treatment options for HCV genotypes 1 and 4 that are approved in the European Union are summarized in **Tables 1** and **2**, respectively.

Sofosbuvir + ribavirin

The combination of NS5B inhibitor sofosbuvir and ribavirin for 24 weeks was the first approved interferon-free treatment regimen in Europe. As sustained virologic response (SVR) rates are low (68% noncirrhotic, 36% cirrhotic), the only indication re-mains the suppression of HCV replication before liver transplant.[59,60]

The 24-week treatment regimen with sofosbuvir and ribavirin is also approved for HCV genotype 4. A small Egyptian trial demonstrated SVR rates of 87% and 100% for treatment-naive and experienced patients, respectively.[61] As shorter therapy pro-tocols are available, the sofosbuvir + ribavirin combination may only be used in selected cases, for example, for HCV suppression before liver transplant.

Sofosbuvir + simeprevir ± ribavirin

The approval of the combination of the NS5B inhibitor sofosbuvir with the NS3/4A in-hibitor simeprevir in the European Union was based on 1 phase 2 trial and is restricted to patients with intolerance to interferon or an urgent therapy indication.[62] The study evaluated the efficacy of the sofosbuvir + simeprevir ± ribavirin combination in pa-tients with and without cirrhosis and in therapy-naive and experienced patients (12 or 24 weeks). Observed SVR rates were more than 90% irrespective of treatment

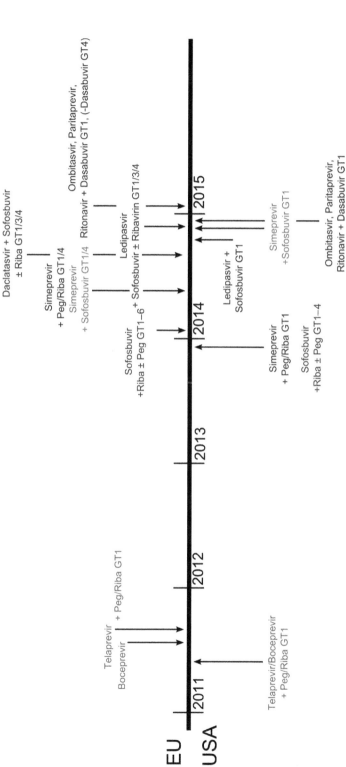

Fig. 4. Time line of HCV drug approvals since 2011 in the European Union (EU) and the United States (USA). The very dense order of approvals within the last year is illustrated. Most therapeutic regimens were approved in close succession in the United States and Europe; only for daclatasvir FDA approval is still pending. GT, genotype.

Table 1
Interferon-free treatment regimens for HCV genotype 1 approved in the European Union

Combination	Duration (wk)	Patients
Sofosbuvir + ribavirin	24	All
Sofosbuvir + daclatasvir ± ribavirin	12	Without cirrhosis
	24	With cirrhosis
Sofosbuvir + simeprevir ± ribavirin	12	All
Paritaprevir/ritonavir + ombitasvir + dasabuvir ± ribavirin	12 − Riba	Subtype 1b without cirrhosis
	12 + Riba	Subtype 1b with cirrhosis
	12 + Riba	Subtype 1a without cirrhosis
	24 + Riba	Subtype 1a with cirrhosis
Sofosbuvir + ledipasvir ± ribavirin	12 − Riba	Without cirrhosis (8 wk selected cases)
	24 − Riba	Cirrhosis (12 wk selected cases[a])
	24 + Riba	Decompensated cirrhosis, pretransplant

[a] 12 wk are preferred in some national guidelines based on Ref.[74]

duration or addition of ribavirin. In 4 of 6 patients with viral relapse, the resistance variant Q80K associated with simeprevir resistance was observed at baseline. Nevertheless, 93% of patients with the Q80K variant achieved an SVR.[62] The standard treatment regimen is the combination of sofosbuvir and simeprevir for 12 weeks. The addition of ribavirin or therapy extension to 24 weeks may be considered in individual patients.

The combination of sofosbuvir + simeprevir ± ribavirin is highly effective against HCV genotype 4 in vitro. Thus, the combination was approved in the European Union for the treatment of HCV genotype 4 (12 weeks), although data from clinical trials is lacking. Trials are ongoing and results expected in 2015.

Sofosbuvir + daclatasvir ± ribavirin

The approval of the first-in-class NS5A inhibitor daclatasvir in combination with NS5B-inhibitor sofosbuvir in the European Union is based on a small phase 2 trial.[63] The combination treatment achieved an SVR rate of 98%, independent of HCV subtype, addition of ribavirin, treatment duration (12 vs 24 weeks), and prior therapies. Because patients with cirrhosis were excluded from the study and thus data are lacking, efficacy and optimal duration for patients with cirrhosis is unknown. Nevertheless, the

Table 2
Interferon-free treatment regimens for HCV genotype 4 approved in the European Union

Combination	Duration (wk)	Patients
Sofosbuvir + ribavirin	24	All
Sofosbuvir + daclatasvir ± ribavirin	12	Without cirrhosis
	24	With cirrhosis
Sofosbuvir + simeprevir ± ribavirin	12	All
Paritaprevir/ritonavir + ombitasvir + ribavirin	12	Without cirrhosis
	24	With cirrhosis
Sofosbuvir + ledipasvir ± ribavirin	12 − Riba	Without cirrhosis
	24 − Riba	With cirrhosis (12 wk selected cases)
	24 + Riba	Decompensated. cirrhosis, pretransplant

EU approval also covers treatment of patients with compensated cirrhosis. Further results from compassionate-use programs and phase 3 trials are expected in 2015. The recommended treatment duration is 12 weeks for patients without cirrhosis. Prolongation to 24 weeks should be considered for patients with prior treatment. For patients with cirrhosis, the treatment duration is 24 weeks. Shortening treatment to 12 weeks may be considered for previously untreated patients with cirrhosis and positive prognostic factors such as low baseline viral load. For patients with advanced liver disease or with other negative prognostic factors such as prior treatment experience, the addition of ribavirin is to be considered.

Daclatasvir is not available in the United States as FDA approval is pending. Recently, a drug application for daclatasvir in combination with sofosbuvir for HCV genotype 3 based on recent phase 3 data was submitted.

The combination of sofosbuvir + daclatasvir ± ribavirin is also highly effective against HCV genotype 4 in vitro. The combination was approved in the European Union for the treatment of HCV genotype 4 (no cirrhosis, 12 weeks; cirrhosis, 24 weeks), although data from clinical trials are lacking. Trials are ongoing and results expected in 2015.

Paritaprevir/ritonavir + ombitasvir + dasabuvir ± ribavirin
The combination of the ritonavir-boosted NS3/4A inhibitor paritaprevir with NS5A-inhibitor ombitasvir and the nonnucleotide polymerase inhibitor dasabuvir represents the first approved interferon-free treatment option without a nucleotide polymerase inhibitor. Approval for the so called 3D regimen was granted based on excellent results of several phase 3 trials. Two placebo-controlled trials investigated the 3D combination with ribavirin for 12 weeks in treatment-naive and experienced HCV genotype 1–infected patients without cirrhosis. SVR rates were as high as 96.2% and 96.3%, respectively, irrespective of HCV subtype as well as prior treatment status.[64,65]

The open-label TURQUOISE-II trial examined the treatment response of previously untreated and previously treated patients with compensated liver cirrhosis and randomized these patients to 12 versus 24 weeks of 3D combination therapy plus ribavirin. SVR rates were 91.8% (12 weeks) and 95.9% (24 weeks). Patients with prior null response achieved an SVR in 80% and 92.9% after 12 and 24 weeks, respectively.[66]

Two further trials examined the impact of ribavirin on the 3D combination treatment response. Concomitant treatment with ribavirin was associated with higher response rates in HCV genotype 1a–infected patients (SVR 97.0% vs 90.2%) but not in patients with HCV genotype 1b infection (99.5% vs 99%).[67]

An additional study in treatment-experienced patients, documented the high response rates of the 3D combination in patients with genotype 1b, irrespective of the addition of ribavirin (with ribavirin 97%, without ribavirin 100%).[68]

The approval in the European Union covers the treatment of HCV genotype 1a/b–infected patients with and without cirrhosis. For genotype 1a–infected patients without cirrhosis and genotype 1b–infected patients with and without cirrhosis, treatment is recommended for 12 weeks. The recommended treatment of cirrhotic patients with genotype 1a is 24 weeks. Concomitant treatment with ribavirin is necessary for patients with genotype 1a infection and for all patients with cirrhosis. A multivariate regression analysis demonstrated that especially cirrhotic patients with genotype 1a infection with platelet count less than $90,000/\mu L$, albumin concentration less than 35 g/L, or an α-fetoprotein level 20 ng/mL or more benefit from the therapy extension to 24 weeks.[69]

The polymerase dasabuvir is not effective against HCV genotype 4 so that only the combination of paritaprevir/ritonavir + ombitasvir ± ribavirin was tested in a small trial.

After 12 weeks of treatment, SVR rates were 91% and 100% with and without ribavirin, respectively.[70] The EU approval covers a 12-week treatment regimen with paritaprevir/ritonavir + ombitasvir + ribavirin for HCV genotype 4–infected patients without cirrhosis and 24 weeks of the combination for genotype 4–infected patients with cirrhosis, although patients with cirrhosis were excluded from the trial.

Sofosbuvir + ledipasvir ± ribavirin

The combination of NS5A inhibitor ledipasvir with sofosbuvir is coformulated in 1 tablet administered once daily. Several phase 3 trials documented SVR rates between 94% and 99% irrespective of treatment duration (12 or 24 weeks) or the addition of ribavirin. However, subgroup analysis demonstrated that patients with cirrhosis achieved significantly higher SVR rates when treated for 24 weeks (99% vs 82%–86%).[71,72] For therapy-naive patients without cirrhosis, the efficacy of the combination of sofosbuvir + ledipasvir ± ribavirin for 8 weeks is equivalent to the 12-week regimen of sofosbuvir + ledipasvir, whereas the addition of ribavirin provided no benefit.[73]

The approval in the European Union covers treatment with sofosbuvir + ledipasvir for 12 weeks for HCV genotype 1–infected patients without cirrhosis. Therapy can be shortened to 8 weeks in selected cases with low viral load (<6 Mio IE/mL) and be extended to 24 weeks in therapy-experienced patients with limited retreatment options. Treatment for 24 weeks is recommended in the European Union for patients with cirrhosis. However, studies show that 12 weeks of sofosbuvir + ledipasvir in combination with ribavirin are sufficient also for patients with cirrhosis.[74] The combination of sofosbuvir + ledipasvir + ribavirin for 24 weeks is approved for patients with decompensated cirrhosis as well as in the pretransplant and posttransplant settings.

As with HCV genotype 1, the combination of sofosbuvir + ledipasvir is approved for a 12-week therapy regimen for HCV genotype 4–infected patients without cirrhosis and for 24 weeks for patients with cirrhosis. The approval was based on a small trial in which 21 genotype 4–infected patients received treatment for 12 weeks without ribavirin (SVR 95%).[75]

Genotype 2

Treatment options for HCV genotype 2 infection that are approved in the European Union are summarized in **Table 3**.

Sofosbuvir + ribavirin

Several phase 3 trials underlined the high efficacy of the sofosbuvir + ribavirin combination therapy for the treatment of patients infected with HCV genotype 2. In therapy-naive and therapy-experienced patients, SVR rates between 90% and 95% were achieved (12-week treatment). SVR rates were slightly lower in pretreated patients with cirrhosis (88%).[76–78] Accordingly, the EU approval covers the 12-week combination of sofosbuvir + ribavirin for all HCV genotype 2–infected patients. In line with some national guidelines, an elongation of treatment to 16 weeks should be considered for treatment-experienced patients with cirrhosis.[79] This recommendation is based on a small study that demonstrated a trend to low SVR rates in this patient

Table 3 Interferon-free treatment regimens for HCV genotype 2 approved in the European Union		
Combination	**Duration (wk)**	**Patients**
Sofosbuvir + ribavirin	12[a]	All

[a] 16 wk should be considered for treatment-experienced patients with cirrhosis according to some national guidelines based on Ref.[76]

group (13 of 18, 72%) that was alleviated by a therapy extension to 16 weeks (7 of 9, 78%).[76]

Sofosbuvir + daclatasvir ± ribavirin

The combination of sofosbuvir + daclatasvir ± ribavirin is not an approved treatment option for patients with HCV genotype 2 infection. Nevertheless, a high SVR rate of 92% in a small phase 2 trial can justify the off-label use in patients with treatment failure to sofosbuvir + ribavirin.[63]

Genotype 3

Treatment options for HCV genotype 3 infection that are approved in the European Union are summarized in **Table 4**.

Sofosbuvir + ribavirin

The combination of sofosbuvir + ribavirin for 24 weeks provides SVR rates of more than 90% for patients without cirrhosis, whereas rates are lower in therapy-naive and experienced patients with cirrhosis (85% and 60%, respectively).[76–78] The approval covers treatment of all patients with HCV genotype 3 infection, but especially for pretreated patients with cirrhosis the combination of sofosbuvir + daclatasvir + ribavirin is preferable.

Sofosbuvir + daclatasvir ± ribavirin

The approval of the sofosbuvir + daclatasvir + ribavirin combination therapy for HCV genotype 3 infection was based on a small phase 2 trial that demonstrated an SVR rate of 89% after 24 weeks of treatment.[63] A larger phase 3 trial reported high SVR rates for treatment-naive and experienced patients after 12 weeks of sofosbuvir + daclatasvir without ribavirin (SVR 96%). The SVR rate was significantly lower in patients with cirrhosis (63%).[80] Whether the addition of ribavirin or therapy extension to 24 weeks can improve results for patients with cirrhosis is subject of further ongoing trials.

Sofosbuvir + ledipasvir + ribavirin

The only data on the efficacy of the sofosbuvir + ledipasvir + ribavirin combination for the treatment of HCV genotype 3 infection derive from small phase 2 trials.[81,82] SVR rates were 100% and 89%, respectively, for therapy-naive and experienced patients after 12 weeks of treatment. Treatment success was much lower in the treatment arm without ribavirin (64%) and in patients with cirrhosis even when ribavirin was added (77%). The combination treatment of 24 weeks of sofosbuvir + ledipasvir + ribavirin was approved for patients with cirrhosis or patients with prior treatment failure, although data are available only for 12 weeks treatment duration. As data are limited and the combination of sofosbuvir + ribavirin is already highly effective, the additional benefit of ledipasvir in combination with sofosbuvir + ribavirin is yet to be clarified.

Table 4
Interferon-free treatment regimens for HCV genotype 3 approved in the European Union

Combination	Duration (wk)	Patients
Sofosbuvir + ribavirin	24	All
Sofosbuvir + daclatasvir + ribavirin	24	Cirrhosis and/or treatment experienced[a]
Sofosbuvir + ledipasvir + ribavirin	24	Cirrhosis and/or treatment experienced

[a] Apart from the approval, 12 wk without ribavirin are preferred for patients without cirrhosis in some national guidelines based on Ref.[80]

SUMMARY

The reduction of the HCV-related health burden in Europe remains a major task even after the approval of highly effective and well-tolerable, all-oral treatment options. Although lot of progress has been made in the field, the patchwork of diverse health systems, political systems, and economic potentials across the European continent still impedes the comprehensive implementation of prevention programs as well as high diagnosis and treatment rates. Although the iatrogenic HCV transmission was reduced enormously during the last 2 decades in most parts of the continent, IDU-related transmission is on the increase especially in parts of Eastern Europe. Another challenge is the high HCV prevalence in the migrant population. The implementation of screening strategies for migrants from high prevalence countries might help to reduce HCV disease burden and long-term complications in the future. Models predict an increase in HCV-related morbidity and mortality in most European countries until 2030. The fact that in countries with high diagnosis and treatments rates such as France or Germany the peak of HCV-related complications will be reached earlier should encourage distinct efforts to reduce the HCV-related health burden across the continent.

Since 2014, an increasing number of highly effective DAAs for the treatment of HCV infection has been approved so that therapeutic regimens with good side-effect profiles and satisfactory SVR rates are available for all HCV genotype infections. However, the high market prices for the new therapeutic regimens impair treatment access for patients in countries with less comprehensive health insurance policies. Concerted efforts are necessary to decrease HCV incidence, increase the diagnosis rate, and guarantee access to treatment on the European continent.

REFERENCES

1. Perz JF, Armstrong GL, Farrington LA, et al. The contributions of hepatitis B virus and hepatitis C virus infections to cirrhosis and primary liver cancer worldwide. J Hepatol 2006;45(4):529–38.
2. Cornberg M, Razavi HA, Alberti A, et al. A systematic review of hepatitis C virus epidemiology in Europe, Canada and Israel. Liver Int 2011;31(Suppl 2):30–60.
3. Gower E, Estes C, Blach S, et al. Global epidemiology and genotype distribution of the hepatitis C virus infection. J Hepatol 2014;61(1 Suppl):S45–57.
4. Mohd Hanafiah K, Groeger J, Flaxman AD, et al. Global epidemiology of hepatitis C virus infection: new estimates of age-specific antibody to HCV seroprevalence. Hepatology 2013;57(4):1333–42.
5. Blachier M, Leleu H, Peck-Radosavljevic M, et al. The burden of liver disease in Europe: a review of available epidemiological data. J Hepatol 2013;58(3):593–608.
6. Bruggmann P, Berg T, Øvrehus ALH, et al. Historical epidemiology of hepatitis C virus (HCV) in selected countries. J Viral Hepat 2014;21(Suppl 1):5–33.
7. Gatselis NK, Rigopoulou E, Stefos A, et al. Risk factors associated with HCV infection in semi-rural areas of central Greece. Eur J Intern Med 2007;18(1):48–55.
8. Davis GL, Alter MJ, El-Serag H, et al. Aging of hepatitis C virus (HCV)-infected persons in the United States: a multiple cohort model of HCV prevalence and disease progression. Gastroenterology 2010;138(2):513–21, 521.e1–6.
9. Deuffic-Burban S, Deltenre P, Buti M, et al. Predicted effects of treatment for HCV infection vary among European countries. Gastroenterology 2012;143(4):974–85.e14.

10. Razavi H, Waked I, Sarrazin C, et al. The present and future disease burden of hepatitis C virus (HCV) infection with today's treatment paradigm. J Viral Hepat 2014;21(Suppl 1):34–59.
11. Krekulova L, Rehak V, Madrigal N, et al. Genotypic and epidemiologic characteristics of hepatitis C virus infections among recent injection drug user and nonuser populations. Clin Infect Dis 2001;33(8):1435–8.
12. Zabransky T, Mravcik V, Korcisova B, et al. Hepatitis C virus infection among injecting drug users in the Czech Republic – prevalence and associated factors. Eur Addict Res 2006;12(3):151–60.
13. European Association for the Study of the Liver. EASL recommendations on treatment of hepatitis C 2014. J Hepatol 2014;61(2):373–95.
14. European Association for Study of the Liver. EASL clinical practice guidelines: management of hepatitis C virus infection. J Hepatol 2014;60(2):392–420.
15. Rantala M, van de Laar MJW. Surveillance and epidemiology of hepatitis B and C in Europe - a review. Euro Surveill 2008;13(21) [pii:18880].
16. Saiz de la Hoya P, Marco A, García-Guerrero J, et al. Hepatitis C and B prevalence in Spanish prisons. Eur J Clin Microbiol Infect Dis 2011;30(7):857–62.
17. Hüppe D, Zehnter E, Mauss S, et al. Epidemiologie der chronischen hepatitis C in Deutschland–Eine Analyse von 10,326 Hepatitis-C-Virus-Infizierten aus Schwerpunktpraxen und -ambulanzen. Z Gastroenterol 2008;46(1):34–44.
18. Hahné SJM, Veldhuijzen IK, Wiessing L, et al. Infection with hepatitis B and C virus in Europe: a systematic review of prevalence and cost-effectiveness of screening. BMC Infect Dis 2013;13:181.
19. Delarocque-Astagneau E, Meffre C, Dubois F, et al. The impact of the prevention programme of hepatitis C over more than a decade: the French experience. J Viral Hepat 2010;17(6):435–43.
20. Kautz A, Chavdarova L, Walker M. Improved hepatitis C screening and treatment in people who inject drugs should be a priority in Europe. BMC Infect Dis 2014; 14(Suppl 6):S3.
21. European Centre for Disease Prevention and Control. Surveillance and prevention of hepatitis B and C in Europe. Stockholm (Sweden): ECDC; 2010.
22. Pomper GJ, Wu Y, Snyder EL. Risks of transfusion-transmitted infections: 2003. Curr Opin Hematol 2003;10(6):412–8.
23. Mauser-Bunschoten EP, Bresters D, van Drimmelen AA, et al. Hepatitis C infection and viremia in Dutch hemophilia patients. J Med Virol 1995;45(3):241–6.
24. Pipe S. Consideration in hemophilia therapy selection. Semin Hematol 2006;43(2 Suppl 3):S23–7.
25. Sauné K, Kamar N, Miédougé M, et al. Decreased prevalence and incidence of HCV markers in haemodialysis units: a multicentric French survey. Nephrol Dial Transplant 2011;26(7):2309–16.
26. Jadoul M, Poignet J, Geddes C, et al. The changing epidemiology of hepatitis C virus (HCV) infection in haemodialysis: European multicentre study. Nephrol Dial Transplant 2004;19(4):904–9.
27. Martínez-Bauer E, Forns X, Armelles M, et al. Hospital admission is a relevant source of hepatitis C virus acquisition in Spain. J Hepatol 2008;48(1):20–7.
28. Deterding K, Wiegand J, Grüner N, et al. The German Hep-Net acute hepatitis C cohort: impact of viral and host factors on the initial presentation of acute hepatitis C virus infection. Z Gastroenterol 2009;47(6):531–40.
29. Cozzolongo R, Osella AR, Elba S, et al. Epidemiology of HCV infection in the general population: a survey in a southern Italian town. Am J Gastroenterol 2009; 104(11):2740–6.

30. Fusco M, Girardi E, Piselli P, et al. Epidemiology of viral hepatitis infections in an area of southern Italy with high incidence rates of liver cancer. Eur J Cancer 2008; 44(6):847–53.
31. Lionis C, Koulentaki M, Biziagos E, et al. Current prevalence of hepatitis A, B and C in a well-defined area in rural Crete, Greece. J Viral Hepat 1997;4(1):55–61.
32. Akcam FZ, Uskun E, Avsar K, et al. Hepatitis B virus and hepatitis C virus sero-prevalence in rural areas of the southwestern region of Turkey. Int J Infect Dis 2009;13(2):274–84.
33. Turhan V, Ardic N, Eyigun CP, et al. Investigation of the genotype distribution of hepatitis C virus among Turkish population in Turkey and various European countries. Chin Med J 2005;118(16):1392–4.
34. Mariano A, Scalia Tomba G, Tosti ME, et al. Estimating the incidence, prevalence and clinical burden of hepatitis C over time in Italy. Scand J Infect Dis 2009;41(9): 689–99.
35. Echevarría JM, León P, Pozo F, et al. Follow-up of the prevalence of hepatitis C virus genotypes in Spain during a nine-year period (1996-2004). Enferm Infecc Microbiol Clin 2006;24(1):20–5.
36. Ramos B, Núñez M, Toro C, et al. Changes in the distribution of hepatitis C virus (HCV) genotypes over time in Spain according to HIV serostatus: implications for HCV therapy in HCV/HIV-coinfected patients. J Infect 2007;54(2):173–9.
37. Diamantis I, Bassetti S, Erb P, et al. High prevalence and coinfection rate of hepatitis G and C infections in intravenous drug addicts. J Hepatol 1997;26(4):794–7.
38. Garfein RS, Vlahov D, Galai N, et al. Viral infections in short-term injection drug users: the prevalence of the hepatitis C, hepatitis B, human immunodeficiency, and human T-lymphotropic viruses. Am J Public Health 1996;86(5):655–61.
39. Hope VD, Eramova I, Capurro D, et al. Prevalence and estimation of hepatitis B and C infections in the WHO European Region: a review of data focusing on the countries outside the European Union and the European Free Trade Association. Epidemiol Infect 2014;142(2):270–86.
40. Nelson PK, Mathers BM, Cowie B, et al. Global epidemiology of hepatitis B and hepatitis C in people who inject drugs: results of systematic reviews. Lancet 2011;378(9791):571–83.
41. Demetriou VL, van de Vijver DA, Hezka J, et al. Hepatitis C infection among intravenous drug users attending therapy programs in Cyprus. J Med Virol 2010; 82(2):263–70.
42. Reimer J, Lorenzen J, Baetz B, et al. Multiple viral hepatitis in injection drug users and associated risk factors. J Gastroenterol Hepatol 2007;22(1):80–5.
43. Camoni L, Regine V, Salfa MC, et al. Continued high prevalence of HIV, HBV and HCV among injecting and noninjecting drug users in Italy. Ann Ist Super Sanita 2010;46(1):59–65.
44. Negro F. Epidemiology of hepatitis C in Europe. Dig Liver Dis 2014;46(Suppl 5): S158–64.
45. Wandeler G, Gsponer T, Bregenzer A, et al. Hepatitis C virus infections in the Swiss HIV Cohort Study: a rapidly evolving epidemic. Clin Infect Dis 2012; 55(10):1408–16.
46. Hurley SF, Jolley DJ, Kaldor JM. Effectiveness of needle-exchange programmes for prevention of HIV infection. Lancet 1997;349(9068):1797–800.
47. Defossez G, Verneau A, Ingrand I, et al. Evaluation of the French national plan to promote screening and early management of viral hepatitis C, between 1997 and 2003: a comparative cross-sectional study in Poitou-Charentes region. Eur J Gastroenterol Hepatol 2008;20(5):367–72.

48. Meffre C, Le Strat Y, Delarocque-Astagneau E, et al. Prevalence of hepatitis B and hepatitis C virus infections in France in 2004: social factors are important predictors after adjusting for known risk factors. J Med Virol 2010;82(4):546–55.
49. Jauffret-Roustide M, Le Strat Y, Couturier E, et al. A national cross-sectional study among drug-users in France: epidemiology of HCV and highlight on practical and statistical aspects of the design. BMC Infect Dis 2009;9:113.
50. Aceijas C, Hickman M, Donoghoe MC, et al. Access and coverage of needle and syringe programmes (NSP) in Central and Eastern Europe and Central Asia. Addiction 2007;102(8):1244–50.
51. European Centre for Disease Prevention and Control. Hepatitis B and C in the EU neighbourhood: prevalence, burden of disease and screening policies. Stockholm (Sweden): ECDC; 2010.
52. Esteban JI, Sauleda S, Quer J. The changing epidemiology of hepatitis C virus infection in Europe. J Hepatol 2008;48(1):148–62.
53. Fattovich G, Stroffolini T, Zagni I, et al. Hepatocellular carcinoma in cirrhosis: incidence and risk factors. Gastroenterology 2004;127(5 Suppl 1):S35–50.
54. Lauer GM, Walker BD. Hepatitis C virus infection. N Engl J Med 2001;345(1):41–52.
55. Mühlberger N, Schwarzer R, Lettmeier B, et al. HCV-related burden of disease in Europe: a systematic assessment of incidence, prevalence, morbidity, and mortality. BMC Public Health 2009;9:34.
56. World Health Organization. WHO Estimates for 2000–2012. Available at: http://www.who.int/healthinfo/global_burden_disease/estimates/en/index1.html. Accessed August 16, 2015.
57. Shepard CW, Finelli L, Alter MJ. Global epidemiology of hepatitis C virus infection. Lancet Infect Dis 2005;5(9):558–67.
58. Adam R, Karam V, Delvart V, et al. Evolution of indications and results of liver transplantation in Europe. A report from the European Liver Transplant Registry (ELTR). J Hepatol 2012;57(3):675–88.
59. Gane EJ, Stedman CA, Hyland RH, et al. Nucleotide polymerase inhibitor sofosbuvir plus ribavirin for hepatitis C. N Engl J Med 2013;368(1):34–44.
60. Osinusi A, Meissner EG, Lee Y, et al. Sofosbuvir and ribavirin for hepatitis C genotype 1 in patients with unfavorable treatment characteristics: a randomized clinical trial. JAMA 2013;310(8):804–11.
61. Ruane PJ, Ain D, Stryker R, et al. Sofosbuvir plus ribavirin for the treatment of chronic genotype 4 hepatitis C virus infection in patients of Egyptian ancestry. J Hepatol 2014;62(5):1040–6.
62. Lawitz E, Sulkowski MS, Ghalib R, et al. Simeprevir plus sofosbuvir, with or without ribavirin, to treat chronic infection with hepatitis C virus genotype 1 in non-responders to pegylated interferon and ribavirin and treatment-naive patients: the COSMOS randomised study. Lancet 2014;384(9956):1756–65.
63. Sulkowski MS, Gardiner DF, Rodriguez-Torres M, et al. Daclatasvir plus sofosbuvir for previously treated or untreated chronic HCV infection. N Engl J Med 2014;370(3):211–21.
64. Zeuzem S, Jacobson IM, Baykal T, et al. Retreatment of HCV with ABT-450/r-ombitasvir and dasabuvir with ribavirin. N Engl J Med 2014;370(17):1604–14.
65. Feld JJ, Kowdley KV, Coakley E, et al. Treatment of HCV with ABT-450/r-ombitasvir and dasabuvir with ribavirin. N Engl J Med 2014;370(17):1594–603.
66. Poordad F, Hezode C, Trinh R, et al. ABT-450/r-ombitasvir and dasabuvir with ribavirin for hepatitis C with cirrhosis. N Engl J Med 2014;370(21):1973–82.
67. Ferenci P, Bernstein D, Lalezari J, et al. ABT-450/r-ombitasvir and dasabuvir with or without ribavirin for HCV. N Engl J Med 2014;370(21):1983–92.

68. Andreone P, Colombo MG, Enejosa JV, et al. ABT-450, ritonavir, ombitasvir, and dasabuvir achieves 97% and 100% sustained virologic response with or without ribavirin in treatment-experienced patients with HCV genotype 1b infection. Gastroenterology 2014;147(2):359–65.e1.
69. Fried MW, Forns X, Reau N, et al. TURQUOISE-II: regimens of ABT-450/r/ombitasvir and dasabuvir with ribavirin achieve high SVR12 rates in HCV genotype 1-infected patients with cirrhosis, regardless of baseline characteristics. Hepatology 2014;60:238A.
70. Pol S, Reddy KR, Baykal T, et al. Interferon-free regimens of ombitasvir and ABT-450/r with or without ribavirin in patients with HCV genotype 4 infection: PEARL-I study results. Hepatology 2014;60:1129A.
71. Afdhal N, Reddy KR, Nelson DR, et al. Ledipasvir and sofosbuvir for previously treated HCV genotype 1 infection. N Engl J Med 2014;370(16):1483–93.
72. Afdhal N, Zeuzem S, Kwo P, et al. Ledipasvir and sofosbuvir for untreated HCV genotype 1 infection. N Engl J Med 2014;370(20):1889–98.
73. Kowdley KV, Gordon SC, Reddy KR, et al. Ledipasvir and sofosbuvir for 8 or 12 weeks for chronic HCV without cirrhosis. N Engl J Med 2014;370(20):1879–88.
74. Reddy KR, Bourlière M, Sulkowski M, et al. Ledipasvir and sofosbuvir in patients with genotype 1 HCV and compensated cirrhosis: an integrated safety and efficacy analysis. Hepatology 2015;62(1):79–86.
75. Kapoor R, Kohli A, Sidharthan S, et al. 240: All oral treatment for genotype 4 chronic hepatitis C infection with sofosbuvir and ledipasvir: interim results from the NIAID SYNERGY trial. Hepatology 2014;60(Suppl 1):91A.
76. Jacobson IM, Gordon SC, Kowdley KV, et al. Sofosbuvir for hepatitis C genotype 2 or 3 in patients without treatment options. N Engl J Med 2013;368(20):1867–77.
77. Lawitz E, Mangia A, Wyles D, et al. Sofosbuvir for previously untreated chronic hepatitis C infection. N Engl J Med 2013;368(20):1878–87.
78. Zeuzem S, Dusheiko GM, Salupere R, et al. Sofosbuvir and ribavirin in HCV genotypes 2 and 3. N Engl J Med 2014;370(21):1993–2001.
79. Sarrazin C, Berg T, Buggisch P, et al. Aktuelle Empfehlung der DGVS und des bng zur Therapie der chronischen Hepatitis C. Z Gastroenterol 2014;52(07):749–56.
80. Nelson DR, Cooper JN, Lalezari JP, et al. All-oral 12-week treatment with daclatasvir plus sofosbuvir in patients with hepatitis C virus genotype 3 infection: ALLY-3 phase III study. Hepatology 2015;61(4):1127–35.
81. Gane EJ, Hyland RH, An D, et al. High efficacy of LDV/SOF regimens for 12 weeks for patients with HCV genotype 3 or 6 infection. Hepatology 2014;60:LB11.
82. Gane EJ, Hyland RH, An D, et al. O6 sofosbuvir/ledipasvir fixed dose combination is safe and effective in difficult-to-treat populations including genotype-3 patients, decompensated genotype-1 patients, and genotype-1 patients with prior sofosbuvir treatment experience. J Hepatol 2014;60(1):S3.

Current and Evolving Treatments of Genotype 1 Hepatitis C Virus

Saleh Alqahtani, MD*, Mark Sulkowski, MD

KEYWORDS

- Hepatitis C • Hepatitis • Sofosbuvir • Simeprevir • Cirrhosis • Ledipasvir antiviral

KEY POINTS

- Direct-acting antivirals (DAAs) have become standard treatment of HCV genotype 1 infection.
- For many treatment regimens, the duration is just 12 weeks.
- Ribavirin may provide additional efficacy for patients with cirrhosis or HCV subtype 1a infection.
- The continued rapid development of DAAs suggests that new regimens will become available for shorter duration of therapy.

INTRODUCTION

There has been a rapid evolution in treatments of hepatitis C virus (HCV) genotype 1 infection. From 1993 until 2011, treatment regimens for HCV included interferon-based therapy. Interferon in combination with ribavirin had not only low success rates but also high discontinuation rates because it was associated with hematologic adverse events (AEs), fatigue, fever, rash, and depression.[1–3]

A better understanding of the life cycle of HCV and of viral protein structure has helped in the design of drugs that act against specific viral targets, in contrast to interferon and ribavirin, which do not specifically target the virus. Drugs that act directly on the HCV are called DAAs. There are 3 major classes of DAAs (**Table 1**): NS3/4A protease inhibitors, NS5B polymerase inhibitors (both nucleoside/nucleotide and nonnucleoside), and NS5A inhibitors.

Potential Conflict of Interest: The authors consults for and received grants from AbbVie, Bristol-Myers Squibb, Gilead, Janssen, and Merck.
Department of Medicine, The Johns Hopkins Hospital, 1830 East Monument Street, Suite 427, Baltimore, MD 21287, USA
* Corresponding author. Department of Medicine, The Johns Hopkins Hospital, 1830 East Monument Street, Suite 427, Baltimore, MD 21287.
E-mail address: salqaht1@jhmi.edu

Gastroenterol Clin N Am 44 (2015) 825–843
http://dx.doi.org/10.1016/j.gtc.2015.06.001
0889-8553/15/$ – see front matter © 2015 Elsevier Inc. All rights reserved.

gastro.theclinics.com

Table 1
The major classes of direct-acting antivirals

NS3/4A Protease Inhibitors	NS5B Polymerase Inhibitors	NS5A Inhibitors
These agents stop HCV replication by inhibiting the HCV NS3/4A serine protease, which is responsible for the cleavage of polyprotein	Two types: nucleoside/ nucleotide analogue inhibitors and nonnucleoside inhibitors. Inhibit the polymerase at a site different from the catalytic site	Thought to inhibit viral replication, assembly, and release, although the exact function of NS5A protein is unknown
Telaprevir Boceprevir Simeprevir Paritaprevir Grazoprevir Asunaprevir	Sofosbuvir (nucleotide) Dasabuvir (nonnucleoside)	Ledipasvir Ombitasvir Daclatasvir Elbasvir

Genotype 1 is the most common HCV genotype in the world and has been difficult to treat with interferon-based regimens. Therefore, treating genotype 1 HCV infection has been a priority for clinical development of DAAs. The recent regulatory approval of interferon-free, HCV treatment regimens including DAAs has increased sustained virologic response (SVR) rates from approximately 40% with interferon-based therapies to more than 90%.[4]

The first-generation DAAs, the NS3/4A protease inhibitors telaprevir and boceprevir, had low genetic barriers to resistance, thrice-daily dosing, and significant adverse effects, including anemia.[5,6] Simeprevir is a next-generation NS3/4A protease inhibitor with greatly improved safety and once-daily dosing.[7] Sofosbuvir became the first nucleotide analogue NS5B polymerase inhibitor to be approved by the US Food and Drug Administration (FDA) and is highly effective in treating all HCV genotypes, including genotype 1.[8–10] In contrast, dasabuvir is a nonnucleoside NS5B inhibitor that is active against genotype 1 and is approved in combination with the protease inhibitor paritaprevir, which is pharmacologically boosted by ritonavir, and the NS5A inhibitor, ombitasvir. Ledipasvir is also an inhibitor of NS5A that is currently approved in combination with sofosbuvir for treating patients with HCV genotype 1 infection. Other NS5A inhibitors, such as daclatasvir, are active against genotype 1 as well as other HCV genotypes, including genotype 3. Daclatasvir has been approved in some regions of the world in combination with sofosbuvir for multiple genotypes, including genotype 3, and in combination with asunaprevir for HCV genotype 1b infection.[11,12] The treatment of HCV/human immunodeficiency virus coinfection, HCV infection post–liver transplant, and HCV-infected patients with renal impairments is not covered in this review.

GOAL OF THERAPY

The aim of treating HCV infection is to cure the chronic viral infection, thereby preventing complications of HCV-related liver disease, including cirrhosis, hepatocellular carcinoma (HCC), and the need for a liver transplant. Cure from HCV infection can be measured by SVR,[13,14] which is defined as the absence of HCV RNA by polymerase chain reaction after cessation of antiviral therapy. Classically, SVR was measured 24 weeks after stopping therapy, but the FDA has accepted the absence of HCV RNA 12 weeks after therapy as the definition of SVR for the approval of HCV treatment regimens.[15]

PATIENT EVALUATION OVERVIEW

Routine laboratory evaluation and assessment of the degree of fibrosis, mostly by noninvasive measures, are extremely important to prioritize patients for treatment and to determine the appropriate treatment regimen and duration. According to the HCV guidance from the American Association for the Study of Liver Diseases (AASLD)/Infectious Diseases Society of America (IDSA), patients with advanced fibrosis, cirrhosis, or with extrahepatic complications of HCV have priority for treatment compared with patients with mild or no liver fibrosis.[16,17] However, treatment is also justified for patients with mild fibrosis and should be prioritized for those at risk of transmitting the infection, regardless of fibrosis stage.[16,17] Treatment is not recommended for patients with limited life expectancy (less than 1 year).[16,17]

The choice of treatment drug and duration of therapy depends largely on 3 factors: the subtype of HCV genotype 1 (a or b) (patients with subtype 1a infection tend to experience treatment failure at higher rates than those with 1b), whether the patient has had previous treatment failure with interferon/ribavirin alone or in combination with a DAA, and whether cirrhosis is present or absent. Guidance for monitoring patients with HCV genotype 1 infection is shown in **Fig. 1**. Before the selection of an HCV treatment regimen, it is also essential that potential drug-drug interactions be evaluated.

TREATMENT OPTIONS

The current HCV treatment guidelines from a joint collaboration of the AASLD, IDSA, and International Antiviral Society USA (IAS-USA)[17] and from the European Association for the Study of the Liver[16] include later-generation DAAs in their recommendations for treatment of genotype 1 infection. Summarized versions of these guidelines can be seen in **Tables 2–4**. Updated and detailed versions of the guidelines should be accessed on their respective Web pages (http://www.HCVguidelines.org) (http://www.easl.eu).[16,17]

These recommendations are based on several clinical trials that have consistently shown strong evidence for the efficacy of DAAs in increasing SVR for patients with HCV genotype 1 infection (**Table 5**).[18–30] The combination of sofosbuvir and ribavirin

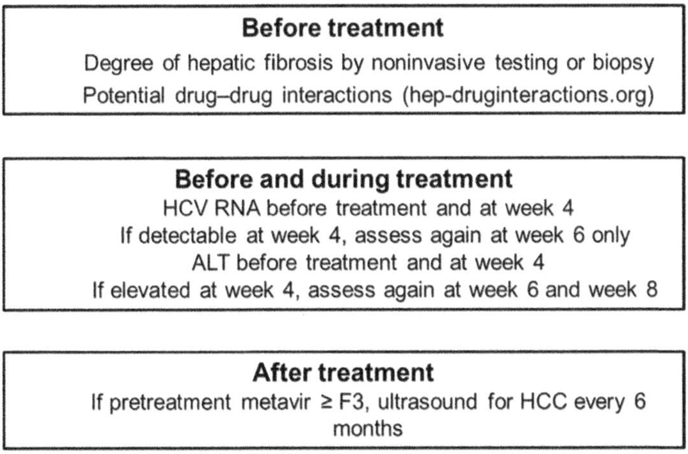

Before treatment
Degree of hepatic fibrosis by noninvasive testing or biopsy
Potential drug–drug interactions (hep-druginteractions.org)

Before and during treatment
HCV RNA before treatment and at week 4
If detectable at week 4, assess again at week 6 only
ALT before treatment and at week 4
If elevated at week 4, assess again at week 6 and week 8

After treatment
If pretreatment metavir ≥ F3, ultrasound for HCC every 6 months

---

Fig. 1. Flow chart of monitoring guidance for treatment of patients with HCV genotype 1 infection. ALT, alanine transaminase.

Table 2
EASL recommendations for treating HCV genotype 1 infection

Regimen	Weeks
Ledipasvir/sofosbuvir	12[a]
OMV/PTV/RTV + DSV ± RBV	12[b]
Simeprevir + sofosbuvir ± RBV	12[c]
Sofosbuvir + daclatasvir	12[c]

Abbreviations: DSV, dasabuvir; EASL, European Association for the Study of the Liver; OMV, ombitasvir; PTV, paritaprevir; RBV, ribavirin; RTV, ritonavir.
   [a] Shorter course can be considered in patients with pretreatment HCV RNA less than 6 million IU/mL. For patients with cirrhosis, RBV should be added or treatment should be extended to 24 wk.
   [b] Subtype 1b with cirrhosis should receive dose plus RBV. Subtype 1a should receive dose plus RBV. Subtype 1a with cirrhosis should receive RBV for 24 wk.
   [c] For patients with cirrhosis, add RBV or extend treatment to 24 wk.
   Data from European Association for the Study of the Liver. EASL recommendations on treatment of hepatitis C 2015. J Hepatol 2015. pii: S0168-8278(15)00208-1. http://dx.doi.org/10.1016/j.jhep.2015.03.025.

is not recommended in patients infected with genotype 1 because of lower efficacy and longer treatment duration.[16,17] In addition, given the substantial toxicity and high discontinuation rates with interferon-containing regimens, they are not recommended for the treatment of HCV genotype 1 and are not discussed in this review.

There are 3 treatment regimens approved by the FDA for treating HCV genotype 1. For the purpose of this review, patients are classified as being treatment naive or treatment experienced, having the absence or presence of cirrhosis, and having failed previous therapy with a DAA.

Treatment-Naive Patients

Ledipasvir plus sofosbuvir
Ledipasvir plus sofosbuvir with and without ribavirin was approved by the FDA for treating HCV genotype 1 infection on October 10, 2014. The approval was based on data from the 2 phase 3 ION trials (ION-1 and ION-3).[22,23] The recommended treatment of treatment-naive patients with HCV genotype 1 infection without cirrhosis is the fixed-dose combination of ledipasvir (NS5A inhibitor) and sofosbuvir (nucleotide

Table 3
AASLD/IDSA/IAS-USA recommendations for treating HCV in treatment-naive patients

	Without Cirrhosis		Compensated Cirrhosis	
Genotype	Regimen	Weeks	Regimen	Weeks
1a or ab	Ledipasvir/sofosbuvir	12[a]	Ledipasvir/sofosbuvir	12
1a	OMV/PTV/RTV + DSV + RBV	12	OMV/PTV/RTV + DSV + RBV	24
1b	OMV/PTV/RTV + DSV	12	OMV/PTV/RTV + DSV + RBV	12
1a	Simeprevir + sofosbuvir ± RBV	12	Simeprevir + sofosbuvir ± RBV	24
1b	Simeprevir + sofosbuvir	12	Simeprevir + sofosbuvir	24

Abbreviations: DSV, dasabuvir; OMV, ombitasvir; PTV, paritaprevir; RBV, ribavirin; RTV, ritonavir.
   [a] An 8-wk course can be considered in patients with pretreatment HCV RNA less than 6 million IU/mL.
   Data from AASLD/IDSA/IAS–USA. Recommendations for testing, managing, and treating hepatitis C. Available at: http://hcvguidelines.org. Accessed May 9, 2015.

Table 4
AASLD/IDSA/IAS-USA recommendations for treating HCV in treatment-experienced patients

| Population | Without Cirrhosis | | Compensated Cirrhosis | |
	Regimen	Weeks	Regimen	Weeks
Prior PEG-IFN/RBV				
GT 1a or b	Ledipasvir/sofosbuvir	12	Ledipasvir/sofosbuvir	24
GT 1a or b	—	—	Ledipasvir/sofosbuvir + RBV	12
GT 1a	OMV/PTV/RTV + DSV + RBV	12	OMV/PTV/RTV + DSV + RBV	24
GT 1b	OMV/PTV/RTV + DSV	12	OMV/PTV/RTV + DSV + RBV	12
GT 1a or b	Simeprevir + sofosbuvir ± RBV	12	Simeprevir + sofosbuvir ± RBV	24
Prior SOF				
GT 1a or b	Defer therapy	—	Ledipasvir/sofosbuvir ± RBV	24
Prior PI				
GT 1a or b	Ledipasvir/sofosbuvir	12	Ledipasvir/sofosbuvir	24
			Ledipasvir/sofosbuvir + RBV	12

Abbreviations: DSV, dasabuvir; GT, genotype; OMV, ombitasvir; PEG-IFN, peginterferon-alfa; PI, protease inhibitor; PTV, paritaprevir; RBV, ribavirin; RTV, ritonavir.
Data from AASLD/IDSA/IAS–USA. Recommendations for testing, managing, and treating hepatitis C. Available at: http://hcvguidelines.org. Accessed May 9, 2015.

analogue NS5B inhibitor) for 12 weeks without ribavirin. According to the US prescribing information, patients with viral load less than 6 million IU/mL can be considered for 8 weeks' therapy. However, the HCV guidance panel favored 12 weeks of therapy as the standard approach for this patient population.

The ION-1 investigators enrolled 865 treatment-naive patients with HCV genotype 1 infection, including 20% who had cirrhosis. Among 4 treatment cohorts, they compared 12 and 24 weeks of therapy with ledipasvir/sofosbuvir with and without ribavirin. SVR12 rates were extremely high: 97% to 99% across all arms. The conclusion from ION 1 was that 12 weeks of therapy was as effective as 24 weeks and that adding ribavirin to ledipasvir/sofosbuvir therapy was not necessary, even for patients with cirrhosis.[22]

In ION-3, investigators enrolled 647 treatment-naive, HCV genotype 1–infected patients without cirrhosis and examined the effect of shortening ledipasvir/sofosbuvir with or without ribavirin therapy to 8 weeks. This was a noninferiority study that showed similar SVR rates between the regimens, with an SVR12 of 94% with 8 weeks of ledipasvir/sofosbuvir, 93% with 8 weeks of ledipasvir/sofosbuvir with ribavirin, and 95% with 12 weeks of ledipasvir/sofosbuvir. However, more patients treated for 8 weeks experienced virologic relapse after stopping therapy (4.6%) compared with those treated for 12 weeks (2%). Post hoc analyses suggested that patients with baseline HCV RNA level less than 6 million IU/mL who received 8 weeks of therapy had a similar relapse rate, 2%, as those who received 12 weeks of therapy. Once again, ribavirin provided no benefit with respect to increasing the SVR rate or decreasing the relapse rate. No sofosbuvir resistance was observed. Most patients (15 of 23 tested) who did not reach SVR because of relapse posttreatment had NS5A resistance-associated variants at the time of relapse.[23]

The results from the ION trials confirmed the safety and tolerability of the ledipasvir/sofosbuvir regimen with and without ribavirin. Fewer than 1% of patients either receiving ribavirin or not discontinued treatment because of an AE. Treatment-related AEs were much less common in the arms without versus with ribavirin (45% vs 71%).[31] Without ribavirin, headache and fatigue were the most common adverse effects.[31]

Table 5
Major clinical trials and studies on which current treatment guidelines are based

Treatment Regimen	Clinical Evidence			
Sofosbuvir plus simeprevir with or without RBV for 12 wk	Phase 2 COSMOS trial.[19] In both treatment-naive and treatment-experienced patients. In the prior null responder group, SVR12 was 96% with RBV and 93% without RBV	Phase 2 COSMOS trial.[20] Included patients with different grades of fibrosis. The SVR12 rate ranged from 79% to 100%	—	—
Ledipasvir/sofosbuvir in combination (FDA approved October 2014)	ELECTRON study in treatment-naive patients with SVR12 rates were 100% for 12 wk, 100% for 8 wk, and 68% for 6 wk[21]	Phase 3 ION-1 trial.[22] SVR12 was 98% with ribavirin and 97% without ribavirin	Phase 3 ION-3 trial.[23] Excluded patients with cirrhosis and investigated shortening therapy from 12 wk to 8 wk. SVR12 was 93%–95%	Phase 2 SIRIUS study.[24] Patients with compensated cirrhosis who failed to achieve an SVR after PEG-IFN, RBV, and either telaprevir or boceprevir. SVR12 rates of 96% and 97%
Paritaprevir/ritonavir/ombitasvir plus dasabuvir with RBV (FDA approved for treating HCV genotype 1a infection in treatment-naive patients)	Phase 3 SAPPHIRE-I trial.[25] SVR12 rate 95%. Higher overall virologic failure for genotype 1a than genotype 1b	Phase 3 PEARL-IV trial.[26] SVR12 was 90% in the RBV-free arm vs 97% in the RBV-containing arm. Confirmed the need for RBV for patients with HCV genotype 1a	Phase 3 TURQUOISE-II trial.[27] Overall, SVR12 rates were 89% in the 12-wk arm and 95% in the 24-wk arm	—
Daclatasvir and sofosbuvir	Phase 2b trial.[28] With 24 wk of therapy, the SVR rates were 100% in treatment-naive patients and 100% and 95% without and with ribavirin, respectively, in patients who did not respond to PEG-IFN, ribavirin, and either telaprevir or boceprevir	—	—	—

Abbreviations: PEG-IFN, peginterferon-alfa; RBV, ribavirin.

Paritaprevir/ritonavir/ombitasvir and dasabuvir

Paritaprevir/ritonavir/ombitasvir and dasabuvir, with or without ribavirin, were approved by the FDA for the treatment of HCV genotype 1 infection on December 19, 2014. The approval was based on data from several phase 3 clinical trials. Paritaprevir is an NS3/4A serine protease inhibitor that is coformulated with ritonavir, an antiretroviral drug that is also a potent inhibitor of CYP3A/4. The addition of low-dose ritonavir allows for high intracellular concentrations of paritaprevir and facilitates once-daily dosing. Paritaprevir/ritonavir is further coformulated with ombitasvir, a NS5A inhibitor. These drugs are also combined with dasabuvir, a nonnucleoside NS5B polymerase inhibitor.

SAPPHIRE-I investigators compared 12 weeks of the paritaprevir/ritonavir/ombitasvir and dasabuvir combination plus ribavirin to matching placebo in 631 treatment-naive patients without cirrhosis.[25] The SVR rates were 95% in patients with HCV genotype 1a infection and 98% in patients with HCV 1b infection. Virologic failure was rare, with only 1 individual experiencing virologic breakthrough during therapy, and 7 patients (<2%) had virologic relapse after the 12-week treatment was discontinued. In the single patient who had breakthrough, resistance-associated variants were observed in the NS3, NS5A, and NS5B domains. In the patients with relapse, all but 1 patient had HCV genotype 1a infection with the presence of NS3 or NS5A resistance-associated variants. The single patient with HCV genotype 1b infection who experienced relapse had resistance-associated variants against the NS3, NS5A, and NS5B domains.[25]

Because this trial was placebo controlled, the combination of DAAs with or without ribavirin could be compared with a no-treatment group. In the active treatment groups, fatigue and headache were the most common AEs; however, their incidence was not different compared with the placebo groups. Other common AEs included pruritus, asthenia, nausea, and insomnia, and these were more commonly observed in the treatment arms. Anemia occurred exclusively in patients taking the active drug regimen and was attributable to ribavirin-induced hemolytic anemia. No patients discontinued treatment because of anemia, which was managed with dose reduction of ribavirin.

The PEARL III and IV studies examined the paritaprevir/ritonavir/ombitasvir and dasabuvir combination with and without ribavirin in treatment-naive patients with HCV genotype 1b (n = 419) (PEARL III) or 1a (n = 305) (PEARL-IV) infection. Patients with cirrhosis were excluded from both studies. The SVR12 rates in HCV genotype 1b participants did not differ between the cohorts, with 99.5% and 99% achieving SVR12 with and without ribavirin, respectively. However, with HCV genotype 1a, the SVR12 rate was 97% with ribavirin and 90% without ribavirin. In the HCV genotype 1a cohort, the rate of virologic failure was higher in the ribavirin-free arm (8% vs 2%). The conclusion from the trial is that ribavirin added benefit for patients infected with HCV genotype 1a but not for those with genotype 1b.[26]

Sofosbuvir plus simeprevir

Simeprevir, an NS3/4A protease inhibitor, was approved by the FDA on November 22, 2013, for the treatment of HCV genotype 1 in combination with peginterferon-alfa and ribavirin. On November 5, 2014, the FDA approved the combination of sofosbuvir/simeprevir as all-oral therapy for HCV genotype 1 infection based on data from the COSMOS trial. COSMOS was a phase 2, open-label trial, in which 167 patients with chronic HCV genotype 1 infection received sofosbuvir plus simeprevir, with or without ribavirin, for either 12 or 24 weeks.[20] Patients were randomly assigned in a 2:1:2:1 ratio to receive simeprevir and sofosbuvir daily for 24 weeks with or without ribavirin or for 12 weeks with or without ribavirin, in 2 cohorts: previous nonresponders with metavir scores F0-F2 (cohort 1) and previous nonresponders and treatment-naive patients with metavir scores F3-F4 (cohort 2). SVR12 was achieved in 92% (154 of 167) of all patients in the study and in 90% (72 of 80) of patients in cohort 1 and 94% (82 of 87) of patients in cohort 2. The most common AEs were fatigue (31%), headache (20%), and nausea (16%). Extending therapy to 24 weeks did not seem to improve SVR rates, except in patients with prior relapse and advanced fibrosis.[20] However, compared with 12 weeks, this longer duration of therapy was associated with lower rates of virologic relapse among patients with cirrhosis who completed therapy, leading to the recommendation that patients with cirrhosis receive 24 weeks of therapy with this combination.

The OPTIMIST-1 study evaluated the efficacy, safety, and quality-of-life outcomes for 8 or 12 weeks of simeprevir plus sofosbuvir without ribavirin in treatment-naive and treatment-experienced patients without cirrhosis. The SVR12 rate was 97% in the 12-week group compared with 83% in the 6-week treatment group. The presence of the NS3/4A protease Q80K mutation, which is a simeprevir resistance-associated variant, did not seem to affect treatment efficacy in these noncirrhotic patients who received 12 weeks of treatment. The 8-week arm resulted in high SVR12 rates only in select patient subgroups: those with genotype 1b (92%), with lower baseline HCV RNA (96%), and with *IL28B* CC genotype (93%).[32]

When simeprevir is combined with peginterferon-alfa and ribavirin, patients with HCV genotype 1a infection and the NS3/4A protease Q80K polymorphism at baseline have higher virologic failure rates than patients with genotype 1b infection or genotype 1a infection without this baseline mutation. Therefore, it was recommended that testing for baseline Q80K be done for all HCV genotype 1a–infected patients before the use of simeprevir with peginterferon-alfa and ribavirin. In contrast, the presence of the Q80K polymorphism does not preclude treatment with simeprevir and sofosbuvir, because of previously mentioned data from the OPTIMIST-1 study and analyses from the COSMOS study, in which the SVR rate was high (88%; 51 of 58) among HCV genotype 1a–infected patients with the NS3/4A Q80K polymorphism.[33] Overall, based on the OPTIMIST-1 study, noncirrhotic, HCV genotype 1–infected patients with or without the Q80K polymorphism should receive 12 weeks of treatment with simeprevir plus sofosbuvir.

Treatment-Experienced Patients

Ledipasvir plus sofosbuvir

In the ION-2 trial, 440 treatment-experienced, HCV genotype 1–infected patients who had failed peginterferon/ribavirin with or without telaprevir or boceprevir were randomized to receive 12 or 24 weeks of treatment with ledipasvir/sofosbuvir with or without ribavirin.[34] The SVR12 rates for 12 weeks of ledipasvir/sofosbuvir were 94% without ribavirin and 96% with ribavirin; for 24 weeks of ledipasvir/sofosbuvir, the SVR12 rates were 99% both with and without ribavirin. Approximately 20% of patients in this trial had cirrhosis (data reviewed in the cirrhosis section).[34] Overall, the recommendation was that noncirrhotic patients who had failed prior treatment (including those nonresponsive to telaprevir or boceprevir) should be treated with ledipasvir/sofosbuvir for 12 weeks without ribavirin.

Paritaprevir/ritonavir/ombitasvir and dasabuvir

The PEARL II study evaluated paritaprevir/ritonavir/ombitasvir and dasabuvir with or without ribavirin for 12 weeks in 179 peginterferon/ribavirin treatment-experienced HCV genotype 1b–infected patients without cirrhosis. Patients who had failed to respond to telaprevir or boceprevir were excluded because cross-resistance with the protease inhibitor, paritaprevir, was anticipated. The SVR rates were 97% with ribavirin and 100% without ribavirin. As expected, reductions in hemoglobin level were more frequently observed in the arms containing ribavirin. This study confirmed that for the combination of paritaprevir/ritonavir/ombitasvir and dasabuvir, ribavirin does not seem to affect clinical efficacy in HCV genotype 1b–infected patients without cirrhosis.[35]

SAPPHIRE-II, a phase 3 randomized controlled trial, examined the efficacy and safety of paritaprevir/ritonavir/ombitasvir and dasabuvir with ribavirin for 12 weeks in 394 HCV genotype 1–infected patients without cirrhosis who had previously failed treatment with peginterferon/ribavirin. Among all patients, 96% achieved SVR12, with similar results observed for HCV genotype 1a (96%) and 1b (97%). The SVR12 rates were similar regardless of prior treatment: 95% for prior relapse, 100% for partial response, and 95% for null response.[36] Thus, among noncirrhotic patients, the type of prior response to peginterferon/ribavirin did not affect the likelihood of SVR with this treatment regimen.

Sofosbuvir plus simeprevir
Data from the COSMOS and OPTIMIST-1 trials indicate the sofosbuvir/simeprevir combination is effective in patients who previously failed peginterferon/ribavirin therapy.[19,32] Patients who failed to respond to telaprevir or boceprevir have been excluded from studies of this regimen because of the likelihood for cross-resistance between these first-generation protease inhibitors and simeprevir. Of the 80 patients in COSMOS with a null response to peginterferon-alfa and ribavirin treatment who had fibrosis (Metavir stage $\leq$F2), 79% to 96% achieved SVR in the ribavirin-containing arms and 93% achieved SVR in both ribavirin-free arms.[19] In OPTIMIST-1 study, which enrolled noncirrhotic patients, rates of SVR12 for treatment-experienced patients were 95% for 12 weeks of therapy and 77% for 8 weeks of therapy. The data suggest that for patients who failed previous therapy, sofosbuvir/simeprevir is effective but only for a period of 12 weeks.[32]

Patients with Established Cirrhosis

Curing HCV infection in patients with cirrhosis has been shown to confer considerable clinical benefit, including stopping the progression of liver disease, reducing the risk of dying, reducing the risk of HCC, decreasing the need for liver transplant, and improving patient-reported quality of life.[37,38]

TURQUOISE-II is phase 3, multicenter, open-label, randomized controlled trial that enrolled treatment-naive and treatment-experienced patients with chronic HCV genotype 1 infection and Child-Turcotte-Pugh class A cirrhosis (n = 380).[27] The investigators evaluated the efficacy of ombitasvir-paritaprevir-ritonavir and dasabuvir plus ribavirin for 12 weeks or 24 weeks. SVR12 rates were 92% for 12 weeks' treatment and 96% for 24 weeks' treatment. For patients with HCV genotype 1a infection, SVR12 rates were 89% for 12 weeks' treatment and 94% for 24 weeks' treatment. For patients with HCV genotype 1b infection, SVR12 rates were 99% for 12 weeks' treatment and 100% for 24 weeks' treatment. Subgroup analysis suggested treatment-experienced patients with HCV genotype 1a infection benefit from extending the treatment duration to 24 weeks. On further post hoc analysis, the observation was made that all HCV genotype 1–infected patients with posttreatment virologic relapse were in the 12-week treatment groups, leading to the recommendation that treatment-naive and treatment-experienced patients with cirrhosis and genotype 1a infection receive 24 weeks of the regimen plus ribavirin. In contrast, 12 weeks of treatment in patients with genotype 1b infection and cirrhosis is sufficient. Because all patients in TURQUOISE-II received ribavirin, the role of ribavirin in these patients with genotype 1b infection is being investigated in a randomized controlled trial. At this time, the recommendation is that ribavirin be included for the treatment of all cirrhotic patients when using this regimen.

In pooled analysis of 513 patients with compensated cirrhosis from phase 2 and 3 clinical trials, in which 70% were treatment experienced, treatment with ledipasvir/ sofosbuvir resulted in an SVR12 rate of 96%.[39] The lowest rate of SVR12 occurred in treatment-experienced patients who received 12 weeks of therapy without ribavirin; further analysis of the data suggested that adding ribavirin and extending the treatment duration from 12 weeks to 24 weeks improved likelihood of reaching SVR. The presence of portal hypertension and severity of liver disease were important predictors for reduced SVR. Based on this analysis, HCV guidance recommended that treatment-naive patients with cirrhosis be treated with 12 weeks of ledipasvir/sofosbuvir alone and that treatment-experienced patients with cirrhosis be treated with 24 weeks of ledipasvir/sofosbuvir alone or with 12 weeks of ledipasvir/sofosbuvir plus ribavirin.

In the SOLAR-1 trial, investigators examined the efficacy and safety of ledipasvir/ sofosbuvir with ribavirin for 12 or 24 weeks in 108 patients with decompensated cirrhosis.[40] Most patients had a baseline model for end-stage liver disease (MELD) score between 10 and 20. SVR12 rates were 87% for 12 weeks of treatment and 89% for 24 weeks of treatment. There were no differences in SVR rates between patients with Child-Turcotte-Pugh B or C cirrhosis. Antiviral therapy was associated with improved MELD scores in most patients (60%–79%). Tolerance was good, and only 3 patients discontinued therapy as a result of AEs.

The SIRUS trail is a phase 2, double-blind trial that compared the efficacy of a 12-week course of ledipasvir-sofosbuvir plus ribavirin versus a 24-week course of ledipasvir-sofosbuvir in treatment-experienced patients with HCV genotype 1 infection and compensated cirrhosis who failed prior treatment with an NS3/4A protease inhibitor.[41] This study suggests that in genotype 1 treatment-experienced patients with cirrhosis, a 12-week course of ledipasvir-sofosbuvir plus ribavirin provides SVR12 rates similar to those of a 24-week course of ledipasvir-sofosbuvir. The 12-week regimen has the advantage of being more cost-effective.

Data from the ALLY-1 phase 3 study suggest that in HCV genotype 1–infected patients with cirrhosis, 12 weeks of sofosbuvir/daclatasvir plus ribavirin has a good safety profile and results in an SVR12 rate of 83%.[42] In the study, the likelihood of SVR12 diminished as severity of cirrhosis increased: more than 90% of patients with Child-Turcotte-Pugh class A and B cirrhosis reached SVR12, whereas only 56% of patients with Child-Turcotte-Pugh class C cirrhosis did. Daclatasvir is currently available in Europe, parts of Asia and Latin America and was recently approved in the US by FDA in July 24, 2015.

The OPTIMIST-2 investigators studied the safety and efficacy of sofosbuvir/sime-previr for 12 weeks in treatment-naive or treatment-experienced patients with chronic HCV genotype 1 infection and cirrhosis.[43] The SVR12 rate was 88%. Further analysis indicated that SVR12 rates were higher in patients who were treatment naive, had genotype 1b infection, or had a higher baseline platelet count. In contrast to the OPTIMIST-1 study, which evaluated this regimen in noncirrhotic patients, patients with genotype 1a infection who had the Q80K polymorphism were less likely to achieve SVR (74%) compared with those with genotype 1b infection (84%) or genotype 1a infection/no Q80K polymorphism (92%). Based on this finding, cirrhotic patients with HCV genotype 1a infection with the Q80K polymorphism should not be treated with simeprevir plus sofosbuvir because other available regimens are expected to yield higher rates of SVR.

Real-life data from the TARGET registry in the United States suggest that sofosbuvir/simeprevir is well tolerated in patients with cirrhosis but that SVR rates are lower in patients with decompensated cirrhosis (83%) than in patients with compensated cirrhosis (93%).[44] In a multivariate analysis, thrombocytopenia, hypoalbuminemia, prior hepatic decompensation, and treatment failure following telaprevir or boceprevir therapy were independent predictors of lower likelihood of SVR.

Although there is firm consensus on the benefit of treatment of patients with compensated cirrhosis (Child-Turcotte-Pugh A) with low MELD score, the risk and benefit of antiviral treatment in patients with more advanced cirrhosis (Child-Turcotte-Pugh B and C) is less clear. Further, many of these patients with advanced disease are on liver transplant waiting lists. In the context of liver transplant, achieving SVR with advanced clinical disease may be disadvantageous if clinical improvements are not enough to avoid liver transplant. The concern is that if a patient has modest improvement in MELD score with SVR, it might delay organ allocation for transplant because the current system is based on MELD score rather than on clinical signs and symptoms, such as ascites and encephalopathy. Further research is needed to define the role of antiviral therapy in patients with Child-Turcotte-Pugh B and C disease before transplant. Nonetheless, there is consensus around one patient population that is expected to benefit greatly from treatment before liver transplant, patients with HCC, because these patients are often well compensated and DAAs can result in a high cure rate. Because of the diagnosis of HCC, these patients can receive a transplant in many regions regardless of their native MELD score. However, in all patient groups, including those with HCC, viral cure before liver transplant may limit the available pool of organs because patients with HCV cure should not receive livers from an anti-HCV-positive donor. In regions with a high prevalence of anti-HCV-positive donors, this may lead to prolonged wait time. Thus, although DAA therapy is safe and highly effective, it is transformative in the context of advanced liver disease, and more studies are needed to determine the best approach for using DAAs for HCV before liver transplant.

In summary, available data suggest that the likelihood of reaching SVR with DAA therapy is lower for patients with decompensated cirrhosis than for those with compensated cirrhosis, and this is particularly true for treatment-experienced patients. Approaches to improving SVR rates in patients with decompensated cirrhosis include extending the duration of therapy, adding ribavirin, and possibly adding another DAA. Based on several studies, the presence of severe thrombocytopenia and hypoalbuminemia may be important predictors of patients for whom the benefits of HCV cure may be limited.

Patients Who Failed Previous Therapy Including a Direct-Acting Antiviral

Sofosbuvir and daclatasvir in combination for 24 weeks has been investigated in 41 HCV genotype 1–infected treatment-naive patients who were nonresponsive to prior treatment, including the first-generation protease inhibitors telaprevir or boceprevir.[28] Among these patients, 98% had an SVR12. Patients who failed telaprevir and boceprevir were also included in the ION-2 and SIRIUS studies of ledipasvir/sofosbuvir with or without ribavirin. Unexpectedly, prior protease inhibitor failure did not adversely affect the likelihood of HCV cure with retreatment with sofosbuvir plus ledipasvir, an inhibitor of NS5A.

Similarly, an open-label trial studied the efficacy and safety of ledipasvir and sofosbuvir plus ribavirin for 12 weeks in 51 patients with HCV genotype 1 infection who failed previous sofosbuvir-based regimens.[45] Of the 51 patients enrolled, 25 had previously received sofosbuvir plus peginterferon-alfa and ribavirin, 20 had received sofosbuvir and ribavirin, 5 had received sofosbuvir placebo plus peginterferon-alfa and ribavirin, and 1 (2%) had received monotherapy with GS-0938, an NS5B polymerase inhibitor. SVR12 was achieved by 50 of the 51 patients (98%) treated.[45] This study established the proof of principle that sofosbuvir can be used to re-treat patients who failed a prior sofosbuvir-based regimen; this is likely due to this agent's high barrier to the emergence of HCV variants with resistance during and after treatment. In vitro, sofosbuvir-resistant HCV variants that harbor the S282T mutation in the NS5B region are markedly less fit than wild-type variants, which may explain the successful reuse of this drug.

In contrast, patients who fail to respond to regimens that include NS5A inhibitors, including ledipasvir/sofosbuvir and paritaprevir/ritonavir/ombitasvir + dasabuvir, are likely to have HCV variants that are resistant to NS5A inhibitors that are selected during treatment and can persist for years. In one study, of 41 HCV genotype 1–infected patients who previously failed ledipasvir/sofosbuvir therapy, 71% achieved SVR12 after retreatment with ledipasvir and sofosbuvir for 24 weeks.[46] SVR12 rates were lower in patients with versus without baseline NS5A resistance-associated variants. Four patients with NS5A resistance-associated variants developed evidence of sofosbuvir resistance, suggesting that they had been re-treated with functional sofosbuvir monotherapy. This result suggests that, unlike sofosbuvir, NS5A inhibitors should not be reused in patients who harbor a resistant variant after prior treatment with these agents.

The question of whether any HCV protease inhibitor–based therapy is effective in persons who failed prior treatment with drugs in the same class was investigated in the C-SALVAGE study, which evaluated combination therapy with the NS3/4A protease inhibitor grazoprevir, the NS5A inhibitor elbasvir, and ribavirin in 79 patients with genotype 1 HCV infection and previous failure with boceprevir, simeprevir, or telaprevir plus peginterferon-alfa and ribavirin therapy.[47] The SVR12 rate was 96%, with similar efficacy regardless of previous virologic failure or presence of baseline resistance-associated variants to boceprevir, simeprevir, or telaprevir. Of the 3 patients who did not reach SVR12, all experienced relapse posttreatment and had resistance-associated variants to NS3 or NS5A or both at baseline. Grazoprevir and elbasvir are being investigated in phase 3 clinical trials and are not yet approved for market.

DRUG INTERACTIONS

A summary of drug interactions from the AASLD/IDSA/IAS-USA guidelines[17] is presented in **Table 6**.

Sofosbuvir

Inducers of intestinal P-glycoprotein (P-gp), such as rifampin and St. John's wort, may significantly lower sofosbuvir levels. In addition, there is a potential for cardiovascular toxicity in patients receiving amiodarone and sofosbuvir.

Additional drug-drug interactions are described in the sofosbuvir (Sovaldi) full prescribing information (http://www.gilead.com/~/media/Files/pdfs/medicines/liver-disease/sovaldi/sovaldi_pi.pdf).

Ledipasvir/Sofosbuvir

The combination of ledipasvir and sofosbuvir has significant drug-drug interactions with P-gp inducers (eg, St. John's wort and rifampin). Because acid-reducing agents can reduce the absorption of ledipasvir, these should be avoided. Additional drug-drug interactions are described in the ledipasvir-sofosbuvir (Harvoni) full prescribing information (http://www.gilead.com/~/media/Files/pdfs/medicines/liver-disease/harvoni/harvoni_pi.pdf).

Table 6
Potential drug-drug interactions with direct-acting antivirals

Concomitant Medications	Ledipasvir	Paritaprevir/ Ritonavir/ Ombitasvir + Dasabuvir	Simeprevir	Sofosbuvir
Acid-reducing agents[a]	X	X	—	—
Alfuzosin/tamsulosin	—	X	—	—
Amiodarone	X[b]	—	—	X
Anticonvulsants	X	X	X	X
Antiretrovirals[a]	Not available	Not available	Not available	Tipranavir/ ritonavir only
Azole antifungals[a]	—	X	X	—
Buprenorphine/naloxone	—	X	—	—
Calcineurin inhibitors[a]	—	X	X	—
Calcium channel blockers[a]	—	X	X	
Cisapride	—	X	X	—
Digoxin	X	—	X	—
Ergot derivatives	—	X	—	—
Ethinyl estradiol– containing products	—	X	—	—
Furosemide	—	X	—	—
Gemfibrozil	—	X	—	—
Glucocorticoids	—	X (inhaled, intranasal)	X	—
Herbals				
St. John's wort	—	X	X	X
Milk thistle	—	—	X	—
Macrolide antimicrobials[a]	—	—	X	—
Other antiarrhythmics[a]	—	X	X	—
Phosphodiesterase type 5 inhibitors[a]	—	X	X	—
Pimozide	—	X	—	—
Rifamycin antimicrobials[a]	X	X	X	X
Salmeterol	—	X	—	—
Sedatives[a]	—	X	X	—
Simeprevir	X	—	—	—
Statins[a]	X	X	X	—

[a] Some drug interactions are not class specific; see product prescribing information for specific drugs within a class.
[b] As coformulated with sofosbuvir.
Adapted from AASLD/IDSA/IAS–USA. Recommendations for testing, managing, and treating hepatitis C. Available at: http://hcvguidelines.org. Accessed May 9, 2015; with permission.

Simeprevir

Simeprevir is primarily metabolized via cytochrome P450 3A (CYP3A) enzymes. Therefore, administering simeprevir with medications that induce CYP3A may significantly reduce levels of simeprevir (eg, rifampin, St. John's wort, and most anticonvulsants).

See the simeprevir (Olysio) full prescribing information for a detailed description of drug interactions (https://www.olysio.com/shared/product/olysio/prescribing-information.pdf).

Ombitasvir/Paritaprevir/Ritonavir plus Dasabuvir

The combination of ombitasvir/paritaprevir/ritonavir plus dasabuvir can potentially cause significant drug-drug interactions, primarily because ritonavir is a potent inhibitor of CYP3A4 enzyme. Detailed drug-drug interactions are described in Viekira Pak prescribing information (http://www.rxabbvie.com/pdf/viekirapak_pi.pdf).

MONITORING DURING THERAPY

Response guided therapy, which was standard of care for interferon-based regimens, is not applicable with all-oral treatment regimens for HCV genotype 1 infection. All-oral treatments of HCV genotype 1 infection are highly effective; data from clinical trials indicate that in 95% to 100% of patients with HCV genotype 1 infection, HCV RNA becomes undetectable during treatment. Virologic failure because of drug resistance is extremely rare. Patients who do not achieve SVR usually experience relapse after treatment, and HCV RNA monitoring during treatment has not been found to be predictive of relapse. Even though evaluating HCV RNA during treatment is no longer needed for response-guided therapy, it can be helpful to monitor patient compliance. For some patients, seeing viral load drop during therapy is a motivating factor for continuing treatment; HCV viral load is usually tested at week 4 of therapy and at the end of the treatment (see **Fig. 1**).

Monitoring safety of treatment through blood tests during treatment is important, especially in ribavirin-containing regimens.

SAFETY OF DIRECT-ACTING ANTIVIRALS

As interferon-based regimens become less common, the complications due to treatment have decreased, and tolerance of current all-oral regimens is excellent.[48] However, ribavirin is associated with adverse hematologic events, fatigue, rash, sinusitis, and gout.[49] Ribavirin is also contraindicated for patients with a history of significant cardiac disease and in women who are pregnant because of significant teratogenic and embryocidal effects.[50] That said, even with ribavirin included, all-oral, DAA-based regimens result in few adverse effects, and the effects that do occur, such as fatigue, headache, nausea, insomnia, indigestion, irritability, skin rash, cough, and pruritus, are generally considered mild or moderate.

FUTURE THERAPY

Several novel DAAs for HCV are in clinical development, making it likely that treatment outcomes for patients with genotype 1 HCV infection will continue to improve.

In the C-WORTHY phase 2 study, HCV genotype 1–infected treatment-naive patients with cirrhosis (cohort 1) and treatment-experienced patients without cirrhosis (cohort 2) received 12 or 18 weeks of grazoprevir (NS3/4A protease inhibitor) and elbasvir (an NS5A inhibitor) with or without ribavirin. SVR12 rates ranged from 90% (28 of 31; 95% confidence interval [CI], 74–98) among treatment-naive patients with cirrhosis receiving 12 weeks of therapy with ribavirin to 100% (33 of 33, 95% CI, 89–100) among treatment-experienced patients without cirrhosis receiving 18 weeks of therapy with ribavirin.[51] Among patients treated for 12 weeks with grazoprevir plus elbasvir without ribavirin, 97% (28 of 29, 95% CI, 82–100) of patients in cohort 1 and 91% (30 of 33, 95% CI, 76–98) of patients in cohort 2 achieved SVR12.

The efficacy of a fixed-dose combination of grazoprevir and elbasvir for 12 weeks was evaluated in 421 treatment-naive patients with HCV genotype 1, 4, or 6 infection.[52] In the study population, 22% of patients had cirrhosis. Patients were stratified by genotype and fibrosis level in a 3:1 ratio to receive immediate or delayed treatment with grazoprevir/elbasvir once daily for 12 weeks. The delayed treatment group received placebo for 12 weeks and at study week 16 received the open-label, active drug. Among patients receiving immediate treatment, SVR12 rates were 95% overall, 92% for HCV genotype 1a–infected patients, 99% for HCV genotype 1b–infected patients, 97% for patients with cirrhosis, and 94% for patients without cirrhosis.[52]

The UNITY-1 study is an open-label study in which 415 patients with HCV genotype 1 infection without cirrhosis received 12 weeks of the 3-drug combination of daclatasvir (NS5A inhibitor), asunaprevir (an NS3 protease inhibitor), and beclabuvir (a nonnucleoside NS5B inhibitor). SVR12 rates were 91% overall, 92% for treatment-naive patients, and 89% for treatment-experienced patients.[53] In UNITY-2, the same 3-drug regimen was administered for 12 weeks to 202 patients with compensated cirrhosis. In treatment-naive patients, the SVR12 rate was 93% without ribavirin and 98% with ribavirin; in treatment-experienced patients, SVR12 was 87% without ribavirin and 93% with ribavirin.[54]

Whether the duration of ledipasvir/sofosbuvir-based therapy can be shortened was examined by Kohli and colleagues[55] in an open-label phase 2A trial, in which 60 treatment-naive patients with HCV genotype 1 infection received the following regimens: 12 weeks of ledipasvir/sofosbuvir, 6 weeks of ledipasvir/sofosbuvir plus GS-9669 (a nonnucleoside NS5B thumb site 3 inhibitor of HCV polymerase), or 6 weeks of ledipasvir/sofosbuvir plus GS-9451 (HCV NS3/4A protease inhibitor). In the 12-week ledipasvir/sofosbuvir group, the SVR12 rate was 100%, and in the two 6-week groups SVR12 was 95%. This proof-of-concept study suggests that adding a third DAA to ledipasvir/sofosbuvir could lead to excellent cure rates with only 6 weeks of therapy.[55]

In a recent phase 2 study, the investigational fixed-dose coformulation of sofosbuvir and GS-5816 (NS5A inhibitor) was administered with GS-9857 (NS3/4A protease inhibitor) for 4 or 6 weeks in patients with HCV genotype 1 infection.[56] The study population included treatment-naive patients with and without cirrhosis, as well as DAA-experienced patients. For 6 weeks of treatment, the SVR12 rate was 93% in patients without cirrhosis and 87% in patients with cirrhosis. The SVR12 rate was lower in DAA-experienced patients receiving the 6-week regimen (67%) and substantially lower in treatment-naive patients receiving the 4-week regimen (27%).[56]

The current wave of DAAs generally target RNA replication, but other points in the viruses' life cycle, such as entry, assembly, egress, and infectivity, provide alternative targets for novel inhibitors that could be important components of potent DAA combinations. Thus, many different DAAs are under investigation, and it is hoped that they will provide alternative antiviral treatment methods.[57]

SUMMARY

In the past 2 years, the HCV therapeutic landscape has shifted from difficult-to-tolerate regimens with low rates of response to shorter, better-tolerated, all-oral regimens with rates of SVR greater than 95%. As more DAAs are approved for use in patients, the focus for future clinical trials will be on treating various patient populations, such patients with advanced fibrosis, post–liver transplant patients, and patients with kidney disease.

REFERENCES

1. Ghany MG, Strader DB, Thomas DL, et al, American Association for the Study of Liver Diseases. Diagnosis, management, and treatment of hepatitis C: an update. Hepatology 2009;49:1335–74.
2. Fattovich G, Giustina G, Favarato S, et al. A survey of adverse events in 11,241 patients with chronic viral hepatitis treated with alfa interferon. J Hepatol 1996;24:38–47.
3. Lotrich FE. Psychiatric clearance for patients started on interferon-alpha-based therapies. Am J Psychiatry 2013;170:592–7.
4. Lawitz E, Lalezari JP, Hassanein T, et al. Sofosbuvir in combination with peginterferon alfa-2a and ribavirin for non-cirrhotic, treatment-naive patients with genotypes 1, 2, and 3 hepatitis C infection: a randomised, double-blind, phase 2 trial. Lancet Infect Dis 2013;13:401–8.
5. Jacobson IM, McHutchison JG, Dusheiko G, et al, ADVANCE Study Team. Telaprevir for previously untreated chronic hepatitis C virus infection. N Engl J Med 2011;364:2405–16.
6. Poordad F, McCone J Jr, Bacon BR, et al, SPRINT-2 Investigators. Boceprevir for untreated chronic HCV genotype 1 infection. N Engl J Med 2011;364:1195–206.
7. Manns M, Reesink H, Berg T, et al. Rapid viral response of once-daily TMC435 plus pegylated interferon/ribavirin in hepatitis C genotype-1 patients: a randomized trial. Antivir Ther 2011;16:1021–33.
8. Lawitz E, Mangia A, Wyles D, et al. Sofosbuvir for previously untreated chronic hepatitis C infection. N Engl J Med 2013;368:1878–87.
9. Gane EJ, Stedman CA, Hyland RH, et al. Nucleotide polymerase inhibitor sofosbuvir plus ribavirin for hepatitis C. N Engl J Med 2013;368:34–44.
10. Spach DH, Kim HN. Medications to treat HCV. In: Spach DH, editor. Hepatitis C online. Available at: http://www.hepatitisc.uw.edu/page/treatment/drugs. Accessed May 15, 2015.
11. Giroux S, Bilimoria D, Cadilhac C, et al. Discovery of thienoimidazole-based HCV NS5A inhibitors. Part 1: C2-symmetric inhibitors with diyne and biphenyl linkers. Bioorg Med Chem Lett 2015;25:936–9.
12. Giroux S, Bilimoria D, Cadilhac C, et al. Discovery of thienoimidazole-based HCV NS5A inhibitors. Part 2: non-symmetric inhibitors with potent activity against genotype 1a and 1b. Bioorg Med Chem Lett 2015;25:940–3.
13. Cammà C, Di Bona D, Craxì A. The impact of antiviral treatments on the course of chronic hepatitis C: an evidence-based approach. Curr Pharm Des 2004;10: 2123–30.
14. Singal AG, Waljee AK, Shiffman M, et al. Meta-analysis: re-treatment of genotype I hepatitis C nonresponders and relapsers after failing interferon and ribavirin combination therapy. Aliment Pharmacol Ther 2010;32:969–83.
15. Chen J, Florian J, Carter W, et al. Earlier sustained virologic response end points for regulatory approval and dose selection of hepatitis C therapies. Gastroenterology 2013;144:1450–5.
16. European Association for the Study of the Liver, Electronic address: easloffice@easloffice.eu. EASL recommendations on treatment of hepatitis C 2015. J Hepatol 2015. http://dx.doi.org/10.1016/j.jhep.2015.03.025.
17. AASLD/IDSA/IAS–USA. Recommendations for testing, managing, and treating hepatitis C. 2014. Updated April 9, 2015. Available at: http://hcvguidelines.org. Accessed May 9, 2015.
18. Kowdley KV, Lawitz E, Crespo I, et al. Sofosbuvir with pegylated interferon alfa-2a and ribavirin for treatment-naive patients with hepatitis C genotype-1 infection

(ATOMIC): an open-label, randomised, multicentre phase 2 trial. Lancet 2013; 381:2100–7.

19. Sulkowski MS, Jacobson IM, Ghalib R, et al. Once-daily simeprevir (TMC435) plus sofosbuvir (GS-7977) with or without ribavirin in HCV genotype-1 prior null responders with metavir F0-2: COSMOS study subgroup analysis. Gastroenterol Hepatol (N Y) 2014;9:1–18.

20. Lawitz E, Sulkowski MS, Ghalib R, et al. Simeprevir plus sofosbuvir, with or without ribavirin, to treat chronic infection with hepatitis C virus genotype 1 in non-responders to pegylated interferon and ribavirin and treatment-naïve patients: the COSMOS randomised study. Lancet 2014;384:1756–65.

21. Gane EJ, Stedman CA, Hyland RH, et al. Efficacy of nucleotide polymerase inhibitor sofosbuvir plus the NS5A inhibitor ledipasvir or the NS5B non-nucleoside inhibitor GS-9669 against HCV genotype 1 infection. Gastroenterology 2014;146: 736–43.e1.

22. Afdhal N, Zeuzem S, Kwo P, et al, ION-1 Investigators. Ledipasvir and sofosbuvir for untreated HCV genotype 1 infection. N Engl J Med 2014;370:1889–98.

23. Kowdley KV, Gordon SC, Reddy KR, et al, ION-3 Investigators. Ledipasvir and sofosbuvir for 8 or 12 weeks for chronic HCV without cirrhosis. N Engl J Med 2014;370:1879–88.

24. Bourlière M, Bronowicki JP, de Ledinghen V, et al. Ledipasvir-sofosbuvir with or without ribavirin to treat patients with HCV genotype 1 infection and cirrhosis non-responsive to previous protease-inhibitor therapy: a randomised, double-blind, phase 2 trial (SIRIUS). Lancet Infect Dis 2015;15:397–404.

25. Feld JJ, Kowdley KV, Coakley E, et al. Treatment of HCV with ABT-450/r-ombitasvir and dasabuvir with ribavirin. N Engl J Med 2014;370:1594–603.

26. Ferenci P, Bernstein D, Lalezari J, et al, PEARL-III Study, PEARL-IV Study. ABT-450/r-ombitasvir and dasabuvir with or without ribavirin for HCV. N Engl J Med 2014;370:1983–92.

27. Poordad F, Hezode C, Trinh R, et al. ABT-450/r-ombitasvir and dasabuvir with ribavirin for hepatitis C with cirrhosis. N Engl J Med 2014;370:1973–82.

28. Sulkowski MS, Gardiner DF, Rodriguez-Torres M, et al, AI444040 Study Group. Daclatasvir plus sofosbuvir for previously treated or untreated chronic HCV infection. N Engl J Med 2014;370:211–21. Available at: http://www.nejm.org/doi/full/10.1056/NEJMoa1306218.

29. Jacobson I, Dore GJ, Foster GR, et al. 1425 Simeprevir (TMC435) with peginterferon/ribavirin for chronic HCV genotype 1 infection in treatment naïve patients: results from QUEST-1, a phase III trial. J Hepatol 2013;58:S574.

30. Manns M, Marcellin P, Poordad FP, et al. 1413 Simeprevir (TMC435) with peginterferon/ribavirin for chronic HCV genotype 1 infection in treatment naïve patients: results from QUEST-2, a phase III trial. J Hepatol 2013;58:S568.

31. Alqahtani SA, Afdhal N, Zeuzem S, et al. Safety and tolerability of ledipasvir/sofosbuvir with and without ribavirin in patients with chronic HCV genotype 1 infection: analysis of phase 3 ION trials. Hepatology 2015. http://dx.doi.org/10.1002/hep.27890.

32. Kwo P, Gitlin N, Nahass R, et al. A phase 3, randomised, open-label study to evaluate the efficacy and safety of 12 and 8 weeks of simeprevir (SMV) plus sofosbuvir (SOF) in treatment-naive and -experienced patients with chronic HCV genotype 1 infection without cirrhosis: OPTIMIST-1. Program and abstracts of the 50th Annual Meeting of the European Association for the Study of the Liver. Vienna (Austria), April 22–26, 2015. Abstract LB14. Available at: https://ilc-congress.eu/scientific-info/abstracts/.

33. Jacobson IM, Ghalib RH, Rodriguez-Torres M, et al. SVR results of a once-daily regimen of simeprevir (TMC435) plus sofosbuvir (GS-7977) with or without ribavirin in cirrhotic and non-cirrhotic HCV genotype 1 treatment-naive and prior null responder patients: the COSMOS study. Hepatology 2013;58:1379A.

34. Afdhal N, Reddy KR, Nelson DR, et al. Ledipasvir and sofosbuvir for previously treated HCV genotype 1 infection. N Engl J Med 2014;370:1483–93. Available at: http://www.nejm.org/doi/full/10.1056/NEJMoa1316366.

35. Andreone P, Colombo MG, Enejosa JV, et al. ABT-450, ritonavir, ombitasvir, and dasabuvir achieves 97% and 100% sustained virologic response with or without ribavirin in treatment-experienced patients with HCV genotype 1b infection. Gastroenterology 2014;147:359–65.e1.

36. Zeuzem S, Jacobson IM, Baykai T, et al. Retreatment of HCV with ABT-450/r–ombitasvir and dasabuvir with ribavirin. N Engl J Med 2014;370:1604–14. Available at: http://www.nejm.org/doi/full/10.1056/NEJMoa1401561.

37. van der Meer AJ, Veldt BJ, Feld JJ, et al. Association between sustained virological response and all-cause mortality among patients with chronic hepatitis C and advanced hepatic fibrosis. JAMA 2012;308:2584–93.

38. Iacobellis A, Perri F, Valvano MR, et al. Long-term outcome after antiviral therapy of patients with hepatitis C virus infection and decompensated cirrhosis. Clin Gastroenterol Hepatol 2011;9:249–53.

39. Bourlière M, Sulkowski MS, Omata M, et al. An integrated safety and efficacy analysis of >500 patients with compensated cirrhosis treated with ledipasvir/sofosbuvir with or without ribavirin. Program and abstracts of the 65th Annual Meeting of the American Association for the Study of Liver Diseases. Boston (MA), November 7–11, 2014. Abstract 82.

40. Flamm SL, Everson GT, Charlton MR, et al. Ledipasvir/sofosbuvir with ribavirin for the treatment of HCV in patients with decompensated cirrhosis: preliminary results of a prospective, multicenter study. Program and abstracts of the 2014 Annual Meeting of the American Association for the Study of Liver Diseases. Boston (MA), November 7–11, 2014. Abstract 239.

41. Bourliere M, Bronowicki J, de Ledinghen V, et al. Ledipasvir/sofosbuvir fixed dose combination is safe and efficacious in cirrhotic patients who have previously failed protease-inhibitor based triple therapy. Program and abstracts of the 65th Annual Meeting of the American Association for the Study of Liver Diseases. Boston (MA), November 7–11, 2014. Abstract LB-6.

42. Poordad F, Schiff ER, Vierling JM, et al. Daclatasvir, sofosbuvir, and ribavirin combination for HCV patients with advanced cirrhosis or post-transplant recurrence: ALLY-1 phase 3 study. Program and abstracts of the 50th Annual Meeting of the European Association for the Study of the Liver. Vienna (Austria), April 22–26, 2015. Abstract L08. Available at: https://ilc-congress.eu/scientific-info/abstracts/.

43. Lawitz E, Matusow G, DeJesus E, et al. A phase 3, open-label, single-arm study to evaluate the efficacy and safety of 12 weeks of simeprevir (SMV) plus sofosbuvir (SOF) in treatment-naive or –experienced patients with chronic HCV genotype 1 infection and cirrhosis: OPTIMIST-2. Program and abstracts of the 50th Annual Meeting of the European Association for the Study of the Liver. Vienna (Austria), April 22–26, 2015. Abstract LP04. Available at: https://ilc-congress.eu/scientific-info/abstracts/.

44. Saxena V, Koraishy FM, Sise M, et al. Safety and efficacy of sofosbuvir-containing regimens in hepatitis C infected patients with reduced renal function: real world experience from HCV-TARGET. Program and abstracts of the 50th Annual Meeting of the European Association for the Study of the Liver. Vienna (Austria),

April 22–26, 2015. Abstract LP08. Available at: https://ilc-congress.eu/scientific-info/abstracts/.

45. Wyles D, Pockros P, Morelli G, et al. Ledipasvir-sofosbuvir plus ribavirin for patients with genotype 1 hepatitis C virus previously treated in clinical trials of sofosbuvir regimens. Hepatology 2015;61(6):1793–7.

46. Lawitz E, Flamm S, Yang JC, et al. Retreatment of patients who failed 8 or 12 weeks of ledipasvir/sofosbuvir-based regimens with ledipasvir/sofosbuvir for 24 weeks. Program and abstracts of the 50th Annual Meeting of the European Association for the Study of the Liver. Vienna (Austria), April 22–26, 2015. Abstract O005. Available at: https://ilc-congress.eu/scientific-info/abstracts/.

47. Forns X, Gordon SC, Zuckerman E, et al. Grazoprevir/elbasvir plus ribavirin for chronic HCV genotype-1 infection after failure of combination therapy containing a direct-acting antiviral agent. J Hepatol 2015. http://dx.doi.org/10.1016/j.jhep.2015.04.009.

48. Ravi S, Nasiri-Toosi M, Karimzadeh I, et al. Pattern and associated factors of anti-hepatitis C virus treatment-induced adverse reactions. Expert Opin Drug Saf 2014;13:277–86.

49. Koh C, Liang TJ. What is the future of ribavirin therapy for hepatitis C? Antivir Res 2014;104:34–9.

50. Rebetol [package insert]. Whitehouse station (NJ): Merck & Co, Inc; 2014.

51. Lawitz E, Gane E, Pearlman B, et al. Efficacy and safety of 12 weeks versus 18 weeks of treatment with grazoprevir (MK-5172) and elbasvir (MK-8742) with or without ribavirin for hepatitis C virus genotype 1 infection in previously untreated patient with cirrhosis and patients with previous null response with or without cirrhosis (C-WORTHY): a randomised, open-label phase 2 trial. Lancet 2014; 385(9973):1075–86. Available at: http://www.jwatch.org/na36381/2014/12/04/promising-all-oral-hcv-regimen-difficult-treat-groups#sthash.upvkVlyJ.dpuf.

52. Zeuzem S, Ghalib R, Reddy KR, et al. Grazoprevir-elbasvir combination therapy for treatment-naive cirrhotic and noncirrhotic patients with chronic HCV genotype 1, 4, or 6 infection: a randomized trial. Ann Intern Med 2015. http://dx.doi.org/10.7326/M15-0785.

53. Poordad F, Sievert W, Mollison L, et al, UNITY-1 Study Group. Fixed-dose combination therapy with daclatasvir, asunaprevir, and beclabuvir for noncirrhotic patients with HCV genotype 1 infection. JAMA 2015;313:1728–35.

54. Muir AJ, Poordad F, Lalezari J, et al. Daclatasvir in combination with asunaprevir and beclabuvir for hepatitis C virus genotype 1 infection with compensated cirrhosis. JAMA 2015;313:1736–44.

55. Kohli A, Osinusi A, Sims Z, et al. Virological response after 6 week triple-drug regimens for hepatitis C: a proof-of-concept phase 2A cohort study. Lancet 2015; 385:1107–13.

56. Gane EJ, Hyland RH, Tang Y, et al. Safety and efficacy of short-duration treatment with GS-9857 combined with sofosbuvir/GS-5816 in treatment-naive and DAA-experienced genotype 1 patients with and without cirrhosis. Program and abstracts of the 50th Annual Meeting of the European Association for the Study of the Liver. Vienna (Austria), April 22–26, 2015. Abstract LP03. Available at: https://ilc-congress.eu/scientific-info/abstracts/.

57. Bush CO, Pokrovskii MV, Saito R, et al. A small-molecule inhibitor of hepatitis C virus infectivity. Antimicrob Agents Chemother 2014;58(1):386–96.

Hepatitis C Virus
Current and Evolving Treatments for Genotypes 2 and 3

Javier Ampuero, MD, PhD, Manuel Romero-Gómez, MD, PhD*

KEYWORDS

- Hepatitis C • Genotype 2 • Genotype 3 • Direct-acting antiviral
- Sustained virologic response

KEY POINTS

- With the advent of new direct-acting antivirals, sustained virologic response (SVR) rates have dramatically increased, and with fewer adverse effects.
- In genotype 2, SVR rates of 90% are achieved with interferon-free regimens based on sofosbuvir and ribavirin.
- The outlook for genotype 3 is slightly different. Patients without cirrhosis and treatment-naive patients with cirrhosis have high SVR rates, whereas treatment-experienced patients with cirrhosis achieve around 60% with 24-week therapies. As such, new treatments are needed for genotype 3 because these have become the most difficult-to-treat patients.
- New drugs have enabled most of the host and viral factors with decreased SVR rates to be resolved. However, new challenges have emerged, such as ribavirin use and duration of therapy, and special populations, such as patients with chronic renal failure.

INTRODUCTION

Hepatitis C virus (HCV) is a pandemic affecting more than 150 million people worldwide. Genotype 3 is the most common in east Asian countries like Pakistan and northern Europe, whereas genotype 2 is the most common on the West Africa coast. In the past, HCV genotypes 2 and 3 have been classified as easy-to-treat genotypes because sustained virologic response (SVR) has been achieved in 75% to 80% of cases with a 24-week therapy period using peginterferon and ribavirin.[1] However,

Disclosure: Advisory Board for Merck, Roche, Gilead, Abbvie, Janssen, BMS; research support from Merck, Roche (M. Romero-Gómez).
Unit for the Clinical Management of Digestive Diseases & CIBERehd, Virgen Macarena - Virgen del Rocio University Hospitals, Avenida Manuel Siurot, s/n, Sevilla 41017, Spain
* Corresponding author.
E-mail address: mromerogomez@us.es

Gastroenterol Clin N Am 44 (2015) 845–857
http://dx.doi.org/10.1016/j.gtc.2015.07.009
0889-8553/15/$ – see front matter © 2015 Elsevier Inc. All rights reserved.

gastro.theclinics.com

recent studies have shown relevant differences between HCV genotypes 2 and 3.[2] Therapy for hepatitis C virus infection is evolving rapidly, with direct-acting antivirals (DAAs) transforming the treatment of hepatitis C such that interferon-free regimens have become a new reality. Serious side effects have been substantially reduced. This article reviews the currently available therapies for HCV genotypes 2 and 3, and summarizes the special features of these genotypes.

HEPATITIS C VIRUS GENOTYPE 2

HCV genotype 2 represents around 13% of all HCV infections, with a major prevalence in sub-Saharan African countries and Asia. This genotype has been strongly associated with acupuncture using nondisposable material.[3] Until 2013, the standard of care for HCV-2 treatment-naive as well as treatment-experienced patients was a combination of peginterferon plus ribavirin for 24 weeks. With this combination, SVR rates up to 80% could be achieved. More recently, the launch of DAAs has resulted in treatments that have been shorter as well as better tolerated (**Table 1**).[4]

Table 1
Studies of sofosbuvir (SOF)-based therapy in HCV genotype 2

Population	Study	Combination	SVR (%)
Treatment naive	PROTON	SOF + IFN + RBV 12 wk	No cirrhosis: 96
	FISSION	SOF + RBV 12 wk	Overall: 95
			No cirrhosis: 97
			Cirrhosis: 83
	POSITRON	SOF + RBV 12 wk	Overall: 93
			No cirrhosis: 92
			Cirrhosis: 94
	VALENCE	SOF + RBV 12 wk	Overall: 99
			No cirrhosis: 97
			Cirrhosis: 100
	PHOTON-1	SOF + RBV 12 wk	Overall: 88
	Japanese trial	SOF + RBV 12 wk	Overall: 98
			No cirrhosis: 97
			Cirrhosis: 100
	AI444-40	SOF + DCV 24 wk	No cirrhosis: 96
		SOF + DCV + RBV 24 wk	
Treatment experienced	LONESTAR-2	SOF + IFN + RBV 12 wk	Overall: 96
			No cirrhosis: 100
			Cirrhosis: 93
	FUSION	SOF + RBV 12 wk	Overall: 82
			No cirrhosis: 90
			Cirrhosis: 60
		SOF + RBV 16 wk	Overall: 88
			No cirrhosis: 92
			Cirrhosis: 78
	VALENCE	SOF + RBV 12 wk	Overall: 90
			No cirrhosis: 91
			Cirrhosis: 88
	PHOTON-1	SOF + RBV 12 wk	Overall: 92
	Japanese trial	SOF + RBV 12 wk	Overall: 96
			No cirrhosis: 95
			Cirrhosis: 89

Abbreviations: IFN, interferon; RBV, ribavirin; SOF, sofosbuvir; wk, weeks.

Treatment Options for Hepatitis C Virus Genotype 2

Treatment-naive patients: direct-acting antivirals in combination with peginterferon/ ribavirin

Sofosbuvir is a potent nucleotide polymerase inhibitor analogue that acts at the catalytic site of Nonstructural protein 5B (NS5B) polymerase.[5] The PROTON trial evaluated the combination of sofosbuvir with peginterferon and ribavirin treatment over 12 weeks. A SVR rate of 96% (25 out of 26) was achieved.[6] Daclatasvir is a NS5A inhibitor that shows pangenotypic activity.[7] Eighty patients with HCV genotype 2 (23% with cirrhosis) were enrolled randomly to 3 treatment arms: (1) daclatasvir, peginterferon, and ribavirin over 12 weeks (n = 24); (2) the same combination over 16 weeks (n = 23); (3) placebo, peginterferon, and ribavirin over 24 weeks (n = 24). SVR, 24 weeks after treatment has ended (SVR24) was higher in groups receiving daclatasvir (83% [20 out of 24] and 82% [19 out of 23], respectively) compared with placebo (63%; 15 out of 24).[8] Simeprevir is a second-wave NS3/4A protease inhibitor with potent antiviral activity in HCV genotypes 1, 4, 5, and 6. A phase 2a study closed early and prevented further development of simeprevir, with or without peginterferon and ribavirin in HCV genotype 2. The study included 6 treatment-naive patients receiving simeprevir in monotherapy (200 mg/d for 7 days); only half of the patients showed antiviral activity.[9]

Treatment-naive patients: interferon-free regimen with direct-acting antivirals

Most studies have evaluated the combination of sofosbuvir plus ribavirin. The FISSION study was a phase 3 trial that compared sofosbuvir plus ribavirin for 12 weeks (n = 73) versus peginterferon plus ribavirin for 24 weeks (n = 67) in 140 previously untreated patients with HCV infection. Patients receiving sofosbuvir plus ribavirin achieved 95% (69 out of 73) SVR compared with 78% (52 out of 67) in those receiving peginterferon plus ribavirin. Patients with cirrhosis had lower SVR rates than those without in both treatment groups (sofosbuvir plus ribavirin, 83% [10 out of 12] vs 97% [59 out of 61]; peginterferon plus ribavirin, 62% [8 out of 13] vs 81% [44 out of 54]).[10] POSITRON was a randomized trial that included patients chronically infected with HCV genotype 2 and for whom treatment with peginterferon was not an option. They were assigned to receive sofosbuvir plus ribavirin (n = 109) or placebo (n = 34) for 12 weeks. Those treated with sofosbuvir plus ribavirin achieved SVR of 93% (101 out of 109), whereas the rate was 0% in those receiving placebo, regardless of the presence of liver cirrhosis (94% [16 out of 17] vs 92% [85 out of 92], respectively).[11] The VALENCE trial evaluated sofosbuvir plus ribavirin or placebo for 12 weeks in treatment-naive patients (n = 32). The treated patients achieved SVR of 97% (29 out of 30) in those who did not have cirrhosis and 100% (2 out of 2) in those with cirrhosis.[12] In the PHOTON-1 study, the combination of sofosbuvir plus ribavirin was evaluated in treatment-naive patients with HCV genotype 2 and concurrent Human immunodeficiency virus (HIV). The SVR achieved was 88% (23 out of 26).[13] In addition, a phase 3 study conducted in Japan assessed the efficacy and safety of sofosbuvir plus ribavirin in treatment-naive patients with chronic genotype 2 HCV infection. The SVR obtained was 97% (80 out of 82) in patients without cirrhosis and 100% (8 out of 8) in those with cirrhosis.[14] Sofosbuvir was also evaluated in combination with daclatasvir, with or without ribavirin, over 24 weeks in 26 HCV-2 treatment-naive patients. Overall, 96% achieved SVR (24 out of 26).[15] Other combinations have been addressed but efficacy has continued to be suboptimal. A combination of ombitasvir and paritaprevir with ritonavir, with or without ribavirin, has been evaluated in treatment-naive patients and adults without cirrhosis with chronic HCV genotype 2. HCV RNA was undetectable from week 4 to 12 in 90% (9 out of 10) receiving the ribavirin-containing regimen and 80% (8 out of 10) receiving the ribavirin-free regimen, whereas SVR12 was achieved by 80% (8 out of 10) receiving the ribavirin-containing regimen, and 60% (6 out of 10) receiving the ribavirin-free regimen.[16]

Treatment-experienced patients: direct-acting antivirals in combination with peginterferon/ribavirin

The LONESTAR-2 trial evaluated sofosbuvir plus peginterferon and ribavirin in combination over 12 weeks in 23 treatment-experienced patients. SVR was 100% (9 out of 9) in patients without cirrhosis and 93% (13 out of 14) in those with cirrhosis.[6] Daclatasvir plus peginterferon and ribavirin combination has been tested in HCV genotype 2. Patients were enrolled into 3 arms: (1) daclatasvir and peginterferon plus ribavirin over 12 weeks (n = 26); (2) the same combination over 16 weeks (n = 27); (c) placebo, peginterferon plus ribavirin over 24 weeks (n = 27). SVR24 was higher in groups receiving daclatasvir (69% [18 out of 26] and 67% [18 out of 27] for 16 and 12 weeks of therapy, respectively) compared with those receiving placebo (59%; 16 out of 27).[8]

Treatment-experienced patients: interferon-free regimen with direct-acting antivirals

All studies described thus far were also conducted in treatment-experienced patients having genotype 2. The treatment regimens were with sofosbuvir and were interferon free. The FUSION trial included patients who had not had a response to previous interferon therapy. Patients received sofosbuvir plus ribavirin for 12 weeks (n = 39) or 16 weeks (n = 35). SVR rates were 90% (26 out of 29) in patients without cirrhosis receiving treatment over 12 weeks, and 92% (24 out of 26) in those treated for 16 weeks; lower SVR was observed in those with cirrhosis (60%; 6 out of 10) and 78% (7 out of 9), respectively.[11] The VALENCE trial evaluated sofosbuvir plus ribavirin or placebo for 12 weeks in patients with HCV who were treatment experienced (n = 41). In patients receiving treatment, the SVR rate was 91% (30 out of 33) in patients without cirrhosis and 88% (7 out of 8) in those patients with cirrhosis.[12] In the PHOTON-1 study, sofosbuvir plus ribavirin was evaluated in treatment-experienced patients with HCV genotype 2, and with concurrent HIV. The SVR rate was 92% (22 out of 24).[13] The Japanese study evaluating sofosbuvir plus ribavirin was also performed in treatment-experienced patients. The SVR12 was 95% (52 out of 54) in patients without cirrhosis and 89% (8 out of 9) in those with cirrhosis.[14]

HEPATITIS C VIRUS GENOTYPE 3

This genotype represents around 20% of overall HCV infections worldwide. The probable origin of HCV genotype 3 has been placed in Asia, where it is more prevalent (south and east Asia, and India). From molecular studies, HCV genotype 3, in particular subtype 3a, is significantly associated with transmission via intravenous drug abuse in industrialized countries (especially North and South America and Europe).[17] HCV genotype 3 has some special features that differ from the other viral genotypes (**Fig. 1**).[18] First, it is associated with the highest rate of steatosis, including a morphologic expression of a viral cytopathic effect.[19] The magnitude of HCV-3 infection–related steatosis correlates with the level of viral replication, and is independent of other well-documented steatogenic factors such as PNPLA3.[20] Second, genotype 3 is associated with a more accelerated fibrosis progression.[21] The mechanism of accelerated fibrogenesis in patients infected with HCV genotype 3 is under debate because some investigators have failed to identify steatosis as an independent factor of fibrosis in these patients.[22] There may be genotype-dependent fibrogenetic effects with respect to proinflammatory cytokines or the hepatic stellate cells. Third, HCV genotype 3 has been found to increase the risk of developing hepatocellular carcinoma, relative to other viral genotypes.[23] Steatosis and fibrosis attributed to the genotype

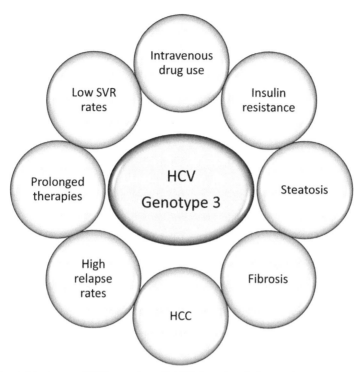

Fig. 1. Special features of HCV genotype 3. HCC, hepatocellular carcinoma.

are, perhaps, the main factors explaining this association. Fourth, genotype 3 seems to interact with the immune response, compared with other HCV genotypes. Haplotype BTN3A3 rs13220495 CC plus IL28B genotype CC were observed to be universally present in patients with genotype 3a.[24] This interaction could explain the 2 critical aspects of the genotype: higher rates of spontaneous viral clearance and higher rates of disease progression.

Treatment Options for Hepatitis C Virus Genotype 3

Treatment-naive patients: direct-acting antivirals in combination with peginterferon/ribavirin

Sofosbuvir has been evaluated in combination with peginterferon and ribavirin over 12 weeks in the PROTON trial. SVR rate was achieved in 96% (38 out of 39) (**Table 2**).[6] The BOSON study also evaluated this combination. This study included 94 (overall SVR, 95%) treatment-naive patients, with SVR rates of 96% (68 out of 71) in noncirrhotic and 91% (21 out of 23) in cirrhotic patients.[25] Daclatasvir together with peginterferon and ribavirin has been used in genotype 3. Seventy-one patients (1% with cirrhosis) were enrolled and randomly assigned to groups to receive 12 or 16 weeks of daclatasvir, or 24 weeks of placebo, all in combination with peginterferon and ribavirin. SVR24 rates were 69%, 67%, and 59%, respectively.[8]

Treatment-naive patients: interferon-free regimen with direct-acting antivirals

Most of the studies in patients of this kind evaluated the combination of sofosbuvir and ribavirin. The FISSION study was a phase 3 trial that compared sofosbuvir plus ribavirin for 12 weeks (n = 183) versus peginterferon plus ribavirin for 24 weeks

Table 2
Studies of sofosbuvir-based therapy in HCV genotype 3

Population	Study	Combination	SVR (%)
Treatment naive	PROTON	SOF + IFN + RBV 12 wk	No cirrhosis: 96
	FISSION	SOF + RBV 12 wk	Overall: 56
			No cirrhosis: 61
			Cirrhosis: 34
	POSITRON	SOF + RBV 12 wk	Overall: 61
			No cirrhosis: 68
			Cirrhosis: 21
	VALENCE	SOF + RBV 24 wk	Overall: 93.3
			No cirrhosis: 94
			Cirrhosis: 92
	BOSON	SOF + IFN + RBV 12 wk	Overall: 95
			No cirrhosis: 96
			Cirrhosis: 91
		SOF + RBV 16 wk	Overall: 77
			No cirrhosis: 83
			Cirrhosis: 57
		SOF + RBV 24 wk	Overall: 88
			No cirrhosis: 90
			Cirrhosis: 82
	PHOTON-1	SOF + RBV 12 wk	Overall: 67
	AI444-40	SOF + DCV 24 wk	No cirrhosis: 89
		SOF + DCV + RBV 24 wk	
	ALLY-3	SOF + DCV 12 wk	Overall: 90
			No cirrhosis: 97
			Cirrhosis: 58
	ELECTRON-2	SOF + LDV 12 wk	No cirrhosis: 64
		SOF + LDV + RBV 12 wk	No cirrhosis: 100
Treatment experienced	LONESTAR-2	SOF + IFN + RBV 12 wk	Overall: 83
			No cirrhosis: 83
			Cirrhosis: 83
	FUSION	SOF + RBV 12 wk	Overall: 30
			No cirrhosis: 37
			Cirrhosis: 19
		SOF + RBV 16 wk	Overall: 62
			No cirrhosis: 63
			Cirrhosis: 61
	VALENCE	SOF + RBV 24 wk	Overall: 70
			No cirrhosis: 85
			Cirrhosis: 60
	BOSON	SOF + IFN + RBV 12 wk	Overall: 91
			No cirrhosis: 94
			Cirrhosis: 86
		SOF + RBV 16 wk	Overall: 64
			No cirrhosis: 76
			Cirrhosis: 47
		SOF + RBV 24 wk	Overall: 80
			No cirrhosis: 82
			Cirrhosis: 77
	ELECTRON-2	SOF + LDV + RBV 12 wk	Overall: 82
			No cirrhosis: 89
			Cirrhosis: 73

(n = 176) in previously untreated patients. Patients receiving sofosbuvir plus ribavirin had an SVR of 56% (102 out of 183), compared with 63% (110 out of 176) in those receiving peginterferon plus ribavirin. Patients with cirrhosis showed lower SVR rates than those without cirrhosis in both treatment groups: sofosbuvir plus ribavirin, 34% (13 out of 38) versus 61% (89 out of 145); and peginterferon plus ribavirin, 30% (11 out of 37) versus 71% (99 out of 139).[10] The POSITRON study included patients chronically infected with HCV genotype 3, for whom treatment with peginterferon was not an option. The patients were assigned to receive sofosbuvir plus ribavirin (n = 98) or placebo (n = 37) for 12 weeks. Those treated with sofosbuvir plus ribavirin achieved a 61% (60 out of 98) SVR rate (0% in those receiving placebo). Note that there was a large difference between those with cirrhosis (21%; 3 out of 14) and those without cirrhosis (68%; 57 out of 84).[11] The VALENCE trial evaluated sofosbuvir plus ribavirin, or placebo, for 24 weeks in HCV treatment-naive patients (n = 105). In those patients receiving treatment, the SVR rate was 94% (86 out of 92) in those without cirrhosis and 92% (12 out of 13) in those with cirrhosis.[12] The BOSON study evaluated sofosbuvir plus ribavirin during 16 versus 24 weeks. Overall results were higher in longer therapy, because overall SVR rate was 88% (83 out of 94) and 90% (65 out of 72) in cirrhotics and 82% (18 out of 22) versus 77% (70 out of 91), 83% (58 out of 70), and 57% (12 out of 21), respectively, in noncirrhotics.[25] In the PHOTON-1 study, the combination of sofosbuvir plus ribavirin over 12 weeks was evaluated among treatment-naive patients with HCV genotype 3 and concurrent HIV infection. The SVR achieved was 67% (28 out of 42) irrespective of the presence of cirrhosis.[13] Sofosbuvir has also been combined with other DAAs. Two studies have added daclatasvir to sofosbuvir. The first study assessing this combination with (n = 5) or without (n = 13) ribavirin over 24 weeks in treatment-naive patients achieved an 89% SVR (16 out of 18).[15] The ALLY-3 phase III study included treatment-naive patients with genotype 3 (n = 101) receiving treatment with sofosbuvir and daclatasvir over 12 weeks. SVR12 rates were 90% (91 out of 101), with patients with cirrhosis showing reduced SVR rates compared with noncirrhotic patients: 58% (11 out of 19) versus 97% (73 out of 75), respectively.[26] In contrast, the ELECTRON-2 trial in comparing the combination of sofosbuvir and ledipasvir with (n = 26) or without (n = 25) ribavirin over 12 weeks achieved SVR rates of 64% and 100% respectively.[27] The combination of ombitasvir and paritaprevir with ritonavir, with or without ribavirin, was evaluated in treatment-naive adults without cirrhosis with chronic HCV genotype 3. Results were suboptimal; SVR12 was achieved in 50% (5 out of 10) of patients receiving the ribavirin-containing regimen, and 9% (1 out of 11) receiving the ribavirin-free regimen.[16]

Data about new experimental drugs have been shown in International Congress. GS-5816 has been evaluated plus sofosbuvir, with or without ribavirin, in naive patients without cirrhosis during 8 weeks in phase 2 study. Four arms were performed: (1) sofosbuvir plus GS-5816 25 mg; (2) sofosbuvir plus GS-5816 25 mg and ribavirin; (3) sofosbuvir plus GS-5816 100 mg; (4) sofosbuvir plus GS-5816 100 mg and ribavirin. SVR rates were 100%, 88%, 96%, and 100%, respectively.[28]

Treatment-experienced patients: direct-acting antivirals in combination with peginterferon/ribavirin

There are few studies evaluating a DAA with peginterferon and ribavirin. In the LONESTAR-2 trial, sofosbuvir was used together with previously used drugs over 12 weeks. The study included 24 treatment-experienced patients and achieved SVR of 83% in patients with cirrhosis (10 out of 12) and in those without (10 out of 12).[6] Recently, the phase 3 BOSON study confirmed these results. This study included

87 (91% overall SVR) treatment-experienced patients, with SVR rates of 94% (49 out of 52) in noncirrhotic patients and 86% (30 out of 35) in cirrhotic patients.[25]

Treatment-experienced patients: interferon-free regimen with direct-acting antivirals
The FUSION trial included patients who had not had a response to previous interferon therapy. Patients received sofosbuvir and ribavirin for 12 weeks (n = 64) or 16 weeks (n = 63). SVR rates were 37% (14 out of 38) in patients without cirrhosis receiving treatment over 12 weeks, and 63% (25 out of 40) over 16 weeks, with a lower SVR of 19% (5 out of 26) in those with cirrhosis and 61% (14 out of 23) in those without.[11] The VALENCE trial evaluated sofosbuvir and ribavirin or placebo over 24 weeks in treatment-experienced patients with HCV (n = 145). In those patients receiving treatment, the SVR rate was 85% (85 out of 100) in patients without cirrhosis and 60% (27 out of 45) in those with cirrhosis.[12] The BOSON study evaluated sofosbuvir plus ribavirin during 16 versus 24 weeks in treatment-experienced patients. Overall results were higher in longer therapy, because SVR rate was 80% overall (70 out of 88), 82% (44 out of 54) in cirrhotics, and 77% (26 out of 34) in noncirrhotics; versus 64% (58 out of 90), 76% (41 out of 54), and 47% (17 out of 36), respectively.[25] In the PHOTON-1 study, sofosbuvir and ribavirin over 24 weeks was evaluated in treatment-experienced patients with HCV genotype 3, and concurrent HIV. The SVR rate was 92% (12 out of 13).[13] The ALLY-3 phase III study included treatment-experienced patients with genotype 3 (n = 51) receiving sofosbuvir and daclatasvir over 12 weeks. SVR12 rates were 86% (44 out of 51). Again, patients with cirrhosis had reduced SVR rates of 69% (9 out of 13) versus 94% (32 out of 34) in those with cirrhosis.[26] In contrast, the ELECTRON-2 trial evaluated the combination of sofosbuvir and ledipasvir plus ribavirin (n = 50) for 12 weeks. The overall SVR rates achieved were 82% (73% in patients with cirrhosis and 89% in those without).[29] GS-5816 has been evaluated plus sofosbuvir, with or without ribavirin, in treatment-experienced patients with cirrhosis during 12 weeks in a phase 2 study. Four arms were performed: (1) sofosbuvir plus GS-5816 25 mg; (2) sofosbuvir plus GS-5816 25 mg and ribavirin; (3) sofosbuvir plus GS-5816 100 mg; (4) sofosbuvir plus GS-5816 100 mg and ribavirin. SVR rates were 85%, 96%, 100%, and 100% in noncirrhotic patients, and 58%, 85%, 88%, and 96% in cirrhotic patients, respectively.[30]

COST-EFFECTIVENESS OF NOVEL REGIMENS

New HCV therapies have increased SVR rates considerably, irrespective of liver fibrosis, have dramatically decreased the occurrence of serious adverse effects, and have shortened the treatment regimens. However, they are extremely expensive compared with the combination of peginterferon and ribavirin. These novel regimens have been evaluated in cost-effectiveness studies. Najafzadeh and colleagues[31] compared peginterferon and ribavirin versus sofosbuvir plus ribavirin or plus daclatasvir or plus daclatasvir and ribavirin. Assuming a price of $7000 for sofosbuvir, $5500 for daclatasvir, and $875 for ledipasvir per week, sofosbuvir plus ribavirin and sofosbuvir plus daclatasvir cost $110,000 and $691,000 per quality-adjusted life year (QALY), respectively for genotype 2. For genotype 3, sofosbuvir plus ledipasvir and ribavirin cost $73,000 per QALY, whereas sofosbuvir plus daclatasvir cost more than $396,000 per QALY. The investigators concluded that the novel treatments for HCV are cost-effective compared with usual care for genotype 3 but not for genotype 2. Similarly, Linas and colleagues[32] estimated the cost-effectiveness of sofosbuvir-based treatments for HCV genotype 2 or 3 infection in the United States. The incremental cost-effectiveness ratio of sofosbuvir-based treatment was less than $100,000 per QALY in patients with cirrhosis (regardless of genotype or whether treatment naive or treatment experienced) as well as in treatment-experienced patients without cirrhosis. However, the cost was more than $200,000 per QALY in treatment-naive patients without cirrhosis. The investigators concluded that sofosbuvir provides good value for money for treatment-experienced patients with HCV genotype 2 or 3 infection, and those with cirrhosis.

NEW CHALLENGES TO OPTIMIZE THERAPY FOR HEPATITIS C VIRUS 2 AND 3

Therapies including DAAs are associated with high rates of SVR among patients with characteristics that were previously known to be associated with a poor response. Both host factors (IL28B polymorphism,[33] insulin resistance,[34] or previous treatment[35]) and viral factors (baseline viral load[36]) have decreased in importance. In contrast, virologic breakthrough is extremely rare and is usually associated with a suboptimal therapy caused by erroneous HCV genotyping.[37] Also, no cross-resistance has been observed,[38] and serious adverse effects have been anecdotal. New challenges have appeared in the treatment of hepatitis C (**Fig. 2**). End-of-treatment virologic response seems similar among patients treated with or without ribavirin in most combinations. This finding may indirectly reflect the antiviral potency and high resistance barrier. Relapse rates represent the main cause of treatment failure. Because ribavirin shows some adverse effects,[39] a ribavirin-free regimen is desirable. However, ribavirin contributes toward shortening treatments and decreasing costs, as well as reducing relapse rates. Optimal treatment duration continues to be debatable. For genotype 2, a 12-week course of sofosbuvir and ribavirin seems to be sufficient for patients without cirrhosis, whereas this combination needs to be extended to 16 weeks for patients with cirrhosis. This situation is similar for genotype 3 because those patients with cirrhosis have lower SVR rates. Thus, increasing the duration of therapy from 12 to 24 weeks is required to achieve better

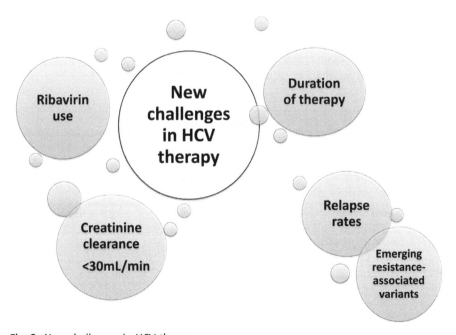

Fig. 2. New challenges in HCV therapy.

Table 3
Characteristics of currently available DAAs and host targeting antivirals

	First-wave Protease Inhibitors	Second-wave Protease Inhibitors	Polymerase Inhibitors (NA)	Polymerase Inhibitors (NNA)	NS5A Inhibitors
Drugs	Telaprevir Boceprevir	Simeprevir Asunaprevir Paritaprevir/r	Sofosbuvir	Dasabuvir	Daclatasvir Ledipasvir[a] Ombitasvir[a]
Barrier to resistance	Low	Low	High	Very Low	Low
Efficacy in HCV-2	No	No	Yes	No	Yes
Efficacy in HCV-3	No	No	Yes	No	Yes

Abbreviations: NA, nucleoside analogues; NNA, non-nucleoside analogues; Paritaprevir/r, paritaprevir/ritonavir.
[a] Low activity in vitro.

SVR rates, irrespective of treatment combination. However, treatment-experienced patients with cirrhosis have become the group that is most difficult to treat, with SVR rates of 19% to 60% with interferon-free regimens. The highest SVR rate (85%) was achieved with interferon-based therapy, including sofosbuvir and ribavirin. However, many patients are ineligible for peginterferon so this combination is restricted. In addition, sofosbuvir plus ledipasvir and ribavirin for 12 weeks[27] showed high SVR rates (75%), but ledipasvir has shown very low in vitro activity against genotype 3 (**Table 3**). Hence, and bearing in mind the ELECTRON-2 trial, neither the American Association for the Study of Liver Diseases (AASLD) nor the European Association for the Study of the Liver (EASL) guidelines[40] include sofosbuvir plus ledipasvir within the recommended options for HCV genotype 3 (**Table 4**). In addition, sofosbuvir-based regimens are contraindicated in patients with creatinine clearance less than 30 mL/min because of the potential toxicity caused by the accumulation of metabolites cleared by kidney.[41] As such, there are no effective drugs available for this subgroup of patients because the therapies that work in genotype 3 are contraindicated in chronic renal failure, whereas the drugs that could be administrated in this situation have no effect in genotype 3.

Table 4
Current IFN-free options for genotypes 2 and 3, according to EASL and AASLD guidelines

	EASL	AASLD
Genotype 2		
No cirrhosis	SOF + RBV 12 wk SOF + DCV 12 wk	SOF + RBV 12 wk
Compensated cirrhosis	SOF + RBV 16–20 wk SOF + DCV 12 wk	SOF + RBV 16 wk
Decompensated cirrhosis	SOF + RBV 16–20 wk SOF + DCV + RBV 12 wk	SOF + RBV 24–48 wk
Genotype 3		
No cirrhosis	SOF + RBV 24 wk SOF + DCV 12 wk	SOF + RBV 24 wk
Compensated cirrhosis	SOF + DCV + RBV 24 wk	SOF + RBV 24 wk
Decompensated cirrhosis	SOF + DCV + RBV 24 wk	SOF + RBV 24–48 wk

SUMMARY

With the advent of new DAAs, SVR rates have dramatically increased, and with fewer adverse effects. In genotype 2, SVR rates of 90% are achieved with interferon-free regimens based on sofosbuvir and ribavirin. The outlook for genotype 3 is slightly different. Patients without cirrhosis and treatment-naive patients with cirrhosis have high SVR rates, whereas treatment-experienced patients with cirrhosis achieve around 60% with 24-week therapies. As such, new treatments are needed for genotype 3 because they have become the most difficult-to-treat patients. New drugs have enabled most of the host and viral factors that previously had decreased SVR rates to be resolved. However, new challenges have emerged, such as ribavirin use, duration of therapy, or special populations such as patients with chronic renal failure. In addition, the data presented need to be interpreted with caution. The small number of patients (particularly those with cirrhosis) that have been included in some studies precludes a clear assessment of efficacy and the possibility of detecting adverse events.

REFERENCES

1. Marcellin P, Cheinquer H, Curescu M, et al. High sustained virologic response rates in rapid virologic response patients in the large real-world PROPHESYS cohort confirm results from randomized clinical trials. Hepatology 2012;56: 2039–50.
2. Zeuzem S, Hultcrantz R, Bourliere M, et al. Peginterferon alfa-2b plus ribavirin for treatment of chronic hepatitis C in previously untreated patients infected with HCV genotypes 2 or 3. J Hepatol 2004;40:993–9.
3. Bourlière M, Barberin JM, Rotily M, et al. Epidemiological changes in hepatitis C virus genotypes in France: evidence in intravenous drug users. J Viral Hepat 2002;9:62–70.
4. Bourlière M, Benali S, Ansaldi C, et al. Optimal therapy of genotype-2 chronic hepatitis C: what's new? Liver Int 2015;35(Suppl 1):21–6.
5. Herbst DA Jr, Reddy KR. Sofosbuvir, a nucleotide polymerase inhibitor, for the treatment of chronic hepatitis C virus infection. Expert Opin Investig Drugs 2013;22:527–36.
6. Lawitz E, Lalezari JP, Hassanein T, et al. Sofosbuvir in combination with peginterferon alfa-2a and ribavirin for non-cirrhotic, treatment-naive patients with genotypes 1, 2, and 3 hepatitis C infection: a randomized, double-blind, phase 2 trial. Lancet Infect Dis 2013;13:401–8.
7. Herbst DA, Reddy KR. NS5A inhibitor, daclatasvir, for the treatment of chronic hepatitis C virus infection. Expert Opin Investig Drugs 2013;22:1337–46.
8. Dore GJ, Lawitz E, Hézode C, et al. Daclatasvir plus peginterferon and ribavirin is noninferior to peginterferon and ribavirin alone, and reduces the duration of treatment for HCV genotype 2 or 3 infection. Gastroenterology 2015;148:355–66.
9. Moreno C, Berg T, Tanwandee T, et al. Antiviral activity of TMC435 monotherapy in patients infected with HCV genotypes 2–6: TMC435-C202, a phase IIa, open-label study. J Hepatol 2012;56:1247–53.
10. Lawitz E, Mangia A, Wyles D, et al. Sofosbuvir for previously untreated chronic hepatitis C infection. N Engl J Med 2013;368:1878–87.
11. Jacobson IM, Gordon SC, Kowdley KV, et al. Sofosbuvir for hepatitis C genotype 2 or 3 in patients without treatment options. N Engl J Med 2013;368:1867–77.
12. Zeuzem S, Dusheiko GM, Salupere R, et al. Sofosbuvir and ribavirin in HCV genotypes 2 and 3. N Engl J Med 2014;370:1993–2001.

13. Sulkowski MS, Naggie S, Lalezari J, et al. Sofosbuvir and ribavirin for hepatitis C in patients with HIV coinfection. JAMA 2014;312:353–61.

14. Omata M, Nishiguchi S, Ueno Y, et al. Sofosbuvir plus ribavirin in Japanese patients with chronic genotype 2 HCV infection: an open-label, phase 3 trial. J Viral Hepat 2014;21:762–8.

15. Sulkowski MS, Gardiner DF, Rodriguez-Torres M, et al. Daclatasvir plus sofosbuvir for previously treated or untreated chronic HCV infection. N Engl J Med 2014; 370:211–21.

16. Lawitz E, Sullivan G, Rodriguez-Torres M, et al. Exploratory trial of ombitasvir and ABT-450/r with or without ribavirin for HCV genotype 1, 2, and 3 infection. J Infect 2015;70:197–205.

17. Gower E, Estes CC, Hindman S, et al. Global epidemiology and genotype distribution of the hepatitis C virus infection. J Hepatol 2014;61:45–57.

18. Ampuero J, Romero-Gómez M, Reddy KR. HCV genotype 3 – the new treatment challenge. Aliment Pharmacol Ther 2014;39:686–98.

19. Rubbia-Brandt L, Quadri R, Abid K, et al. Hepatocyte steatosis is a cytopathic effect of hepatitis C virus genotype 3. J Hepatol 2000;33:106–15.

20. Ampuero J, Del Campo JA, Rojas L, et al. PNPLA3 rs738409 causes steatosis according to viral & IL28B genotypes in hepatitis C. Ann Hepatol 2014;13:356–63.

21. Bochud PY, Cai T, Overbeck K, et al. Genotype 3 is associated with accelerated fibrosis progression in chronic hepatitis C. J Hepatol 2009;51:655–66.

22. Leandro G, Mangia A, Hui J, et al. Relationship between steatosis, inflammation, and fibrosis in chronic hepatitis C: a meta-analysis of individual patient data. Gastroenterology 2006;130:1636–42.

23. Nkontchou G, Ziol M, Aout M, et al. HCV genotype 3 is associated with a higher hepatocellular carcinoma incidence in patients with ongoing viral C cirrhosis. J Viral Hepat 2011;18:516–22.

24. Ampuero J, Del Campo JA, Rojas L, et al. Fine-mapping butyrophilin family genes revealed several polymorphisms influencing viral genotype selection in hepatitis C infection. Genes Immun 2015;16:297–300.

25. Foster G, Pianko S, Cooper C, et al. Sofosbuvir + peginterferon/ribavirin for 12 weeks vs sofosbuvir + ribavirin for 16 or 24 weeks in genotype 3 HCV infected patients and treatment-experienced cirrhotic patients with genotype 2 HCV: the BOSON study. J Hepatol 2015;S1:1–186.

26. Nelson DR, Cooper JN, Lalezari JP, et al. All-oral 12-week treatment with daclatasvir plus sofosbuvir in patients with hepatitis C virus genotype 3 infection: ALLY-3 phase III study. Hepatology 2015;61:1127–35.

27. Gane EJ, Hyland RH, An D, et al. Sofosbuvir/ledipasvir fixed dose combination is safe and effective in HCV infected populations including decompensated patients and patients with prior sofosbuvir treatment experience. Gastroenterology 2014;146:S904–5.

28. Gane EJ, Hyland R, An D, et al. Once daily sofosbuvir with GS-5816 for 8 weeks with or without ribavirin in patients with HCV genotype 3 without cirrhosis result in high rates of SVR12: the Electron2 study. Hepatology 2014;60:1045–695.

29. Gane EJ, Hyland RH, An D, et al. High efficacy of LDV/SOF regimens for 12 weeks for patients with HCV genotype 3 or 6 infection. Hepatology 2014;60:1042–695.

30. Pianko S, Flamm S, Shiffman M, et al. High efficacy of treatment with sofosbuvir + GS-5816 ± ribavirin for 12 weeks in treatment experienced patients with genotype 1 or 3 HCV infection. Hepatology 2014;60:1045–695.

31. Najafzadeh M, Andersson K, Shrank WH, et al. Cost-effectiveness of novel regimens for the treatment of hepatitis C virus. Ann Intern Med 2015;162:407–19.

32. Linas BP, Barter DM, Morgan JR, et al. The cost-effectiveness of sofosbuvir-based regimens for treatment of hepatitis C virus genotype 2 or 3 Infection. Ann Intern Med 2015;162(9):619–29.
33. Eslam M, Leung R, Romero-Gomez M, et al. IFNL3 polymorphisms predict response to therapy in chronic hepatitis C genotype 2/3 infection. J Hepatol 2014;61:235–41.
34. Romero-Gómez M, Viloria MM, Andrade RJ, et al. Insulin resistance impairs sustained response rate to peginterferon plus ribavirin in chronic hepatitis C patients. Gastroenterology 2005;128:636–41.
35. Ferenci P. Treatment of hepatitis C in difficult-to-treat patients. Nat Rev Gastroenterol Hepatol 2015;12(5):284–92.
36. Romero-Gómez M, Turnes J, Ampuero J, et al. Prediction of week 4 virological response in hepatitis C for making decision on triple therapy: the Optim study. PLoS One 2015;10:e0122613.
37. Quer J, Gregori J, Rodríguez-Frias F, et al. High-resolution hepatitis C virus subtyping using NS5B deep sequencing and phylogeny, an alternative to current methods. J Clin Microbiol 2015;53:219–26.
38. Harvoni (ledipasvir/sofosbuvir) prescribing information. Foster City (CA): Gilead Sciences; 2014.
39. Romero-Gómez M, Berenguer M, Molina E, et al. Management of anemia induced by triple therapy in patients with chronic hepatitis C: challenges, opportunities and recommendations. J Hepatol 2013;59:1323–30.
40. European Association for the Study of the Liver. EASL recommendations on treatment of hepatitis C 2015. J Hepatol 2015;63(1):199–236.
41. Abraham GM, Spooner LM. Sofosbuvir in the treatment of chronic hepatitis C: new dog, new tricks. Clin Infect Dis 2014;59:411–5.

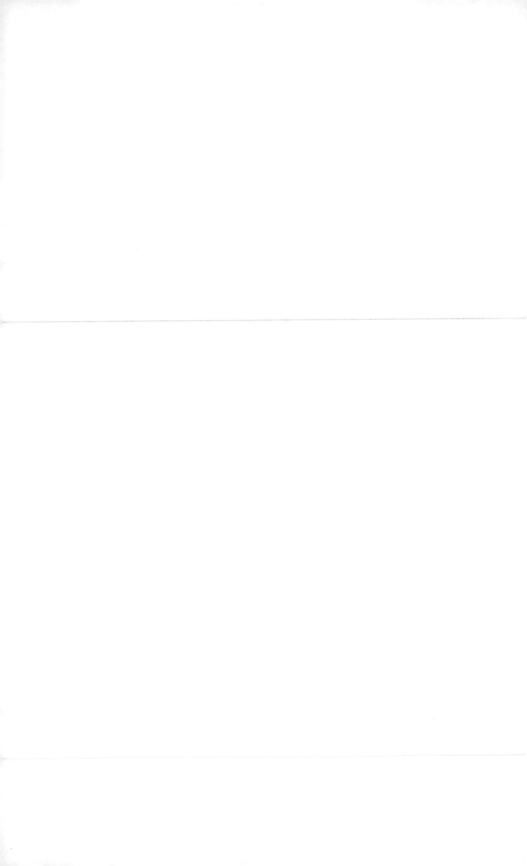

Hepatitis C Virus

Current and Evolving Treatments for Genotype 4

Tarik Asselah, MD, PhD[a],*, Marc Bourlière, MD[b]

KEYWORDS

- Direct-acting antivirals • Sofosbuvir • Ledipasvir • Paritaprevir • Ombitasvir • Egypt
- Access to treatment • Screening

KEY POINTS

- Hepatitis C virus (HCV) genotype 4 (GT4) accounts for approximately 20% of all cases of HCV among the 170 million of HCV-infected subjects worldwide (approximately 34 million).
- HCV infection has high prevalence in the Middle East and sub-Saharan Africa regions, and has recently been increasing in southern Europe.
- A major predictor of response to pegylated interferon and ribavirin therapy in patients with HCV GT4 was the interleukin (IL)-28B genotype. Sustained virological response (SVR) rates for patients with IL-28B rs12979860 CC ranged from more than 80% to approximately 30% for patients with genotype TT.
- In patients infected with HCV GT4, SVR with different direct-acting antivirals appears to provide high SVR rates and good tolerability. The primary limitations of these clinical trials on HCV GT4 are their small sample size and the relatively mild stage of liver disease of the patients included.
- Sofosbuvir plus ledipasvir and the combination of paritaprevir/r plus ombitasvir plus ribavirin have demonstrated high SVR rates in small clinical studies. Grazoprevir and elbasvir with and without ribavirin has shown promising response in GT4-infected patients.

Disclosure: T. Asselah is a speaker and investigator for AbbVie, BMS, Janssen, Gilead, Roche, and Merck. M. Bourlière is a speaker and investigator for AbbVie, BMS, Janssen, Gilead, Roche, and Merck.
[a] Department of Hepatology, Beaujon Hospital, UNITY, INSERM, UMR1149, Team Viral hepatitis, Centre de Recherche sur l'inflammation, Labex INFLAMEX, Université Denis Diderot Paris 7, 100 Bd du Général Leclerc, Clichy, Cedex 92110, France; [b] Saint Joseph Hospital, Marseilles 13008, France
* Corresponding author. Hepatology, Centre de Recherche sur l'Inflammation (CRI), UMR 1149 Inserm, Université Paris Diderot, Service d'Hépatologie, AP-HP Hôpital Beaujon, 100 Bd du Général Leclerc, Clichy 92110, France.
E-mail address: tarik.asselah@aphp.fr

Gastroenterol Clin N Am 44 (2015) 859–870
http://dx.doi.org/10.1016/j.gtc.2015.07.013
gastro.theclinics.com

HEPATITIS C VIRUS GENOTYPE 4 EPIDEMIOLOGY AND VIRUS DIVERSITY

Hepatitis C virus (HCV) genotype 4 (GT4) accounts for approximately 20% among the 170 millions of HCV-infected subjects worldwide (approximately 34 million). This population accounts for most new infections that have limited access to therapy. Although HCV GT4 is responsible for 1% to 2% of HCV infections in the United States, it is the main cause of HCV infection in the Middle East and sub-Saharan Africa regions, and has recently been increasing in southern Europe.[1–3] However, only limited country-specific estimates of HCV prevalence are available. In Egypt, where the prevalence of HCV is the highest in the world, the reuse of glass syringes during the parenteral therapy campaigns to control endemic schistosomiasis is widely held to be responsible for a very large number of iatrogenic transmissions.[4] GT4 has a large diversity with numerous subtypes.[5] In Egypt, GT4a is predominant, and in sub-Saharan Africa subtypes non-4a and non-4d account for most infections. In France and southern Europe, all the subtypes are represented, depending on country where patients immigrated and also the source of contamination.

PEGYLATED INTERFERON PLUS RIBAVIRIN: HISTORICAL PERSPECTIVES

HCV GT4 has been considered "difficult to treat" with pegylated interferon (PEG) and ribavirin (RBV), with sustained virological response (SVR) rates of approximately 50%. Large real-life cohort data have been published and provide interesting information,[6,7] regarding proportion of patients with HCV GT4, and SVR. In the real-life cohort Prophesys, HCV GT4 has been underrepresented with approximately 7% of the total number of patients treated (317/4520 = 7%).[6] The SVR rate was 41% (130/317) (**Fig. 1**A). In a German real-life cohort, HCV GT4 prevalence was low (474/7835) = 6%, with an SVR rate of 44% (207/474)[7] (see **Fig. 1**B).

A major predictor of response to PEG-RBV therapy in patients with HCV GT4 was the interleukin (IL)-28B genotype.[8,9] SVR rates for patients with IL-28B rs12979860 CC ranged from more than 80% to approximately 30% for patients with genotype TT. Egyptian patients infected with HCV GT4 treated with PEG-RBV in Europe responded better than French/European or African patients infected with the same genotype[8] (**Fig. 2**). An overall better response was observed in patients infected with the HCV GT4 subtype 4a, which was the predominant subtype among patients infected in Egypt compared with patients from sub-Saharan Africa. IL-28B polymorphism distribution among different ethnicities may be the explanation for this difference in terms of SVR: rs12979860 CC is more frequent among Egyptian than among Caucasian, and even more than among black Africans.[8]

NEW HOPE WITH DATA AVAILABLE WITH DIRECT-ACTING ANTIVIRALS FOR HEPATITIS C VIRUS GENOTYPE 4

The introduction of all-oral, interferon (IFN)-free regimens that combine direct-acting antiviral (DAA) agents has significantly advanced the treatment of HCV, especially for patients with HCV GT1 infection.[10,11] High efficacy rates (greater than 95%), short treatment duration (12 weeks), and favorable adverse event (AE) profiles have been demonstrated with multiple regimens, both with and without RBV. Several original articles reporting efficacy of DAAs for the treatment of chronic GT4 HCV infection have been published recently. However, we have to recognize that the total number of trials with DAAs in patients with HCV GT4 infection is limited and with a small number of patients.

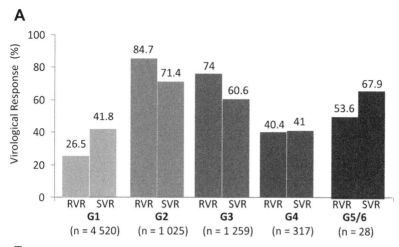

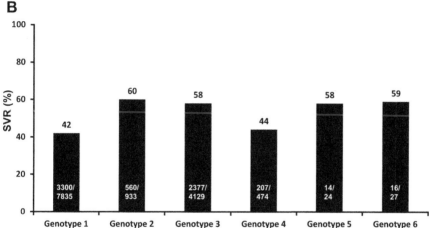

Fig. 1. (*A*) SVR with PEG-IFN plus RBV in the real-life cohort Prophesys. HCV GT4 has been underrepresented with approximately 7% of the total number of patients treated (317/4520 = 7%). SVR rate was 41% (130/317). (*B*) SVR with PEG-IFN plus RBV in a German real-life cohort, HCV-GT4 prevalence was low (474/7835) = 6%, with an SVR rate of 44% (207/474). (*Data from* [*A*] Marcellin P, Cheinquer H, Curescu M, et al. High sustained virologic response rates in rapid virologic response patients in the large real-world PROPHESYS cohort confirm results from randomized clinical trials. Hepatology 2012;56(6):2039–50; and Mauss S, Berger F, Vogel M, et al. Treatment results of chronic hepatitis C genotype 5 and 6 infections in Germany. Z Gastroenterol 2012;50(5):441–4; [*B*] Mauss S, Berger F, Vogel M, et al. Treatment results of chronic hepatitis C genotype 5 and 6 infections in Germany. Z Gastroenterol 2012;50(5):441–4.)

DIRECT-ACTING ANTIVIRALS PLUS PEGYLATED INTERFERON PLUS RIBAVIRIN

Data from several studies with PEG-IFN have recently become available, and the data are summarized in **Fig. 3**.[12–15]

SOFOSBUVIR PLUS PEGYLATED INTERFERON PLUS RIBAVIRIN (NEUTRINO STUDY)

Sofosbuvir is the first-in-class, potent nucleotide analogue polymerase inhibitor that acts as a chain terminator within the catalytic site of the NS5B polymerase.[16]

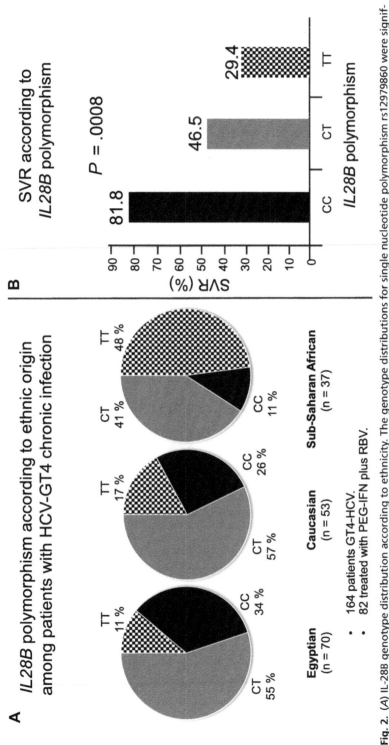

Fig. 2. (A) IL-28B genotype distribution according to ethnicity. The genotype distributions for single nucleotide polymorphism rs12979860 were significantly different among the 3 ethnic groups: Egyptian, Caucasian, and sub-Saharan African. (B) IL-28B rs12979860 CC genotype was associated with a better treatment response rate. The response rates were 81.8%, 46.5%, and 29.4% for genotype CC, CT, and TT, respectively. (Data from [B] Asselah T, De Muynck S, Broët P, et al. IL28B polymorphism is associated with treatment response in patients with genotype 4 chronic hepatitis C. J Hepatol 2012;56(3):527–32.)

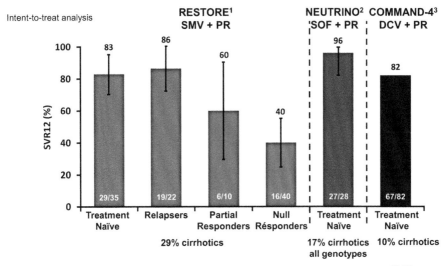

Fig. 3. Results (SVR12) in studies involving DAAs with PEG-IFN. (*Data from* Refs.[12–15])

The Neutrino trial was a single-group, open-label phase III study of sofosbuvir (SOF) plus PEG-IFN/RBV in 327 naïve patients infected with HCV GT 1, 4, 5, or 6.[13] Most of the patients who were included in the study had HCV GT1 (89%), 9% had GT4, and 2% had GT5 or 6. All patients received SOF, PEG-IFN/RBV for 12 weeks. Sofosbuvir was given orally at a dose of 400 mg, once a day, along with RBV, also given orally in a dose based on body weight. A total of 295 (90%) of the 327 patients had an SVR12. According to the HCV genotype: 89% for patients with HCV GT1 and 96% (27/28) of those with GT4 had SVR.

Almost all the patients with HCV GT4 had HCV GT4a subtypes (Egyptian ancestry). The single patient with G5 and all 6 patients with G6 in this trial had an SVR. Treatment discontinuation because of AEs was uncommon among patients receiving SOF regimens, with rates of 2%. The most common AEs in all patient groups were fatigue, headache, nausea, and insomnia.

SIMEPREVIR PLUS PEGYLATED INTERFERON PLUS RIBAVIRIN (RESTORE STUDY)

Simeprevir is a second-wave first-generation NS3/4A protease inhibitor with potent antiviral activity in HCV GT1, GT2, and GT4.

The Restore study was an open-label, single-arm study to assess the efficacy and safety of simeprevir (SMV) with PEG-IFN-α-2a/RBV in patients with chronic HCV GT4 infection (NCT01567735).[14] A total of 107 patients that included, treatment-naïve (n = 35) and prior relapsers (n = 22) received SMV 150 mg every day + PEG-IFN/RBV (12 weeks), followed by PEG-IFN/RBV alone (12 or 36 weeks, response-guided [HCV RNA <25 IU/mL detectable/undetectable at week 4 and <25 IU/mL undetectable at week 12]). Previous nonresponders (partial, n = 10; null, n = 40) received SMV/PEG-IFN/RBV (12 weeks), followed by PEG-IFN/RBV for 36 weeks. Overall, 65.4% (70/107) of patients achieved SVR12 (82.9% [29/35] treatment-naïve, 86.4% [19/22] prior relapsers, 60.0% [6/10] prior partial responders, 40.0% [16/40] prior null responders). In treatment-naïve and prior relapser patients fulfilling response-guided criteria for 24 weeks of treatment (88.6% [31/35] and 90.9% [20/22]), SVR12 rates were high: 93.5% (29/31) and 95.0% (19/20), respectively. Overall on-treatment failure and relapse rates were 23.4% (25/107) and 14.6% (12/82), respectively. AEs were mainly grade 1/2; serious AEs were infrequent (4.7%) and considered unrelated to SMV. The SVR12 rate in patients with METAVIR score F4 was 46.7% (14/30); of note, most of these patients (63%; 19/30) were prior partial and null responders. The SVR12 rate in patients with METAVIR score F0 to F2 was 76.3% (45/59) compared with 66.7% (10/15) in patients with F3; 37% (22/59) of patients with METAVIR F0 to F2 and 13% (2/15) of those with F3 were prior partial or null responders. The effectiveness of protease inhibitor–based regimens in combination with PEG-IFN/RBV may be limited in patients who are nonresponders to previous PEG-IFN/RBV therapy. The investigators concluded that efficacy and safety of SMV 150 mg every day for 12 weeks with PEG-IFN/RBV in treatment-naïve or experienced patients with chronic HCV GT4 infection were in line with previous reports for HCV GT1 infection. These results support the use of an response guided therapy-based approach to individualize the duration of treatment in HCV GT4–infected patients. Shortening of treatment duration in these patients may be beneficial, as it would reduce overall drug exposure and minimize therapy costs. A 12-week trial with SMV and PEG-IFN/RBV is ongoing (NCT01846832).

DACLATASVIR PLUS PEGYLATED INTERFERON PLUS RIBAVIRIN (COMMAND STUDY)

Daclatasvir (DCV) is a potent first-in-class NS5A inhibitor that has been shown to have pangenotypic activity.[17,18]

The addition of the NS5A inhibitor DCV to a 24-week course of PEG-IFN/RBV improved SVR rates in patients with HCV to 67% with a single oral daily dose of 20 mg, and to 100% with a 60-mg dose compared with 50% with standard 48-week PEG-IFN/RBV treatment.[15]

In a phase 2b double-blind, placebo-controlled study, treatment-naïve adults with HCV GT4 (n = 30) infection were randomly assigned (2:2:1) to DCV 20 mg or 60 mg, or placebo once daily plus weekly PEG-IFN-α-2a and twice-daily RBV. DCV recipients achieving protocol-defined response (PDR; HCV-RNA < lower limit of quantitation at week 4 and undetectable at week 10) were rerandomised at week 12 to continue DCV/ PEG-IFN-α-2a/RBV for 24 weeks' total duration or to placebo/PEG-IFN-α-2a/ RBV for another 12 weeks. Patients without PDR and placebo patients continued PEG-IFN-α/RBV through week 48. Primary efficacy endpoints were undetectable HCV-RNA at weeks 4 and 12 (extended rapid virologic response) and at 24 weeks after treatment (SVR24).

High proportions of GT4-infected patients receiving DCV 20 mg (66.7%; 8/12) or 60 mg (100.0%; 12/12) achieved SVR24 versus placebo (50.0%; 3/6). Most DCV-treated patients achieved PDR and experienced less virologic failure and higher SVR24 rates with a shortened 24-week treatment duration. AEs occurred with similar frequency across all treatment groups.

The investigators concluded that the combination of DCV/PEG-IFN-α/RBV was generally well tolerated and achieved higher SVR24 rates compared with placebo/ PEG-IFN-α/RBV among patients infected with HCV GT4.

INTERFERON-FREE REGIMEN
Sofosbuvir Plus Ribavirin

An open-label phase 2 study was done to assess the efficacy and safety of SOF in combination with RBV in patients of Egyptian ancestry chronically infected with GT4 HCV (ClinicalTrials.gov Identifier NCT01713283).[19] Treatment-naïve (n = 30) and previously treated patients (n = 30) with GT4 HCV were randomly allocated in a 1:1 ratio to receive SOF 400 mg and weight-based RBV for 12 or 24 weeks. SVR12 was achieved by 68% of patients (95% confidence interval [CI] 49%–83%) in the 12-week group and 93% of patients (95% CI 77%–99%) in the 24-week group. This study suggested that 24 weeks of SOF plus RBV is an efficacious and well-tolerated treatment in patients with HCV GT4 infection. No viable resistance-associated variants were detected in any of the patients who did not achieve SVR. Overall and in nearly every patient subgroup, patients receiving 24 weeks of treatment had substantially higher rates of SVR12 than patients receiving 12 weeks of treatment. In this study, the number of patients overall was small. Especially for difficult-to-treat patients with cirrhosis, efficacy of this regimen will be defined only by future trials.

A recent trial performed in Egypt provided similar results.[20] Treatment-naïve or treatment-experienced patients with GT4 HCV infection (n = 103) were randomly assigned to receive either 12 or 24 weeks of SOF 400 mg and RBV 1000 to 1200 mg daily. Randomization was stratified by previous treatment experience and by presence or absence of cirrhosis. Among all patients, 52% had received previous HCV treatment and 17% had cirrhosis at baseline. SVR12 rates were 90% (46/51) with 24 weeks and 77% (40/52) with 12 weeks of SOF and RBV therapy. Patients with cirrhosis at baseline had lower rates of SVR12 (63% 12 weeks, 78% 24 weeks) than those without cirrhosis (80% 12 weeks, 93% 24 weeks).

There is a very large national Egyptian program ongoing with the use of this regimen, and we hope data will soon become available. Nevertheless, compared with other regimens, the SVR rate with 24 weeks of SOF and RBV appears to be suboptimal in particular among the patients with cirrhosis and should be considered only if no other options are available.

SOFOSBUVIR PLUS LEDIPASVIR (SYNERGY STUDY AND TRIAL GS 1119)

Synergy is a single-center, open-label, phase 2a trial of LDV/SOF for 12 weeks in 20 patients with HCV GT 4. SVR12 was 95% (19/20) (**Fig. 4**A).[21] Thirty-eight percent of the participants had been treated before, but none of them with DAAs. Ten percent had advanced fibrosis and 33% had compensated cirrhosis. Twenty participants achieved a sustained virologic response 12 weeks after completing therapy (SVR12, considered a cure), for a cure rate of 95%. The one person who was not cured stopped treatment after the first dose. The regimen was generally safe and well tolerated.

An open-label phase 2 study of SOF/LDV conducted in France (Study GS-US-337–1119, O056), noted high SVR rates in both treatment-naïve and treatment-experienced patients with chronic HCV GT4 or GT5 infection, 50% of whom had cirrhosis (NCT02081079).[22] Ninety-three percent of patients with GT4 (41/44) and 95% of patients with GT5 (39/41) achieved SVR12 (see **Fig. 4**B). GT4 subtypes were well represented: 4a (n = 25), 4d (n = 10), non-4a non-4d (n = 9). Response rates were similar among both treatment-naïve and treatment-experienced patients and regardless of cirrhosis. The most common AEs (affecting more than 10% of patients) were asthenia, headache, and fatigue. This regimen appears to be highly effective with an SVR of more than 90% in the patients with HCV GT4.

SOFOSBUVIR AND SIMEPREVIR

In the French HEPATHER real-life cohort, 34 patients with HCV GT4 (28 with compensated cirrhosis) were treated with SOF plus simeprevir (SIM) for 12 or 24 weeks with RBV in 7 patients. Only 2 patients with cirrhosis relapsed in the group treated without

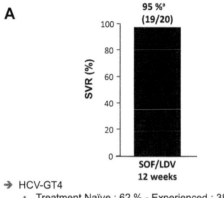

→ HCV-GT4
  • Treatment Naïve : 62 % - Experienced : 38 %
  • Fibrosis F3-F4 : 43 %

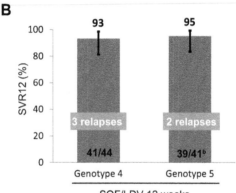

SOF/LDV 12 weeks

Fig. 4. (*A*) Single-center, open-label, phase 2a trial of LDV/SOF for 12 weeks in 20 patients with HCV GT4. SVR12 was 95% (Synergy). [a] 1 Withdrew consent. 1 patient did not reach SVR12 time point. (*B*) Open-label phase 2 study of SOF/LDV conducted in France (Study GS-US-337–1119, O056). Ninety-three percent of patients with GT4 (41/44) and 95% of patients with GT5 (39/41) achieved SVR12. [b] 1 GT 5 supposed to have reached SVR12 with the result of SVR24. (*Data from* [A] Kapoor R, Kohli A, Sidharthan S, et al. All oral treatment for genotype 4 chronic hepatitis C infection with sofosbuvir and ledipasvir: interim results from the NIAID synergy trial. [abstract]. Hepatology 2014;60:321A; [B] Abergel A, Loustaud-Ratti V, Metivier S, et al. Ledipasvir/sofosbuvir treatment results in high SVR rates in patients with chronic genotype 4 and 5 HCV infection. EASL; 2015.)

RBV. All patients treated with RBV achieved an SVR.[23] Therefore, this regimen appears to be a valuable IFN-free options in patients with HCV GT4.

SOFOSBUVIR AND DACLATASVIR

In the French HEPATHER real-life cohort, 48 patients with HCV GT4 (39 with compensated cirrhosis) were treated with SOF plus DCV for 12 or 24 weeks with RBV in 15 patients. Only 1 patient with cirrhosis relapsed in the group treated without RBV. All patients treated with RBV achieved an SVR.[23] Therefore, this regimen appears to be another IFN-free option in patients with HCV GT4.

OMBITASVIR/PARITAPREVIR/RITONAVIR (PEARL STUDY)

Ombitasvir/paritaprevir/ritonavir (OBV/PTV/r) represents an efficient regimen for HCV-GT4. OBV (formerly ABT-267) is a potent NS5A inhibitor. PTV (formerly ABT-450) is a potent NS3/4A protease inhibitor (identified by AbbVie and Enanta) that is coadministered with low-dose ritonavir (PTV/r) to increase the peak, trough, and overall drug exposures of PTV/r and thus enabling once-daily dosing. OBV/PTV/r is coformulated as a tablet, taken as 2 tablets once daily with weight-based RBV.

The PEARL-I study enrolled subjects with HCV GT4 infection (**Fig. 5**). Eighty-six treatment-naïve patients were enrolled and randomized to receive 12 weeks of OBV/PTV/r with RBV (42) or without RBV (44). Forty-nine treatment-experienced patients were enrolled and treated with 12 weeks of OBV/PTV/r plus RBV.[24] SVR was achieved in 40/44 (91%) patients who received 12 weeks of OBV/PTV/r without RBV. All treatment naïve or treatment-experienced patients who received OBV/PTV/r with RBV for 12 weeks achieved an SVR. However, in this large study, patients with cirrhosis were not included. Treatment was well tolerated, with low rates of treatment discontinuation. Thus this regimen appeared to be very effective in patients without cirrhosis. An ongoing study is being conducted to determine if 24 weeks' treatment duration can achieve the same results in patients with cirrhosis.

DACLATASVIR, ASUNAPREVIR, AND BECLABUVIR

A randomized, open-label, phase 2a study that included 21 HCV GT4 naïve patients, explored the efficacy and safety of the oral combination of DCV (NS5A inhibitor),

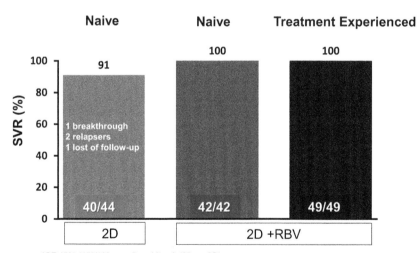

ABT-450/r (150/100 mg qd); ombitasvir (25 mg QD)
RBV (weight-based 1000 or 1200 mg/day divided BID)

Fig. 5. The PEARL-I study enrolled subjects with HCV GT1b and GT4 infection; those with GT4 were treated for 12 weeks with OBV/PTV/r.[20] A sustained virologic response (HCV RNA <25 IU/mL) rate 12 weeks posttreatment (SVR12) of 100% was achieved among treatment-naïve and prior PEG-IFN and RBV-experienced HCV GT4–infected subjects without cirrhosis who received OBV/PTV/r with RBV. BID, twice a day; QD, every day. (*Data from* Hézode C, Asselah T, Reddy KR, et al. A randomized, open-label study of ombitasvir and ABT-450/r with or without ribavirin in treatment-naïve and treatment-experienced patients with chronic hepatitis C virus infection (PEARL-I): results in patients with genotype 4 infection. Lancet 2015;385(9986):2502–9.)

asunaprevir (NS3 protease inhibitor), and beclabuvir (non-nucleoside NS5B polymerase inhibitor) (NCT01455090).[25] The patients (n = 21) were enrolled at 9 sites in the United States as an expansion of a larger study, and were randomized 1:1 to receive a twice-daily oral regimen comprising 75 mg or 150 mg of beclabuvir, each with DCV (30 mg) and asunaprevir (200 mg), for 12 weeks with 48 weeks of posttreatment follow-up. HCV-RNA decline was rapid: median (range) log10 change from baseline at day 7 was −4.39 (−4.91, −2.95) IU/mL in the 75-mg beclabuvir group and −4.01 (−5.03, −3.47) IU/mL in the 150-mg group. All patients had less than 25 IU/mL by week 2 of treatment. Two patients, one in each treatment arm, had missing data at posttreatment week 12, but were confirmed to have HCV RNA less than 25 IU/mL after week 12, and therefore all patients achieved an SVR. Concordance between SVR12 and SVR24 was 100% in the 9 patients in each arm with available HCV-RNA data at both these posttreatment time points. Although baseline resistance associated variants in NS5A were observed in just fewer than half of the patients assessed, there were no on-treatment virologic failures, and no posttreatment relapses through the primary endpoint or in any patient for whom post-SVR12 data were available at time of analysis. There were no notable safety or tolerability issues, consistent with previous data for this regimen with GT1. The use of a fixed-dose combination tablet currently is under phase 3 evaluation.

The efficacy of grazoprevir (100 mg) and elbasvir (50 mg) with and without RBV was evaluated in GT4-infected patients in the phase 2/3 clinical program. Data from a total of 66 treatment-naïve and 37 treatment-experienced GT4 subjects, including 17 patients with cirrhosis, were analyzed. Overall, 64 (97%) of 66 treatment-naïve (including 6 of 6 patients with cirrhosis) and 32 (86%) of 37 treatment-experienced GT4 subjects achieved SVR12.

SUMMARY

Despite the small number of HCV GT4 patients included in most studies and real-life cohorts, several IFN-free DAA combinations with high efficacy are now available. Twelve weeks' treatment duration appears sufficient in patients without cirrhosis. The use of RBV for SOF/DCV, SOF/SIM, or SOF/LDV regimen is useful in those with cirrhosis and with a 12-week treatment duration. In case of RBV intolerance, the duration of treatment may need to be increased to 24 weeks (especially in patients with predictors of nonresponse). For the OBV/PTV/r regimen, the use of RBV is recommended.

We will need to increase the knowledge regarding HCV GT4 infection and to perform more studies. Finally, the primary limitations of the available clinical trials on HCV GT4 are their small sample size and the relatively mild stage of liver disease of the patients included. In real life, we first treat the patients with advanced fibrosis (F3/F4) and we need particular data for this population. Moreover, the large number of HCV GT4 subtypes may be of importance in terms of antiviral activities of DAAs (NS5A inhibitors and especially non-nucleoside NS5B inhibitors). With the limited available data, we face difficulties providing advice or guidance to help physicians with their patients. Finally, there is optimism for patients with GT4 HCV infection, with several promising ongoing trials.[26,27] With these excellent data, the next steps will be to improve screening and access to therapy.[28]

REFERENCES

1. Abdel-Razek W, Waked I. Optimal therapy in genotype 4 chronic hepatitis C: finally cured? Liver Int 2015;35(Suppl 1):27–34.

2. Messina JP, Humphreys I, Flaxman A, et al. Global distribution and prevalence of hepatitis C virus genotypes. Hepatology 2015;61(1):77–87.
3. Gower E, Estes C, Blach S, et al. Global epidemiology and genotype distribution of the hepatitis C virus infection. J Hepatol 2014;61(Suppl 1):S45–57.
4. Frank C, Mohamed MK, Strickland GT, et al. The role of parenteral antischistosomal therapy in the spread of hepatitis C virus in Egypt. Lancet 2000;355(9207): 887–91.
5. Smith DB, Bukh J, Kuiken C, et al. Expanded classification of hepatitis C virus into 7 genotypes and 67 subtypes: updated criteria and genotype assignment web resource. Hepatology 2014;59:318–27.
6. Marcellin P, Cheinquer H, Curescu M, et al. High sustained virologic response rates in rapid virologic response patients in the large real-world PROPHESYS cohort confirm results from randomized clinical trials. Hepatology 2012;56(6):2039–50.
7. Mauss S, Berger F, Vogel M, et al. Treatment results of chronic hepatitis C genotype 5 and 6 infections in Germany. Z Gastroenterol 2012;50(5):441–4.
8. Asselah T, De Muynck S, Broët P, et al. IL28B polymorphism is associated with treatment response in patients with genotype 4 chronic hepatitis C. J Hepatol 2012;56(3):527–32.
9. Estrabaud E, Vidaud M, Marcellin P, et al. Genomics and HCV infection: progression of fibrosis and treatment response. J Hepatol 2012;57:1110–25.
10. Schinazi R, Halfon P, Marcellin P, et al. HCV direct-acting antiviral agents: the best interferon-free combinations. Liver Int 2014;34(Suppl 1):69–78.
11. Wendt A, Adhoute X, Castellani P, et al. Chronic hepatitis C: future treatment. Clin Pharmacol 2014;6:1–17.
12. Asselah T. Optimism for patients with genotype 4 HCV infection: clinical trials with direct-acting antivirals finally available. J Hepatol 2015;62(5):996–9.
13. Lawitz E, Mangia A, Wyles D, et al. Sofosbuvir for previously untreated chronic hepatitis C infection. N Engl J Med 2013;368:1878–87.
14. Moreno C, Hezode C, Marcellin P, et al. Efficacy and safety of simeprevir with PegIFN/ribavirin in naïve or experienced patients infected with chronic HCV genotype 4. J Hepatol 2015;62(5):1047–55.
15. Hézode C, Hirschfield GM, Ghesquiere W, et al. Daclatasvir plus peginterferon alfa and ribavirin for treatment-naive chronic hepatitis C genotype 1 or 4 infection: a randomised study. Gut 2015;64(6):948–56.
16. Asselah T. Sofosbuvir for the treatment of hepatitis C virus. Expert Opin Pharmacother 2014;15:121–30.
17. Gao M, Nettles RE, Belema M, et al. Chemical genetics strategy identifies an HCV NS5A inhibitor with a potent clinical effect. Nature 2010;465:96–100.
18. Asselah T. NS5A inhibitors: a new breakthrough for the treatment of chronic hepatitis C. J Hepatol 2011;54:1069–72.
19. Ruane PJ, Ain D, Stryker R, et al. Sofosbuvir plus ribavirin for the treatment of chronic genotype 4 hepatitis C virus infection in patients of Egyptian ancestry. J Hepatol 2015;62(5):1040–6.
20. Doss W, Shiha G, Hassany M, et al. Sofosbuvir plus ribavirin for treating Egyptian patients with hepatitis C genotype 4. J Hepatol 2015;63(3):581–5.
21. Kapoor R, Kohli A, Sidharthan S, et al. All oral treatment for genotype 4 chronic hepatitis C infection with sofosbuvir and ledipasvir: interim results from the NIAID Synergy Trial [abstract]. Hepatology 2014;60:321A.
22. Abergel A, Loustaud-Ratti V, Metivier S, et al. Ledipasvir/sofosbuvir treatment results in high SVR rates in patients with chronic genotype 4 and 5 HCV infection. J Hepatol 2015;62(Suppl 2):S219.

23. Fontaine H, Hézode C, Zoulim F, et al. Efficacy of the oral sofosbuvir-based combinations in HCV genotype 4-mono-infected patients from the French observational cohort ANRS CO22 HEPATHER. J Hepatol 2015;62(Suppl 2):S278.

24. Hézode C, Asselah T, Reddy KR, et al. Ombitasvir plus paritaprevir plus ritonavir with or without ribavirin in treatment-naive and treatment-experienced patients with genotype 4 chronic hepatitis C virus infection (PEARL-I): a randomized, open-label trial. Lancet 2015;385(9986):2502–9.

25. Hassanein T, Sims KD, Bennett M, et al. A randomized trial of daclatasvir in combination with asunaprevir and beclabuvir in patients with chronic hepatitis C virus genotype 4 infection. J Hepatol 2015;62(5):1204–6.

26. Asselah T, Hassanein T, Qaqish RB, et al. A randomized, open-label study to evaluate efficacy and safety of ombitasvir/paritaprevir/ritonavir co-administered with ribavirin in adults with genotype 4 chronic hepatitis C infection and cirrhosis. J Hepatol 2015;62(Suppl 2):S1345.

27. Asselah T, Charlton M, Feld J, et al. The ASTRAL studies: evaluation of SOF/GS-5816 single tablet regimen for the treatment of genotype 1–6 HCV infection. J Hepatol 2015;62(Suppl 2):S1332.

28. Asselah T, Perumalswami PV, Dieterich D. Is screening baby boomers for HCV enough? A call to screen for hepatitis C virus in persons from countries of high endemicity. Liver Int 2014;34(10):1447–51.

Current Treatment Options in Patients with Hepatitis C Virus Genotype 6

Nghia H. Nguyen, MD, MAS[a,b], Mindie H. Nguyen, MD, MAS[c,*]

KEYWORDS

• Genotype 6 • SVR • Treatment • Direct-acting agents • Hepatitis C

KEY POINTS

- Hepatitis C virus (HCV) genotype 6 is geographically limited to countries in southeast Asia and the surrounding regions, where there is limited access to newer anti-HCV medications.
- Preliminary small clinical studies with direct-acting agents (ledipasvir with sofosbuvir fixed-dosed combination; grazoprevir plus elbasvir combination) have reported high sustained virologic response (SVR) rates in patients with HCV genotype 6 (>90%).
- The mainstays of therapy for these patients are currently pegylated interferon and ribavirin, which also lead to high SVR rates (approximately 80%).
- Additional studies are needed on the clinical effectiveness and tolerability of new direct-acting agents in patients with HCV-6.

INTRODUCTION

Hepatitis C virus (HCV) chronically infects more than 175 million people globally and is also one of the leading causes of liver cirrhosis and hepatocellular carcinoma worldwide.[1,2] HCV genotype 6 (HCV-6) is a subtype of HCV that is largely restricted to southeast Asia, its surrounding areas, and migrants coming from this region. In addition, the prevalence of HCV is also particularly high in several countries in southeast Asia and the surrounding regions (~6%–7% in Vietnam and Thailand) compared with a prevalence of 1.8% in the United States.[1–5]

It is widely recognized that HCV genotype is a major independent predictor of treatment response, measured by sustained virologic response (SVR; defined as undetectable HCV RNA, at 12 weeks [SVR12] or 24 weeks after end of treatment, which is

[a] School of Medicine, University of California, San Diego, La Jolla, CA, USA; [b] Division of Gastroenterology and Hepatology, Stanford University Medical Center, Palo Alto, CA, USA; [c] Liver Transplant Program, Division of Gastroenterology and Hepatology, Stanford University Medical Center, 750 Welch Road, #210, Palo Alto, CA 94304, USA
* Corresponding author.
E-mail address: mindiehn@stanford.edu

Gastroenterol Clin N Am 44 (2015) 871–881
http://dx.doi.org/10.1016/j.gtc.2015.07.010
0889-8553/15/$ – see front matter © 2015 Elsevier Inc. All rights reserved.
gastro.theclinics.com

considered to be a surrogate of virologic cure).[3-6] As mentioned previously, HCV-6 is geographically restricted to southeast Asia and the surrounding regions (China, Taiwan, Macau, Vietnam, Thailand, and Myanmar) and can often be the most common genotype in patients infected with HCV from this region, with a prevalence of approximately 30% to 40%.[1,3-5] However, the prevalence of HCV-6 in these countries also ranges widely: 18% in Thailand, 23.6% in Hong Kong, and 49% in Myanmar.[1,7,8] Studies of southeast Asian Americans showed HCV-6 prevalence of 41% in a sample cohort of 308 consecutive clinic-based patients.[9,10] Another important difference in the epidemiology of HCV infection in this region is that most patients contracted HCV via iatrogenic exposure with conventional medical care as well as with traditional remedies such as acupuncture, cupping, tattooing, and piercing, and this is the most likely route of HCV transmission for most patients with HCV-6 infection.[1,4,8]

The current standard of care for the treatment of patients with HCV-6 in the past decade or so has been pegylated interferon and ribavirin (PEG-IFN and RBV). Data from older studies with mostly Asian patients suggest that patients with HCV-6 respond better to PEG-IFN and RBV therapy (SVR ~80%) compared with patients with HCV-1 (SVR ~50%).[10-12] Previously, the question of the optimal treatment duration for patients with HCV-6 treated with PEG-IFN and RBV was unanswered, because results from older studies had been inconclusive because of small sample sizes. More recently, a meta-analysis on this topic found significantly lower SVR with 24 weeks compared with 48 weeks of PEG-IFN + plus RBV in patients with HCV-6 except for those with rapid virologic response (RVR; undetectable HCV RNA at 4 weeks after initiation of treatment) who may be treated with a shorter duration of 24 weeks.[13]

Although there has been a rapid growth of new direct-acting antiviral agents (DAAs) in recent years, and with them high rates of SVR, most of the data have been derived from clinical trials conducted in Western countries, where HCV-6 is rare.[14-18]

This article summarizes the currently available data for the treatment of patients with HCV-6 (**Box 1**).

PHARMACOLOGIC TREATMENT OPTIONS
Pegylated Interferon and Ribavirin

Combination therapy with PEG-IFN and RBV has been the mainstay therapy for patients with HCV-6 for more than a decade. Previous studies examining the treatment response of PEG-IFN and RBV reported a wide range of SVR rates and were unable to definitely assess the optimal treatment duration with this regimen.[1,5] Results from these studies were also limited by their small sample sizes and heterogeneous study methodologies.

A recent meta-analysis on PEG-IFN and RBV in HCV-6 was conducted to assess the effectiveness and optimal duration (48 vs 24 weeks) with this treatment regimen.[13] The meta-analysis included 13 studies (10 observational studies and 3 randomized controlled trials) with a total of 640 patients with HCV-6. The investigators observed a pooled overall SVR estimate of 77% (95% confidence interval [CI], 70%–83%), which suggested that patients with HCV-6 generally have a more favorable treatment response compared with historical results with PEG-IFN and RBV combination for other genotypes, such as genotypes 1 and 4. This favorable treatment response could partly be explained by the single-polynucleotide polymorphisms near the gene *IL-28B* on chromosome 19 that influences interferon (IFN) sensitivity and thus SVR rates in patients treated with IFN-based therapies. The more treatment-favorable *IL-28B* polymorphism (CC genotype) has been shown to be selectively distributed by geographic region and is more common in areas with a high prevalence of HCV-6.[19-21]

> **Box 1**
> **Patient evaluation overview**
>
> - Patients with the following risk factors should be tested and treated for HCV (per American Association for the Study of Liver Diseases guideline).
>   - Persons who were born between 1945 and 1965 should receive a 1-time HCV test.
>   - Men who have sex with men who undertake risky sexual behaviors.
>   - Persons who are actively injecting drugs or using illicit drugs via intranasal route.
>   - Persons who are incarcerated.
>   - Persons who received tattoos in an unregulated setting.
>   - Women who are wishing to become pregnant and are known to be infected with HCV.
>   - Health care workers who are infected with HCV who perform procedures that may expose patients to the risk of acquiring HCV.
>   - Persons who received blood transfusions, blood products, or any organ transplants before 1992. In addition, persons who received blood clotting factor concentrates that were produced before 1987 should also receive HCV testing.
>   - Persons with human immunodeficiency virus infection.
> - If patients are suspected to have HCV infection, then they should receive testing with an anti-HCV test. If the result is positive, then current HCV infection should be confirmed with an HCV RNA test.
>   - HCV RNA should be quantitatively measured before starting treatment to establish the baseline level of viremia.
>   - HCV genotype should also be determined to help guide selection of the most appropriate treatment regimen.
> - The goal of anti-HCV treatment is to induce virologic cure (SVR). SVR has been shown to reduce all-cause mortality and deleterious liver-related health outcomes (end-stage liver disease and hepatocellular carcinoma).

Subgroup analysis of 4 studies that had data available for direct comparison of SVR in patients with HCV-6 treated for 48 weeks versus 24 weeks in the meta-analysis mentioned earlier (149 patients treated for 48 weeks and 112 patients treated for 24 weeks) observed pooled SVR estimates of 74% and 59% in patients treated with PEG-IFN for 48 weeks and 24 weeks, respectively.[13] This difference in SVR rates was statistically significant with an odds ratio (OR) of 1.86 (CI, 1.08–3.21; $P = .026$) favoring the 48-week treatment course. In a separate subgroup analysis inclusive of 2 studies with direct comparison of patients with RVR and SVR data treated for 48 versus 24 weeks, there was no statistically significant difference in treatment response rates (85.5% vs 77.6%, respectively; OR, 1.74; CI, 0.65–4.64; $P = .27$). Data from this meta-analysis suggest that patients with PEG-IFN and RBV should be treated for 48 weeks, whereas those who achieve RVR may be treated for a shorter duration.[13] Preliminary results from a more recent randomized controlled trial in patients with HCV-6 with RVR treated for 24 versus 48 weeks with PEG-IFN and RBV further support the observation that there is no significant difference in treatment response rates if patients are treated for 24 versus 48 weeks if they have RVR.[22]

Treatment with PEG-IFN and RBV combination has also been shown to be safe in patients with genotype 6 (GT6) and the side effect profile in GT6 seems to be similar to what has been reported in landmark trials for HCV genotypes 1 to 3.[13,23,24]

Telaprevir-based or Boceprevir-based Regimens

The first-generation DAAs were the NS3/4A protease inhibitors boceprevir (Victrelis, Merck, Kenilworth, NJ) and telaprevir (Incivek, Vertex Pharmaceuticals, Boston, MA). Triple therapy with these protease inhibitors was highly potent with a low to intermediate barrier to resistance, and produced high rates of SVR compared with dual IFN-based therapies.[15,25] In 2011, they were approved for the treatment of HCV in combination with PEG-IFN and RBV but subsequently fell out of favor in the United States because of poor tolerability and the introduction of newer DAAs/second-generation protease inhibitors with fewer side effects, easier dosing schedules, and greater efficacy.[15,17,25]

Sofosbuvir

Sofosbuvir (SOF; GS-7977, Sovaldi, Gilead Sciences Inc, Foster City, CA) is a uridine nucleotide analogue that selectively inhibits HCV NS5B polymerase and has been shown to have intermediate to high potency, pangenotypic coverage, and a high resistance barrier. In the NEUTRINO study, which was an open-label, single-arm, phase III trial, 327 treatment-naive patients with genotypes 1 and 4 to 6 were treated with a 12-week regimen of SOF 400 mg orally daily plus PEG-IFN-2a 180 µg subcutaneously weekly and RBV 1000 to 1200 mg orally daily.[26] Only 6 patients in this study had HV-6 but all 6 achieved SVR12 (undetectable HCV RNA by polymerase chain reaction [PCR] 12 weeks after end of therapy) and the adverse events in these patients were similar to those seen with PEG-IFN and RBV therapy.[26]

In the ATOMIC trial, which was a separate open-label, randomized, multicenter phase II trial, there were 5 patients with HCV-6 who were assigned to 24 weeks of SOF (400 mg) plus PEG-IFN (180 µg weekly) and weight-based ribavirin (1000 mg [<75 kg] to 1200 mg [≥75 kg]).[27] All 5 patients achieved SVR (either at posttreatment week 12 or posttreatment week 24). Adverse event profiles for patients with HCV-6 were not available, but the investigators noted that, for the cohort, the most common adverse events were those typically seen with PEG-IFN and RBV: fatigue, headache, and nausea.[27]

To date, there have been no clinical trials evaluating the treatment and tolerability of SOF plus RBV as a combination therapy in patients with HCV-6. The only available data are from a retrospective study by Vu and colleagues[28] that reported treatment and safety data on patients with SMV-based and SOF-based treatments. A total of 5 patients with HCV-6 were treated with SOF plus weight-based RBV for either 12 or 24 weeks. SVR12 data were not yet available for these patients.

Although there are currently no data for SOF and weight-based RBV plus weekly PEG-IFN for 12 weeks in treatment-experienced patients, the American Association for the Study of Liver Diseases (AASLD) recommends that the same regimen can be used for treatment-experienced patients with HCV-6 infection in whom prior treatment has failed and who are IFN eligible.[6]

In 2014, phase III trial of a new DAA combination with SOF plus GS-5816 for chronic hepatitis C genotypes 1 to 6 was launched, with results expected to be available in late 2015 to early 2016.[29] GS-5816 is a pangenotypic NS5A inhibitor with picomolar potency against HCV genotypes 1 to 6. SOF plus GS-5816 was previously evaluated in an open-label, phase II trial in treatment-naive patients with HCV genotypes 1 to 6. Patients were assigned to 12 weeks of treatment with SOF (400 mg) plus GS-5816 (25 mg) or 12 weeks of treatment with SOF (400 mg) plus GS-5816 (100 mg). All patients were treatment naive and none had cirrhosis. No RBV was administered in this trial. There were a total of 154 patients enrolled in the study, with 9 patients with HCV-6: 4 were assigned to SOF plus GS-5816 25 mg and 5 were assigned to SOF plus GS-5816,100 mg. All 9 patients from both treatment groups achieved SVR12. Adverse event profiles for patients with HCV-6 were not analyzed separately but the treatment was well tolerated by the overall study patient population.[29]

Simeprevir

Simeprevir (SMV; TMC435, Olysio, Janssen Therapeutics, Titusville, NJ) is a second-generation NS3/4A protease inhibitor that was shown in a phase IIa proof-of-concept trial to have potent activity in patients with genotypes 4, 5, and 6 and with higher barriers to resistance compared with the first-generation protease inhibitors.[30] Although this phase II trial showed potent activity with SMV in patients with GT6, this medication was administered as a monotherapy, thus limiting the conclusion of these results. Since that small phase II study and the ensuing phase III clinical trials, SMV has been approved to be coadministered with SOF in the United States for the treatment of patients with HCV-1.[6] However, there have been limited treatment and tolerability data with this regimen in patients with HCV-6, with the only study to investigate this combination therapy a retrospective study by Vu and colleagues.[28] There were 3 patients who were treated with SMV plus SOF combination. RBV was not used in these patients, because they had severe renal insufficiency. Of these 3 patients, 2 had available SVR12 with both achieving SVR12. At present, the combination of SMV plus SOF has not received US Food and Drug Administration (FDA) approval in the United States for the treatment of HCV genotypes none-1, including HCV-6.

Daclatasvir

Daclatasvir (DCV; Daklinza, BMS-790052, Bristol-Myers Squibb, New York, NY) is a pangenotypic NS5A inhibitor that is given as a 60-mg once-daily dosing in combination with other DAAs and has been shown to be effective in patients with non-GT6.[31–33] At present, clinical data on DCV-based regimens in patients with HCV-6 are limited.

Ledipasvir

Ledipasvir (LDV; GS-5885, Gilead Sciences Inc, Foster City, CA) is a once-daily, oral, 90-mg NS5A inhibitor.[34] A small, 2-center, open-label study (NCT01826981) investigated the safety and in vivo efficacy of LDV plus SOF in a fixed-dose combination pill (also known as Harvoni) for 12 weeks in treatment-naive and treatment-experienced patients with HCV-6 infection.[35] The study include 25 patients, most of whom were treatment naive (92%) and Asian (88%) and included 7 different subtypes (32%, 6a; 24%, 6e; 12%, 6l; 8%, 6m; 12%, 6p; 8%, 6q; 4%, 6r). Only 2 patients (8%) had cirrhosis. The SVR12 rate was 96% (n = 24 out of 25), and the 1 patient who experienced relapse was discontinued from treatment at week 8 because of active illicit drug use. No patient discontinued treatment because of adverse events and the treatment was well tolerated (**Table 1**).

In the United States, based on the limited data provided from this small study, the AASLD guideline recommends that treatment-naive patients with HCV-6 be treated with a daily fixed-dose combination of LDV (90 mg)/SOF (400 mg) for 12 weeks.[6] Although there are currently no data on this regimen in treatment-experienced patients, this same combination is also recommended by the AASLD guideline for patients in whom prior treatment has failed.[6]

Table 1
Overall safety summary of LDV and SOF

Patients	HCV GT6 (n = 25); n (%)
Any AE	21 (84)
Grade 3/4 AE	1 (4)
Serious AE	1 (4)
Discontinuation because of AE	0 (0)
Grade 3/4 laboratory abnormality	1 (4)
Hemoglobin	
<10 g/dL	1 (4)
<8.5 g/dL	0 (0)
AEs in >5% of patients in any treatment arm	
AE	**HCV GT6 (n = 25); n (%)**
Fatigue	6 (24)
Headache	2 (8)
Upper respiratory tract infection	6 (24)
Insomnia	0 (0)
Rash	2 (8)
Diarrhea	4 (16)
Nausea	0 (0)
Lethargy	1 (4)
Irritability	0 (0)
Depression	2 (8)
Pruritus	0 (0)
Urinary tract infection	2 (8)

Abbreviation: AE, adverse event.
Data from Gane EJ, RH Hyland, An D, et al. High efficacy of LDV/SOF regimens for 12 weeks for patients with HCV genotype 3 or 6 infection. [abstract]. Hepatology 2014;60(Suppl):LB-11.

Grazoprevir-Elbasvir (Merck, Kenilworth, NJ)

Grazoprevir (100 mg)-elbasvir (50 mg) is an investigational, once-daily single-tablet formulation consisting of grazoprevir (NS3/4A protease inhibitor) and elbasvir (NS5A inhibitor).[36] In the phase III C-EDGE trial (a randomized, blinded, and placebo-controlled study), treatment-naive patients with genotypes 1, 4, and 6 were treated with this combination therapy for 12 weeks.[36] In the study, 13 patients with HCV-6 were enrolled with 10 assigned to the active arm, whereas 3 received placebo. Eight out of 10 patients from the treatment arm achieved SVR12, whereas 2 experienced virologic relapse.[36]

Ritonavir-boosted Paritaprevir, Ombitasvir, and Dasabuvir (Viekira Pak, AbbVie Inc, North Chicago, IL)

Paritaprevir (ABT-450/r) is a protease inhibitor that is coadministered with ritonavir and coformulated with ombitasvir (ABT-267, an NS5A inhibitor) and dasabuvir (ABT-333, a non-nucleoside NS5B polymerase inhibitor).[37,38] In December 2014, this 3-drug combination, in combination with RBV, was FDA approved for the treatment of patients with HCV-1, including those with compensated cirrhosis.[38] However, no efficacy and safety data are currently available for patients with HCV-6.

TREATMENT RESISTANCE/COMPLICATIONS

Many studies have shown that response rates in retreatment of patients with HCV infection in general with PEG-IFN and RBV depend on the initial treatment response of the patient during the previous IFN-based therapy.[39] Patients are classified as either combination therapy relapsers (those who had end-of-treatment response, which is undetectable HCV RNA by PCR at end of treatment) or combination therapy non-responders (patients who never experienced undetectable HCV RNA at any time during treatment). Those who were relapsers could experience SVR when retreated with PEG-IFN, albeit at a lower SVR than those of treatment-naive patients, whereas those who were nonresponders experienced an extremely low SVR rate when retreated with PEG-IFN and RBV.[39]

Although many studies have been conducted in the retreatment of patients infected with HCV who either relapsed or did not respond to PEG-IFN and RBV initially, these studies have only included patients who did not have HCV-6.[39,40] At present, there are no data available to help guide the optimal treatment duration and dosage of PEG-IFN and RBV in patients with HCV-6 who have previously failed IFN-based treatment. Therefore, patients with HCV-6 who have failed IFN-based therapies need to discuss with their physicians the risks and benefits of retreatment and their options, and a decision to retreat should be made on an individualized basis.

Although several studies have examined drug-resistant variants in patients who failed DAAs and were retreated with different DAA regimens, most of these data have been on patients who did not have HCV-6.[41–43] Therefore, and similar to the issue with patients with GT6 who failed IFN-based therapies, treatment decisions for patients with HCV-6 who have failed on DAA regimens need to be made on an individualized patient basis until additional data are available. However, there are currently several pangenotypic DAAs in clinical development and treatment options for patients with HCV-6, at least those not residing in resource-limited regions, are expected to expand in the near future (**Table 2**).

Table 2
Summary of treatment options with available treatment and safety data for patients with HCV-6

Treatment Options	Comments
PEG-IFN and RBV for 48 wk or 24 wk if with RVR	Current standard of care for patients with HCV-6
SOF-based regimens • SOF plus PEG-IFN and weight-based RBV • SOF plus weight-based RBV	Current data are limited to 6 patients treated with SOF plus PEG-IFN and RBV for 12 wk (NEUTRINO trial) and 5 patients treated with SOF plus PEG-IFN and RBV for 24 wk (ATOMIC trial). All 11 patients achieved SVR
SMV plus SOF	Two out of 2 patients achieved SVR12 in a small retrospective study
LDV plus SOF	A small phase II study showed that 12 wk of LDV plus SOF produced SVR in 24 out of 25 patients infected with HCV-6
Grazoprevir-elbasvir	In a phase III study (C-EDGE trial), 8 out of 10 patients with GT6 achieved SVR with this treatment regimen

EVALUATION OF OUTCOMES AND LONG-TERM RECOMMENDATIONS

SVR has been shown to be associated with improved survival, and the risk of all-cause mortality was shown to be much lower in patients with SVR compared with patients without SVR.[44,45] In a large, international, multicenter study with long-term follow-up from 5 large tertiary care hospitals in Europe and Canada with 530 patients with chronic HCV infection, patients who achieved SVR with IFN-based treatment had a lower risk of death compared with their counterparts who did not achieve SVR.[44] In addition, the risk of developing hepatocellular carcinoma, liver failure, or liver-related mortality, or of needing liver transplantation, was also shown to be decreased in patients with SVR.[44]

Although new DAA therapies may not be available for many patients with HCV-6 who reside in resource-poor regions, these patients should still receive antiviral regimens that are available and more affordable in their regions, especially when SVR can be expected to be almost 80% with 48 weeks of the PEG-IFN and RBV combination. In addition, if patients achieve certain on-treatment responses, such as RVR, then the treatment course may be shortened and the exposure to potential side effects and costs could be reduced.[18,46]

SUMMARY/DISCUSSION

The PEG-IFN and RBV combination is highly effective, with an SVR rate of approximately 80% in patients treated for 48 weeks.[46] In patients who achieve RVR with this combination, therapy can be truncated to 24 weeks.

At present, data on DAAs for HCV-6 are still very limited. The largest available source of treatment and safety data on DAA combinations for patients with HCV-6 is a study of 25 patients treated with the fixed-dose combination of LDV and SOF, which produces an SVR rate of 96%.[35] Other DAA combinations have only been investigated in studies with even smaller sample sizes, which limits the applicability of the results from these studies. The cost of new DAAs, such as SOF-based regimens, can lead to additional barriers to care in many areas where HCV-6 is prevalent.[17,47,48]

REFERENCES

1. Wantuck JM, Ahmed A, Nguyen MH. Review article: the epidemiology and therapy of chronic hepatitis C genotypes 4, 5 and 6. Aliment Pharmacol Ther 2014; 39(2):137–47.
2. Global surveillance and control of hepatitis C. Report of a WHO Consultation organized in collaboration with the Viral Hepatitis Prevention Board, Antwerp, Belgium. J Viral Hepat 1999;6(1):35–47.
3. Nguyen LH, Nguyen MH. Systematic review: Asian patients with chronic hepatitis C infection. Aliment Pharmacol Ther 2013;37(10):921–36.
4. Nguyen MH, Keeffe EB. Chronic hepatitis C: genotypes 4 to 9. Clin Liver Dis 2005;9(3):411–26.
5. Nguyen MH, Keeffe EB. Prevalence and treatment of hepatitis C virus genotypes 4, 5, and 6. Clin Gastroenterol Hepatol 2005;3(10 Suppl 2):S97–101.
6. AASLD/IDSA/IAS-USA. Recommendations for testing, managing, and treating hepatitis C. 2015. Available at: http://www.hcvguidelines.org/fullreport. Accessed April 2, 2015.
7. Chao DT, Abe K, Nguyen MH. Systematic review: epidemiology of hepatitis C genotype 6 and its management. Aliment Pharmacol Ther 2011;34(3):286–96.

8. Seong MH, Kil H, Kim JY, et al. Clinical and epidemiological characteristics of Korean patients with hepatitis C virus genotype 6. Clin Mol Hepatol 2013;19(1): 45–50.

9. Nguyen NH, Vutien P, Trinh HN, et al. Risk factors, genotype 6 prevalence, and clinical characteristics of chronic hepatitis C in Southeast Asian Americans. Hepatol Int 2010;4(2):523–9.

10. Nguyen NHVP, Garcia RT, Trinh H, et al. Response to pegylated interferon and ribavirin in Asian American patients with chronic hepatitis C genotypes 1 vs 2/3 vs 6. J Viral Hepat 2010;17(10):691–7.

11. Lam KD, Trinh HN, Do ST, et al. Randomized controlled trial of pegylated interferon-alfa 2a and ribavirin in treatment-naive chronic hepatitis C genotype 6. Hepatology 2010;52(5):1573–80.

12. Thu Thuy PT, Bunchorntavakul C, Tan Dat H, et al. A randomized trial of 48 versus 24 weeks of combination pegylated interferon and ribavirin therapy in genotype 6 chronic hepatitis C. J Hepatol 2012;56(5):1012–8.

13. Nguyen NH, McCormack SA, Yee BE, et al. Meta-analysis of patients with hepatitis C virus genotype 6: 48 weeks with pegylated interferon and ribavirin is superior to 24 weeks. Hepatol Int 2014;8:540–9.

14. Colombo M. Interferon-free therapy for hepatitis C: the hurdles amid a golden era. Dig Liver Dis 2015 [pii:S1590-8658(15) 00276–5].

15. Pawlotsky JM. New hepatitis C therapies: the toolbox, strategies, and challenges. Gastroenterology 2014;146(5):1176–92.

16. Jayasekera CR, Barry M, Roberts LR, et al. Treating hepatitis C in lower-income countries. N Engl J Med 2014;370(20):1869–71.

17. Wei L, Lok AS. Impact of new hepatitis C treatments in different regions of the world. Gastroenterology 2014;146(5):1145–50.e1–4.

18. Papastergiou V, Karatapanis S. Current status and emerging challenges in the treatment of hepatitis C virus genotypes 4 to 6. World J Clin Cases 2015;3(3): 210–20.

19. Seto WK, Tsang OT, Liu K, et al. Role of IL28B and inosine triphosphatase polymorphisms in the treatment of chronic hepatitis C virus genotype 6 infection. J viral Hepat 2013;20(7):470–7.

20. Seto WK, Tanaka Y, Liu K, et al. The effects of IL-28B and ITPA polymorphisms on treatment of hepatitis C virus genotype 6. Am J Gastroenterol 2011;106(5):1007–8.

21. Thomas DL, Thio CL, Martin MP, et al. Genetic variation in IL28B and spontaneous clearance of hepatitis C virus. Nature 2009;461(7265):798–801.

22. Cai Qing-Xian ZZ, Lin C, Min Xu, et al. Shortened treatment duration in treatment-naive genotype 6 chronic hepatitis C patients with rapid virological response: a randomized controlled trial. Hepatology 2013;58(S1):1855.

23. Nguyen NH, McCormack SA, Vutien P, et al. Meta-analysis: superior treatment response in Asian patients with hepatitis C virus genotype 6 versus genotype 1 with pegylated interferon and ribavirin. Intervirology 2015;58(1):27–34.

24. Fried MW, Shiffman ML, Reddy KR, et al. Peginterferon alfa-2a plus ribavirin for chronic hepatitis C virus infection. N Engl J Med 2002;347(13):975–82.

25. Vo KP, Vutien P, Akiyama MJ, et al. Poor sustained virological response in a multicenter real-life cohort of chronic hepatitis C patients treated with pegylated interferon and ribavirin plus telaprevir or boceprevir. Dig Dis Sci 2015;60(4):1045–51.

26. Lawitz E, Lalezari JP, Hassanein T, et al. Sofosbuvir in combination with peginterferon alfa-2a and ribavirin for non-cirrhotic, treatment-naive patients with genotypes 1, 2, and 3 hepatitis C infection: a randomised, double-blind, phase 2 trial. Lancet Infect Dis 2013;13(5):401–8.

27. Kowdley KV, Lawitz E, Crespo I, et al. Sofosbuvir with pegylated interferon alfa-2a and ribavirin for treatment-naive patients with hepatitis C genotype-1 infection (ATOMIC): an open-label, randomised, multicentre phase 2 trial. Lancet 2013; 381(9883):2100–7.
28. Vu V, Chang CY, Trinh HN, et al. Treatment response and tolerability of simeprevir (SMV)-based or sofosbuvir (SOF)-based therapy for the treatment of genotype 6 (HCV-6) chronic hepatitis C infection [abstract]. Gastroenterology 2015;148(4 Supplement 1):S-1088.
29. Everson GT, Tran TT, Towner WJ, et al. Safety and efficacy of treatment with interferon-free, ribavirin-free combination of sofosbuvir + GS-5816 for 12 weeks in treatment-naive patients with genotypes 1-6 HCV infection [abstract]. J Hepatol 2014;60(1):S46.
30. Moreno C, Berg T, Tanwandee T, et al. Antiviral activity of TMC435 monotherapy in patients infected with HCV genotypes 2-6: TMC435-C202, a phase IIa, open-label study. J Hepatol 2012;56(6):1247–53.
31. Kumada H, Suzuki Y, Ikeda K, et al. Daclatasvir plus asunaprevir for chronic HCV genotype 1b infection. Hepatology 2014;59(6):2083–91.
32. Sulkowski MS, Gardiner DF, Rodriguez-Torres M, et al. Daclatasvir plus sofosbuvir for previously treated or untreated chronic HCV infection. N Engl J Med 2014; 370(3):211–21.
33. Muir AJ, Poordad F, Lalezari J, et al. Daclatasvir in combination with asunaprevir and beclabuvir for hepatitis C virus genotype 1 infection with compensated cirrhosis. JAMA 2015;313(17):1736–44.
34. Alqahtani SA, Afdhal N, Zeuzem S, et al. Safety and tolerability of ledipasvir/sofosbuvir with and without ribavirin in patients with chronic HCV genotype 1 infection: analysis of phase 3 ION trials. Hepatology 2015;62(1):25–30.
35. Gane EJ, Hyland RH, An D, et al. High efficacy of LDV/SOF regimens for 12 weeks for patients with HCV genotype 3 or 6 infection. Hepatology 2014; 60(Suppl):LB-11 [abstract].
36. Zeuzem S, Ghalib R, Reddy KR, et al. Grazoprevir-elbasvir combination therapy for treatment-naive cirrhotic and noncirrhotic patients with chronic HCV genotype 1, 4, or 6 infection: a randomized trial. Ann Intern Med 2015;163(1):1–13.
37. Minaei AA, Kowdley KV. ABT-450/ritonavir and ABT-267 in combination with ABT-333 for the treatment of hepatitis C virus. Expert Opin Pharmacother 2015;16(6):929–37.
38. Gohil K. Pharmaceutical approval update. P T 2015;40(3):172–3.
39. Jacobson IM, Gonzalez SA, Ahmed F, et al. A randomized trial of pegylated interferon alpha-2b plus ribavirin in the retreatment of chronic hepatitis C. Am J Gastroenterol 2005;100(11):2453–62.
40. Ghany MG, Strader DB, Thomas DL, et al. Diagnosis, management, and treatment of hepatitis C: an update. Hepatology 2009;49(4):1335–74.
41. Nguyen LT, Gray E, Dean J, et al. Baseline prevalence and emergence of protease inhibitor resistance mutations following treatment in chronic HCV genotype 1-infected individuals. Antivir Ther 2015. [Epub ahead of print].
42. Poveda E, Wyles DL, Mena A, et al. Update on hepatitis C virus resistance to direct-acting antiviral agents. Antivir Res 2014;108:181–91.
43. Pol S, Sulkowski MS, Hassanein T, et al. Sofosbuvir plus peginterferon and ribavirin in patients with genotype 1 HCV in whom prior therapy with direct-acting antivirals has failed. Hepatology 2015;62(1):129–34.
44. van der Meer AJ, Veldt BJ, Feld JJ, et al. Association between sustained virological response and all-cause mortality among patients with chronic hepatitis C and advanced hepatic fibrosis. JAMA 2012;308(24):2584–93.

45. Ng V, Saab S. Effects of a sustained virologic response on outcomes of patients with chronic hepatitis C. Clin Gastroenterol Hepatol 2011;9(11):923–30.
46. Nguyen MH, Trinh HN, Garcia R, et al. Higher rate of sustained virologic response in chronic hepatitis C genotype 6 treated with 48 weeks versus 24 weeks of peginterferon plus ribavirin. Am J Gastroenterol 2008;103(5):1131–5.
47. Schiff L. Finding truth in a world full of spin: myth-busting in the case of Sovaldi. Clin Ther 2015;37(5):1092–112.
48. Rein DB, Wittenborn JS, Smith BD, et al. The cost-effectiveness, health benefits, and financial costs of new antiviral treatments for hepatitis C virus. Clin Infect Dis 2015;61(2):157–68.

Treatment of Chronic Hepatitis C in Special Populations

Chalermrat Bunchorntavakul, MD[a],*, Tawesak Tanwandee, MD[b]

KEYWORDS

- Hepatitis C virus • Treatment • Decompensated cirrhosis • Liver transplantation
- HIV coinfection • Chronic kidney disease

KEY POINTS

- The management of hepatitis C virus (HCV) infection in special populations, including patients with decompensated cirrhosis, liver transplantation, human immunodeficiency virus coinfection, and end-stage renal disease, is challenging.
- Interferon-based therapy had reduced efficacy, increased side effects, altered pharmacokinetics, and the potential for drug-drug interactions (DDI), via CYP3A, with boceprevir and telaprevir.
- New-generation direct-acting antivirals (DAA) with high potency and no to minimal DDI are preferred, especially as interferon-free regimens. The efficacy and safety data of the currently approved all-oral DAA combinations, containing sofosbuvir, ledipasvir, daclatasvir, paritaprevir/ritonavir/ombitasvir plus dasabuvir, and ribavirin, is compelling for use is special HCV populations, as has recently been recommended by the AASLD/IDSA and EASL guidelines.

INTRODUCTION

Chronic hepatitis C virus (HCV) infection is a worldwide leading cause of chronic liver disease that affects more than 170 million individuals. Treatment of HCV has been

Conflict of Interest: C. Bunchorntavakul has received research grants from Merck and Biotron; T. Tanwandee has received research grants from FibroGen, Merck, Roche, Bristol-Myers Squibb, Biotron, and Celsion.
Financial Support: None.
[a] Division of Gastroenterology and Hepatology, Department of Internal Medicine, Rajavithi Hospital, College of Medicine, Rangsit University, Rajavithi Road, Ratchathewi, Bangkok 10400, Thailand; [b] Division of Gastroenterology and Hepatology, Department of Internal Medicine, Faculty of Medicine Siriraj Hospital, Mahidol University, 2 Wanglang Road, Bangkoknoi, Bangkok 10700, Thailand
* Corresponding author. Department of Medicine, Rajavithi Hospital, Rajavithi Road, Ratchathewi, Bangkok 10400, Thailand.
E-mail address: dr.chalermrat@gmail.com

evolving rapidly over the past few years, shifting from a combination of pegylated-interferon (PEG-IFN) plus ribavirin (RBV) to an all-oral combination of direct-acting antivirals (DAA) targeting NS3/4A, NS5A, and NS5B HCV proteins. Experiences have shown that the epidemiology, the natural history, and the response to treatment of HCV vary among certain patient populations, especially in those with decompensated cirrhosis, liver transplantation (LT), human immunodeficiency virus (HIV) coinfection, and end-stage renal disease (ESRD). The management of HCV in these populations is challenging, particularly with IFN-based therapy, because of reduced efficacy of treatment, increased treatment-related side effects, altered pharmacokinetics, and the potential for significant drug-drug interactions (DDI) with early-generation protease inhibitors, such as boceprevir, telaprevir, and simeprevir. Accordingly, new-generation DAA with high potency and minimal DDI, especially the IFN-free/RBV-free regimens, are preferred. Recently, the safety and efficacy data of the currently approved all-oral DAA combinations in special HCV populations have been increasingly reported. Although the number of patients is still limited in clinical trials, these data are convincing, which has led to a recommendation for their use in special HCV populations in guidelines published by the American Association for the Study of Liver Diseases (AASLD) and the Infectious Diseases Society of America (IDSA), and the European Association for the Study of the Liver (EASL).[1,2]

This review focuses on the DAA-based management of HCV patients with decompensated cirrhosis, post-LT, HIV coinfection, and ESRD, using the currently available regimens in the United States and Europe. In addition, unique clinical features of these HCV populations and the use of IFN-based therapy are briefly reviewed. Important pharmacokinetic and metabolic properties of the currently available DAA are summarized in **Table 1**.[3,4] In addition, at this evolving stage of HCV management, it is suggested that continuous updates on the more recent recommendations for HCV treatment be obtained from the AASLD and the EASL Web sites.[1,2]

TREATMENT OF HEPATITIS C VIRUS IN PATIENTS WITH END-STAGE RENAL DISEASE
Overview

Epidemiology
The prevalence of HCV infection in patients with ESRD varies among the various geographic areas of the World and dialysis centers, but is clearly higher than in the general population.[5–7] In a national survey (N = 164,845), the prevalence of anti-HCV positivity among United States dialysis centers was 10.4% in 1985 and 7.8% in 2002 (range 5.5%–9.8%).[7] Although the prevalence and incidence of HCV among ESRD patients on dialysis has declined in the past decades, a recent estimated seroconversion rate of 0.2%–15% per year for dialysis continues to be a cause for concern.[5–7] Furthermore, the Centers for Disease Control and Prevention recommend that all ESRD patients on hemodialysis be screened for anti-HCV at baseline, and subsequently semiannually.[8]

Natural history
HCV infection in patients with ESRD is associated with more rapid liver disease progression, more liver-related mortality, and reduced renal graft and patient survival following kidney transplantation (KT).[9–13] A meta-analysis on survival in dialysis patients (7 studies; N = 11,589) showed an estimated relative risk for death in anti-HCV–positive patients of 1.34 (95% confidence interval [CI] 1.13–1.59), with liver-related complications contributing to poorer outcomes.[10]

It should also be noted that serum alanine aminotransferase (ALT) levels in patients with ESRD are lower than in the general population, and there is a weak correlation between ALT levels and liver disease severity in this population.[11,14] Liver biopsy or noninvasive assessment of the stage of liver fibrosis is recommended in all HCV-positive KT candidates. Patients with established cirrhosis and portal hypertension often have poor outcomes after KT, particularly if they failed (or are not suitable for) HCV treatment, so that an isolated KT may be contraindicated in this setting, and consideration should be given for a combined liver and KT.[15,16]

Management

Interferon-based therapy

The pharmacokinetics of IFN and RBV are altered in patients with ESRD. In patients with severe renal impairment (creatinine clearance, CrCl <30 mL/min), the maximum plasma concentration and the area under the curve (AUC) of PEG-IFN α2a and α2b are increased by approximately 90% and the half-life is increased by approximately 40%.[17] RBV has an extensive volume of distribution and is primarily excreted renally, so that its AUC is increased by more than 2-fold in patients with moderate to severe renal impairment.[18,19] Hemodialysis has only a minimal effect on PEG-IFN and RBV clearance. Several studies and meta-analyses have reported that IFN or PEG-IFN monotherapy is effective for HCV patients with ESRD, with overall sustained virological response (SVR) rates of 33% to 41% and withdrawal rates of 17% to 30%.[15] Later, a randomized trial of 205 HCV patients with ESRD revealed that addition of low-dose RBV to PEG-IFN treatment was associated with higher rates of SVR (64% vs 33%, $P<.001$) and anemia (hemoglobin <8.5 g/dL) (72% vs 6%, $P<.001$), with comparable discontinuation rates (7% vs 4%, P not significant).[20] With dose adjustment and careful monitoring, treatment with PEG-IFN plus RBV in HCV patients with ESRD can be associated with SVR rates nearly comparable with those with normal renal function.[11,14,15,18] Of note, in patients with severe renal impairment or ESRD on dialysis, the recommended starting doses are 135 μg/wk for PEG-IFN α2a, 1 μg/kg/wk (or 50% reduction) for PEG-IFN α2b, and 200 mg/d for RBV.[15] However, the Kidney Disease: Improving Global Outcomes (KDIGO) Guideline 2008 does not recommend adding RBV in patients with stage 5 chronic renal disease (CrCl <15 mL/min or dialysis).[21]

It should also be noted that IFN-based treatment is often ineffective in HCV-positive KT recipients and may be associated with a risk of graft rejection (15%–100%).[9,15] Therefore, IFN-based therapy should only be initiated in KT recipients under specific clinical situations, such as fibrosing cholestatic hepatitis (FCH) or severe de novo glomerulonephritis, when DAA are unavailable and the risk of not treating HCV infection outweighs the risk of graft loss.[9,15]

All-oral direct-acting antiviral therapy

Based on the available data, the AASLD/IDSA guidance advised that no dose reduction is needed when using sofosbuvir in HCV patients with mild to moderate renal impairment (CrCl ≥30 mL/min). However, until more data becomes available sofosbuvir is not recommended in patients with severe renal impairment or ESRD (CrCl <30 mL/min) or those who require dialysis. For DAA with primarily hepatic metabolism (eg, boceprevir, simeprevir, daclatasvir, and paritaprevir), no dosage adjustment is required for patients with mild to moderate to severe renal impairment. However, the clinical safety and efficacy of these agents in patients with ESRD, including those requiring dialysis, are still limited. In a preliminary report of the RUBY-1 study, the 3D regimen (without RBV for genotype 1b and with RBV 200 mg/d for genotype 1a) was associated with an SVR_4 (ie, SVR after 4 weeks) rate of 100% in HCV genotype 1 patients with severe renal impairment or ESRD (n = 10).[22] The 3D regimen was well tolerated, and there was 1 case of anemia (hemoglobin <8 g/dL) without the need for blood

Table 1
Pharmacokinetic and metabolic parameters of direct-acting antivirals

Drug	Metabolism/Excretion Route	Interaction with CYP and Substrate Transporters	Dosage Adjustment in Patients with Renal Impairment	Dosage Adjustment in Patients with Liver Impairment
NS3/4A Protease Inhibitors				
Telaprevir	Hepatic (CYP3A)	Strong CYP3A inhibitor, moderate P-gp inhibitor	No dose adjustment is required for any degree of RI (clinical data limited)	No dose adjustment is required in compensated cirrhosis; not recommended for CTP class B/C
Boceprevir	Hepatic (CYP3A, aldoketo-reductase)	Moderate CYP3A inhibitor, weak P-gp inhibitor	No dose adjustment is required for any degree of RI (clinical data limited)	No dose adjustment is required in compensated cirrhosis; not recommended for CTP class B/C
Simeprevir	Hepatic (CYP3A)	Mild CYP1A2 and CYP3A inhibitor, inhibitor of OATP1B1 and MRP2	No dose adjustment is required for mild-severe RI; no data in ESRD	No dose adjustment is required in compensated cirrhosis; not recommended for CTP class C
Paritaprevir (ABT-450)/ritonavir	Hepatic (CYP3A)	Strong CYP3A inhibitor (ritonavir), inhibitor of OATP1B1, substrate of P-gp and BCRP	No dose adjustment is required for mild-moderate RI; no data in severe RI/ESRD	No dose adjustment is required in compensated cirrhosis; not recommended for CTP class C
Asunaprevir	Hepatic (CYP3A)	Weak CYP3A4 inducer, moderate CYP2D6 inhibitor, inhibitor of P-gp and OATP1B1	No dose adjustment is required for any degree of RI (clinical data limited)	No dose adjustment is required in compensated cirrhosis; not recommended for CTP class B/C

NS5A Replication Complex Inhibitors				
Daclatasvir	Hepatic (CYP3A)	Not a CYP3A inducer/inhibitor, moderate inhibitor of P-gp and OATP1B1	No dose adjustment is required for any degree of RI (clinical data is limited)	No dose adjustment is required in compensated cirrhosis; Not recommended for CTP class C
Ledipasvir	Feces (major); hepatic and renal (minor)	Not a CYP inducer/inhibitor, weak inhibitor of P-gp and OATP1B1	No dose adjustment is required for mild-moderate RI; no data in severe RI/ESRD	No dose adjustment is required for any degree of liver impairment
Ombitasvir (ABT-267)	Amide hydrolysis and oxidative metabolism	Not a CYP inducer/inhibitor, substrate of P-gp and BCRP	No dose adjustment is required for mild-moderate RI; no data in severe RI/ESRD	No dose adjustment is required in compensated cirrhosis; not recommended for CTP class C
NS5B Nucleotide Polymerase Inhibitors				
Sofosbuvir	Renal	Not a CYP inducer/inhibitor, substrate of P-gp	No dose adjustment is required for mild-moderate RI; no data in severe RI/ESRD	No dose adjustment is required for any degree of liver impairment
NS5B Non-Nucleoside Polymerase Inhibitors				
Dasabuvir (ABT-333)	Hepatic (CYP2C8 60%, CYP3A4 30%, CYP2D6 10%)	Not a CYP inducer/inhibitor, substrate of P-gp and BCRP	No dose adjustment is required for mild-moderate RI; no data in severe RI/ESRD	No dose adjustment is required in compensated cirrhosis; not recommended for CTP class C

Abbreviations: BCRP, breast cancer resistance protein; CTP, Child-Turcotte-Pugh; CYP, cytochrome P450; ESRD, end-stage renal disease; MRP, multiple drug resistance protein; OATP, organic anion transporting polypeptide; P-gp, P-glycoprotein; RI, renal impairment.

transfusion or treatment discontinuation among 17 patients in this ongoing trial.[22] A phase II clinical study (NCT01958281) is currently under way to assess optimal dosing of sofosbuvir plus RBV for HCV patients with severe renal impairment. Grazoprevir (an NS3/4A inhibitor, formerly MK-5172) and elbasvir (a NS5A inhibitor, formerly MK-8742) are both less than 1% renally excreted, and no dose adjustment is needed for ESRD.[23] A preliminary report (N = 111) of a phase II/III C-SURFER study demonstrated that once-daily grazoprevir plus elbasvir for 12 weeks was well tolerated and highly effective (SVR$_{12}$ 99%) for the treatment of HCV genotype 1 among patients with CrCl less than 30 mL/min (75% on dialysis).[24]

TREATMENT OF HEPATITIS C VIRUS IN PATIENTS WITH DECOMPENSATED CIRRHOSIS
Overview

Chronic HCV infection is generally a slowly progressive disease characterized by persistent hepatic inflammation, leading to the development of cirrhosis in approximately 10% to 40% of patients over 20 to 30 years of infection.[25] Once cirrhosis has developed, the disease progression remains unpredictable with the overall 1% to 5% annual risk of hepatocellular carcinoma (HCC) and 3% to 6% annual risk of hepatic decompensation.[25] Following an episode of decompensation, the risk of death in the following year is between 15% and 20%, and LT generally remains the only life-saving option.

Management

Treatment of HCV is strongly recommended for patients with advanced fibrosis and compensated cirrhosis, as an SVR in this high-risk group is associated with a significant decrease in the incidence of clinical decompensation and HCC, although the risk is not eliminated.[25-27] However, the SVR rates are generally lower with IFN-based therapies, and side effects occur more commonly in patients with advanced fibrosis or cirrhosis in comparison with patients with mild to moderate fibrosis.[26-28] Furthermore, successful viral eradication in patients with decompensated cirrhosis independently reduces portal hypertension, decreases the likelihood of clinical decompensation, and improves survival, which may then facilitate, delay, or, in a small proportion of patients, avoid LT, and prevent HCV recurrence following LT.[26-28] Of note, in patients who achieved SVR before LT, the incidence of HCV recurrence after LT is low (0%–20%).[29] In a meta-analysis that included 2649 HCV patients with advanced liver disease, SVR was associated with a reduction in the overall risk of developing HCC from 17.8% to 4.2%, with a reduction in incidence from 3.3% per person-year to 1.05% (95% CI 0.7%–1.5%) per person-year.[30]

Interferon-based therapy

In the past, the outcome of IFN-based therapy in patients with decompensated cirrhosis had been disappointing because of low efficacy (SVR 7%–30% for genotype 1, and 44%–57% for genotypes 2, 3) and high rates of treatment-related side effects (led to dose reduction in 40%–70% and treatment discontinuation in 13%–40%).[29,31] A French cohort (CUPIC Study Group) of HCV genotype 1 with cirrhosis treated with boceprevir-based or telaprevir-based triple therapy (N = 674) reported a high incidence of serious adverse events, including death, related to a platelet count of less than 100,000/mm^3 and/or albumin less than 3.5 g/dL at baseline.[32] In addition, the real-world experience HCV-TARGET study (N = 2084; all genotype 1, 38% with cirrhosis) revealed that triple therapy was associated with high rate of adverse events (>90%), particularly anemia (66%), and involved frequent treatment modifications.[33] Five deaths occurred in this study and the overall SVR rate was 52%.[33] Therefore, these triple-therapy regimens have no role in patients with decompensated liver disease.

All-oral direct-acting antiviral therapy

The pharmacokinetics of sofosbuvir and daclatasvir do not appear to change significantly in patients with moderate or severe liver impairment.[1,34] A fixed-dose combination of paritaprevir/ritonavir/ombitasvir plus dasabuvir and RBV is safe in patients with compensated cirrhosis, but should not be used in decompensated patients. Similarly, simpeprevir is not recommended in Child-Turcotte-Pugh (CTP) class B and C cirrhosis.[1,34] The AASLD/IDSA guideline recommends that patients with decompensated cirrhosis can be treated with all-oral DAA regimens containing sofosbuvir, ledipasvir, and RBV, according to the HCV genotype[1,2] (**Table 2**). In addition, the EASL panel also recommends sofosbuvir plus daclatasvir and weight-based RBV as an option for patients with decompensated cirrhosis awaiting LT.[2] These recommended all-oral combination regimens are generally associated with SVR rates nearly similar to those of patients without decompensated cirrhosis.[1,2,34] Of note, antiviral therapy should be started at least 3 months before anticipated surgery with a goal of undetectable HCV-RNA for at least 30 days.[35,36] The phase III ALLY-1 study evaluated a 12-week course of daclatasvir 60 mg daily, sofosbuvir 400 mg daily, and RBV (initially 600 mg/d, adjusted to 1000 mg/d based on hemoglobin levels) in patients with HCV genotypes 1 to 6 (about 70% were genotype 1) with advanced cirrhosis (n = 60) or post-LT HCV recurrence (n = 53).[37] In an advanced cirrhosis cohort, SVR_{12} was achieved in 92%, 94%, and 56% of patients with CTP-A (n = 12), CTP-B (n = 32), and CTP-C (n = 16), respectively.[37] Most patients improved their Model for End-Stage Liver Disease (MELD) scores following treatment, although some patients continued to show further increases in MELD score. In the post-LT cohort, SVR_{12} was achieved in 92% of patients without the need for dose modification of immunosuppressive agents. Among patients with genotype 3 (n = 17), the SVR_{12} rate was 83% in advanced cirrhosis and 91% in the post-LT cohort.[37]

Table 2		
Recommended HCV treatment for patients with decompensated cirrhosis		
	AASLD/IDSA	**EASL**
HCV genotype 1	SOF-LDV + RBV (initial dose of 600 mg, increased as tolerated) for 12 wk (consider 24 wk for prior SOF failure) SOF-LDV for 24 wk (if anemia or RBV intolerance)	SOF-LDV + RBV (initial dose of 600 mg, increased as tolerated) for 12 wk SOF + DCV + RBV for 12 wk
HCV genotype 2	SOF + RBV for up to 48 wk	SOF + DCV + RBV for 12 wk SOF + RBV for 12 wk
HCV genotype 3	SOF + RBV for up to 48 wk	SOF + DCV + RBV for 12 wk
HCV genotype 4	SOF-LDV + RBV for 12 wk (consider 24 wk for prior SOF failure) SOF-LDV for 24 wk (if anemia or RBV intolerance)	SOF-LDV + RBV for 12 wk SOF + DCV + RBV for 12 wk

SOF-LDV + RBV and SOF + DCV + RBV are effective for genotypes 5 or 6.
Abbreviations: DCV, daclatasvir; LDV, ledipasvir; RBV, ribavirin; SOF, sofosbuvir.
Data from American Association for the Study of Liver Diseases and Infectious Diseases Society of America. Recommendations for testing, managing, and treating hepatitis C. Available at: http://www.hcvguidelines.org/full-report-view. Accessed June 8, 2015; and European Association for the Study of the Liver. Recommendations on treatment of hepatitis C. 2015. Available at: http://www.easl.eu/research/our-contributions/clinical-practice-guidelines/detail/recommendations-on-treatment-of-hepatitis-c-2015. Accessed June 8, 2015.

In the SOLAR-1 study, 108 treatment-naïve and treatment-experienced patients with HCV genotypes 1 and 4 who had decompensated cirrhosis (59 had CTP-B and 49 had CTP-C) were randomized to receive daily fixed-dose combination sofosbuvir/ledipasvir and RBV (initial dose 600 mg, increased as tolerated) for 12 or 24 weeks.[38] SVR was achieved in 87% and 89% of patients treated for 12 weeks and 24 weeks, respectively.[38] Most patients improved their CTP and MELD scores following treatment, although some patients continued to show further increases in MELD score, demonstrating that there may be a point of no return for recovery of liver function in those who present with late liver disease. There were 5 deaths during the study, none of which were attributed to antiviral treatment. Grade 3 or 4 side effects developed more commonly in the 24-week arm (34%) than in the 12-week arm (15%).[38] In a preliminarily report of the SOLAR-2 study, a fixed-dose combination sofosbuvir/ledipasvir and RBV for 12 to 24 weeks was associated with SVR_{12} rates of 87% to 89% and 72% to 85% in HCV genotype 1 patients with cirrhosis CTP-B (n = 46) and CTP-C (n = 38), respectively.[39] The administration of sofosbuvir plus RBV before LT has been shown to prevent post-LT HCV recurrence in an open-label study of 61 patients with CTP-A and HCV of any genotype who were on wait lists for LT for hepatocellular carcinoma.[35] In addition, a report from the NHS England Early Access Program has confirmed the efficacy of a 12-week course of sofosbuvir plus a NS5A inhibitor, either ledipasvir or daclatasvir, with or without RBV for HCV genotype 1 or 3 in more than 400 patients with decompensated cirrhosis.[40] A preliminary result of the phase II/III C-SALT study revealed that grazoprevir plus elbasvir for 12 weeks was well tolerated and highly effective (SVR_4 93%) in 30 patients with CTP-B and HCV genotype 1.[41] Of note, from all these studies data in patients with more advanced liver disease (CTP score >12 or MELD score >20) are limited. Thus the decision to treat HCV in patients with decompensated cirrhosis to maximize survival should be individualized, together with a consideration of the expected waiting time to LT. It is debatable whether the decompensated patients with MELD greater than 15 should be treated before LT with aim to cure or to prevent post-LT recurrence, or that such patients should be monitored until LT and treatment initiated at the time of established recurrence of HCV.[2]

TREATMENT OF HEPATITIS C VIRUS IN LIVER TRANSPLANT RECIPIENTS
Overview

Epidemiology
HCV infection is the most common indication for LT in the United States, Japan, and many countries in Europe. Based on the United States database (the Organ Procurement and Transplantation Network), among 126,862 new primary registrants for LT between 1995 and 2010, 41% had HCV.[42] Although effective therapies are currently available and the prevalence of HCV has already peaked and is now decreasing, it is predicted that the number of cases of advanced liver disease, HCC, and liver-related deaths will continue to increase through 2030 globally.[43] In addition, there is a trend toward increasing age and occurrence of HCC in HCV-positive LT candidates, which will be a further challenging problem to the transplant community.[42]

Natural history
Liver transplantation in HCV patients is associated with suboptimal graft survival, which is attributable to universal recurrence of HCV in the graft.[29,44,45] The natural course of HCV is accelerated in LT recipients, with more than 40% progressing to cirrhosis within 10 years and approximately 50% developing liver failure shortly thereafter.[29,44,45] (**Fig. 1**) An analysis of the UNOS database (N = 11,036) before the era of effective antiviral therapy (1992–1998) revealed that LT in HCV-positive recipients was

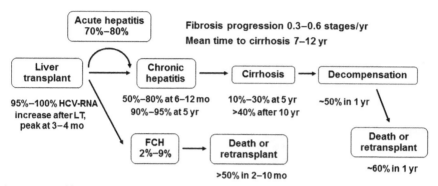

Fig. 1. Natural history of recurrent HCV after liver transplantation. FCH, fibrosing cholestatic hepatitis.

associated with an increased rate of death (hazard ratio [HR] 1.23; 95% CI 1.12–1.35) and allograft failure (HR 1.30; 95% CI: 1.21–1.39), compared with LT for other indications.[46]

A subset of patients (2%–9%) may develop post-LT FCH, which is characterized by persistent cholestasis of at least 4 weeks' duration, high HCV-RNA, hepatocyte ballooning, rapid progression to graft failure, and, in the absence of biliary and hepatic artery complications, sepsis and drug-induced cholestasis.[29,47] This complication is often resistant to antiviral therapy, and leads to death in more than 50% of patients.[29,47]

The benefit of immunosuppressive strategy on the natural history HCV recurrence has not been well elucidated, although there has been evidence to suggest a neutral or small beneficial effect of cyclosporine, mycophenolate mofetil, and sirolimus.[29,44,45]

Management

In the IFN era, the recommended standard of care for LT recipients was treatment of confirmed significant or progressive recurrent HCV disease, based either on persistent, unexplained, elevated ALT levels or on histologically confirmed fibrosis, once rejection, biliary obstruction, vascular complication, and other causes had been excluded.[29,44,45] This recommendation was based on the limited efficacy and increased treatment-related side effects of IFN-based therapy in immunosuppressed patients. When new DAA become widely available, IFN-based therapies will generally no longer be recommended, and all patients with post-LT recurrence of HCV will be considered for therapy.[2] New-generation DAA with higher potency and no/minimal DDI are preferred, ideally as IFN-free/RBV-free regimens.[1,36] The optimal time period to initiate such treatment is before the development of significant fibrosis.

Interferon-based therapy

Treatment with PEG-IFN/RBV has been associated with SVR rates of 24% to 40% in LT recipients, but adverse effects are common (two-thirds of patients required dose reductions and one-fourth discontinued treatment early).[29,45,48] Addition of boceprevir or telaprevir to a PEG-IFN/RBV regimen improves SVR rates but also increases treatment-related side effects, and has a DDI issue with calcineurin inhibitors whereby the immunosuppressive regimens need to be closely monitored and preemptively adjusted during the treatment period.[29,48]

All-oral direct-acting antiviral therapy

The AASLD/IDSA and EASL guidelines recommend that patients who develop recurrent HCV post-LT, including those with compensated cirrhosis, can be treated with all-oral DAA regimens, according to genotype.[1,2] (**Table 3**) Tacrolimus or cyclosporine dose adjustments are not needed when coadministered with regimens that include sofosbuvir, ledipasvir, daclatasvir, and RBV.[2] However, careful monitoring is recommended because of the limited safety data in this group of patients[1] (**Table 4**). In the SOLAR-1 study, 223 LT recipients who had recurrent HCV with genotype 1 or 4 (111 with METAVIR stage F0–F3, 51 with CTP-A, and 61 with CTP-B/C) were randomized to receive a daily fixed-dose combination sofosbuvir/ledipasvir and RBV (weight-based dose for noncirrhotics and CTP-A cirrhosis; and initial dose of 600 mg, increased as tolerated for CTP-B/C), for either 12 or 24 weeks.[38] Overall, SVR was attained in 96% of patients with F0 to F3 and 96% of those with compensated cirrhosis, in both treatment arms.[38] Efficacy of treatment was lower in patients with decompensated cirrhosis (85% in CTP-B and 60% in CTP-C), without the increase in SVR observed in patients treated for 24 weeks.[38] To date, there have been fairly limited data for LT recipients with recurrent HCV genotype 3; however, a 24-week course of sofosbuvir plus RBV was effective, as in non-LT settings.[1,49] In a preliminary report of SOLAR-2, a fixed-dose combination sofosbuvir/ledipasvir and RBV for 12 to 24 weeks was associated with SVR_4 rates of 94% to 100%, 92% to 97%, 100%, and 50% to 100% in LT recipients who had recurrent HCV with genotype 1 or 4 with

Table 3
Recommended HCV treatment for patients with recurrent HCV after liver transplantation

	AASLD/IDSA	EASL
HCV genotype 1	SOF-LDV + RBV for 12 wk (including compensated cirrhosis) SOF-LDV for 24 wk (including compensated cirrhosis)[a] PTV-RTV-OMV + DSV + RBV for 12 wk (for early recurrence: fibrosis stage F0-F2)[a] SOF + SMV ± RBV for 12 wk[a]	SOF-LDV + RBV for 12 wk SOF + DCV + RBV for 12 wk SOF + SMV + RBV for 12 wk PTV-RTV-OMV + DSV + RBV for 12 wk (genotype 1b) or 24 wk (genotype 1a with cirrhosis)
HCV genotype 2	SOF + RBV for 24 wk	SOF + RBV for 12 wk SOF + DCV + RBV for 12 wk
HCV genotype 3	SOF + RBV for 24 wk	SOF + DCV + RBV for 12 wk
HCV genotype 4	SOF-LDV + RBV for 12 wk (including compensated cirrhosis) SOF-LDV for 24 wk (including compensated cirrhosis)[a]	SOF-LDV + RBV for 12 wk SOF + DCV + RBV for 12 wk SOF + SMV + RBV for 12 wk PTV-RTV-OMV + RBV for 12 wk (without cirrhosis) or 24 wk (with cirrhosis)

SOF-LDV + RBV and SOF + DCV + RBV are effective for genotypes 5 or 6.

Abbreviations: DCV, daclatasvir; DSV, dasabuvir; LDV, ledipasvir; OMV, ombitasvir; PTV, paritaprevir; RBV, ribavirin; RTV, ritonavir; SMV, simeprevir; SOF, sofosbuvir.

[a] Alternative regimens.

Data from American Association for the Study of Liver Diseases and Infectious Diseases Society of America. Recommendations for testing, managing, and treating hepatitis C. Available at: http://www.hcvguidelines.org/full-report-view. Accessed June 8, 2015; and European Association for the Study of the Liver. Recommendations on treatment of hepatitis C. 2015. Available at: http://www.easl.eu/research/our-contributions/clinical-practice-guidelines/detail/recommendations-on-treatment-of-hepatitis-c-2015. Accessed June 8, 2015.

Table 4
Recommended dose reduction of calcineurin inhibitors when coadministration with direct-acting antivirals

	Tacrolimus	Cyclosporine
Boceprevir	↓ 5 fold[a]	↓ 2 fold[a]
Telaprevir	↓ 24–35 fold[a]	↓ 3–4 fold[a]
Sofosbuvir	No adjustment	No adjustment
Ledipasvir	No adjustment	No adjustment
Simeprevir	No adjustment	No adjustment[a]
Daclatasvir	No adjustment	No adjustment
Paritaprevir-ritonavir-ombitasvir and dasabuvir	↓ 20–100 fold	↓ 5 fold

[a] Not recommended for concomitant use by the AASLD/IDSA and EASL guidelines.

METAVIR F0 to F3 (n = 100), CTP-A (n = 67), CTP-B (n = 44), and CTP-C (n = 9), respectively.[39]

The phase II CORAL-1 study (N = 34) examined the safety and efficacy of paritaprevir/ritonavir/ombitasvir plus dasabuvir and RBV for 24 weeks in noncirrhotic LT recipients (METAVIR F0–F2) with recurrent HCV genotype 1.[50] The overall SVR rate was 97%, with a low rate of serious adverse events (<15%). Of note, ritonavir is a strong CYP3A inhibitor, and therefore the dose of calcineurin inhibitors should be adjusted (tacrolimus should be reduced to 0.5 mg once weekly or 0.2 mg every 3 days, whereas cyclosporine should be reduced to one-fifth of the daily dose given before HCV treatment; the use of mTOR [mammalian target of rapamycin] inhibitors is not recommended) and closely monitored during the treatment.[2,50] Two retrospective experiences (N = 123[51] and N = 61[52]) have reported that a 12-week course of sofosbuvir plus simeprevir with or without RBV was well tolerated and associated with high SVR rates (90%–93%) in LT recipients with HCV genotype 1.[51,52] However, patients with genotype 1a who had advanced fibrosis in the allograft were more likely to relapse (SVR 66%–71%).[51,52] It should be noted that concomitant use of simeprevir with calcineurin inhibitors at steady state resulted in an increase in plasma concentrations of simeprevir (approximately 2-fold with tacrolimus and 6-fold with cyclosporine); therefore, the coadministration of simeprevir with cyclosporine is not recommended.[1]

Data from the first 104 patients in the sofosbuvir compassionate-use program for LT recipients with severe recurrent HCV, including those with FCH and decompensated cirrhosis who had a life expectancy of less than 1 year, revealed that sofosbuvir plus RBV for 24 to 48 weeks provided significant clinical improvement in 57% of patients.[53] The SVR$_{12}$ rate was 73% in those with severe early recurrence and 43% in those with decompensated cirrhosis. Overall, 57% of patients reported improvement.[53]

TREATMENT OF HEPATITIS C VIRUS IN HUMAN IMMUNODEFICIENCY VIRUS–INFECTED PERSONS
Overview

Epidemiology
Globally it is estimated that 4 to 5 million people are infected with both HIV and HCV owing to shared common routes of transmission.[54] In developed countries, approximately 15% to 25% of HIV-infected persons are chronically infected with HCV.[55–57] The prevalence of HIV/HCV coinfection varies depending on the route of HIV acquisition, being lower among persons reporting high-risk sexual exposures (1%–12% of heterosexuals and 9%–27% of men who have sex with men [MSM]) and higher in

those reporting injection drug use (70%–95%).[54,56,57] The incidence of new HCV infection has decreased dramatically over the last decade; however, cases of acute HCV infection continue to occur among populations in certain settings, such as injection drug users, MSM, persons with high-risk sexual activities, and health care–associated procedures.[58,59] Accordingly, there have been emerging epidemics of acute HCV infection in HIV-infected persons, mainly among MSM, in Europe, Australia, and the United States.[59] Therefore, anti-HCV screening should be conducted in all patients with HIV infection, then tested annually in those who continue high-risk behaviors.

Natural history
HIV infection adversely affects the natural history of HCV, leading to increased viral persistence after acute infection, higher levels of viremia, accelerated progression to cirrhosis and end-stage liver disease, and increased risk of liver-related death.[56,57,60,61] Successful HCV eradication in HIV-infected patients not only prevents progression of liver disease, but is also associated with a reduction in the risk of antiretroviral (ARV)-induced hepatotoxicity, progression of HIV disease, and non–liver-related mortality.[56,57,61–63]

Management

Prompt treatment of HCV should be considered in all HCV patients with HIV coinfection. This approach must also be considered within the context of the faster progression of liver fibrosis in HIV/HCV coinfection, beneficial effects of HCV eradication on liver disease and course of HIV infection, and the improved outcome in such patients treated with DAA.[64] If HCV infection is identified early in the course of HIV (before ARV treatment), treatment of HCV should be initiated so that there is no need to consider DDI.[64] In patients with a CD4$^+$ cell count less than 500 cells/μL, early ARV treatment is recommended and the treatment of HCV can be subsequently initiated.[64] Of note, in patients with CD4$^+$ cell count less than 200 to 350 cells/μL, it may be preferable to improve the CD4$^+$ cell count by starting ARV before HCV treatment.[36]

IFN-based HCV therapy is associated with higher SVR rates in HIV patients with higher CD4$^+$ cell count and completely suppressed HIV replication.[65]

Interferon-based therapy
HCV treatment in HIV-infected patients is sometimes limited because of historically low response rates, patient comorbidities, physician perception, adverse effects associated with IFN-based therapy, and DDIs (with boceprevir and telaprevir). Treatment of chronic HCV in the coinfected population with PEG-IFN plus RBV has been associated with SVR in 14% to 29% of patients with HCV genotype 1 and 44% to 73% of those with HCV genotype 2 or 3.[66] The PEG-IFN/RBV regimen for patients with HIV/HCV coinfection should be 48 weeks in duration regardless of the HCV genotype, and RBV dose should always be weight based.[67] The combined use of RBV and didanosine is contraindicated because of the potential for dangerous interactions resulting in mitochondrial toxicity causing hepatic steatosis, liver failure, peripheral neuropathy, pancreatitis, and lactic acidosis.[68] In addition, the combined use of RBV and zidovudine should also be avoided because of the increased rate of anemia.[69]

All-oral direct-acting antiviral therapy
In the era of DAA, it seems there is no longer any separation between HCV-monoinfected and HIV-coinfected patients for the indications of HCV treatment or regimen choice.[64] However, the treatment still requires awareness of the complex DDIs between DAA and ARV (see **Table 4**). The AASLD//IDSA and EASL guidelines

have recommended that HIV/HCV-coinfected patients be treated and retreated in the manner similar to non-HIV patients, after recognizing and managing interactions with ARV[1,2] (**Table 5**). Although the various regimens have been evaluated in a limited number of patients, these recommended all-oral DAA regimens are generally associated with SVR rates of greater than 90% and are similar to those for non-HIV patients.[1,2]

In a combined analysis of phase III PHOTON-1 and PHOTON-2 studies (N = 332), HIV-coinfected patients with genotypes 1 to 4 were treated with sofosbuvir and weight-based ribavirin for 12 or 24 weeks according to genotype and previous treatment status.[70] High SVR_{12} rates were observed for all HCV genotypes (81% for genotype 1, 89% for genotype 2, 84% each for genotypes 3 and 4).[70] SVR_{12} rates were lower for patients with cirrhosis with HCV genotype 1a and treatment-experienced patients with HCV genotype 3 who were treated for 24 weeks (65% vs 85%, respectively, and 95% vs 79%, respectively).[70] The safety and efficacy of 12 weeks of sofosbuvir/ledipasvir was evaluated in the phase II study (ERADICATE), which included 50 patients with HIV/HCV genotype 1 coinfection. Overall, 98% of patients achieved SVR_{12}.[71] Thirty-seven patients were on ARV, including tenofovir, and the median $CD4^+$ count was 576 cells/μL. Renal function was closely monitored, and there

Table 5	
Important drug-drug interactions between direct-acting antivirals and antiretroviral agents	
Agents	**Potential Interactions and Suggested Dosage Adjustment**
Sofosbuvir-ledipasvir	Because LDV increases tenofovir levels, concomitant use mandates close renal monitoring and should be avoided in those with CrCl <60 mL/min
	Because potentiation of this effect is expected when tenofovir is used with RTV-boosted HIV protease inhibitors, LDV should be avoided with this combination (pending further data) unless ARV cannot be changed and the urgency of treatment is high
Paritaprevir-ritonavir-ombitasvir and dasabuvir	PTV-RTV-OMV + DSV should be used with ARV without substantial interactions including raltegravir (and probably dolutegravir), enfuvirtide, tenofovir, emtricitabine, lamivudine, and atazanavir
	The dose of RTV used for boosting of HIV protease inhibitors may need to be adjusted (or held) when administered with PTV-RTV-OMV + DSV and then restored when HCV treatment is completed
	HIV protease inhibitor should be administered at the same time as the fixed-dose HCV combination
Simeprevir	SMV should only be used with ARV without clinically significant interactions including raltegravir (and probably dolutegravir), rilpivirine, maraviroc, enfuvirtide, tenofovir, emtricitabine, lamivudine, and abacavir
Daclatasvir	DCV dose should be increased to 90 mg/d when coadministered with efavirenz
	DCV dose should be reduced to 30 mg/d when coadministered with atazanavir/ritonavir
	No dose adjustments are required with tenofovir, lamivudine, zidovudine, emtricitabine, abacavir, stavudine, raltegravir, rilpivirine, maraviroc, enfuvirtide, darunavir, and lopinavir
	Owing to lack of data, coadministration of DCV and etravirine or nevirapine is not recommended

Abbreviations: DCV, daclatasvir; DSV, dasabuvir; HIV, human immunodeficiency virus; LDV, ledipasvir; OMV, ombitasvir; PTV, paritaprevir; RTV, ritonavir; SMV, simeprevir; SOF, sofosbuvir.

Data from American Association for the Study of Liver Diseases and Infectious Diseases Society of America. Recommendations for testing, managing, and treating hepatitis C. Available at: http://www.hcvguidelines.org/full-report-view. Accessed June 8, 2015.

were no clinically significant changes in renal parameters during the treatment.[71] Another phase II/III study (TURQUOISE-I) evaluating a combination of paritaprevir/ritonavir/ombitasvir plus dasabuvir and RBV in 63 patients with HIV/HCV genotype 1 coinfection, including those with cirrhosis (19%), for 12 or 24 weeks demonstrated SVR rates of 91% and 94%, respectively.[72] The clinical efficacy of sofosbuvir plus daclatasvir in HIV/HCV-coinfected patients has been evaluated in a phase III study (ALLY-2), which included 151 treatment-naïve patients and 52 treatment-experienced patients with HIV/HCV coinfections (83% genotype 1, 9% genotype 2, 6% genotype 3, and 2% genotype 4).[73] Overall, 97% of patients achieved SVR_{12} after 12 weeks of treatment, compared with 76% in those who were treated for 8 weeks.[73] Factors associated with relapse included high baseline HCV-RNA (>2,000,000 IU/mL), presence of cirrhosis, and coadministration with darunavir-boosted ARV (daclatasvir dose was reduced to 30 mg/d).[73] A preliminary result (N = 315) of the phase III C-EDGE study revealed that once-daily grazoprevir plus elbasvir for 12 weeks was well tolerated and highly effective (SVR_4 97%) for HIV patients coinfected with HCV genotype 1, 4, or 6.[74]

Drug interactions are common, particularly in combinations including HCV protease inhibitors, which are metabolized through the cytochrome P450 pathways, similar to many ARVs. Sofosbuvir, which is not metabolized by cytochrome P450, generally has no to minimal DDI with ARV, but is not recommended for use with tipranavir because of the potential of this drug to induce P-glycoprotein.[1] Updated information regarding DDI between HCV and HIV medications can be found on drug interaction Web sites, such as www.hep-druginteractions.org, and the EASL Web site.[2]

ACKNOWLEDGMENTS

The authors are grateful to Professor K. Rajender Reddy of the University of Pennsylvania for supportive guidance and critical review of the article.

REFERENCES

1. American Association for the Study of Liver Diseases and Infectious Diseases Society of America. Recommendations for testing, managing, and treating hepatitis C. http://www.hcvguidelines.org/full-report-view. Accessed June 8, 2015.
2. European Association for the Study of the Liver Recommendations on Treatment of Hepatitis C. http://www.easl.eu/_newsroom/latest-news/easl-recommendations-on-treatment-of-hepatitis-c-2015. Accessed June 8, 2015.
3. Kiser JJ, Burton JR Jr, Everson GT. Drug-drug interactions during antiviral therapy for chronic hepatitis C. Nat Rev Gastroenterol Hepatol 2013;10(10):596–606.
4. Tischer S, Fontana RJ. Drug-drug interactions with oral anti-HCV agents and idiosyncratic hepatotoxicity in the liver transplant setting. J Hepatol 2014;60(4): 872–84.
5. Jadoul M, Poignet JL, Geddes C, et al. The changing epidemiology of hepatitis C virus (HCV) infection in haemodialysis: European multicentre study. Nephrol Dial Transplant 2004;19(4):904–9.
6. Fabrizi F, Lunghi G, Ganeshan SV, et al. Hepatitis C virus infection and the dialysis patient. Semin Dial 2007;20(5):416–22.
7. Finelli L, Miller JT, Tokars JI, et al. National surveillance of dialysis-associated diseases in the United States, 2002. Semin Dial 2005;18(1):52–61.
8. Recommendations for preventing transmission of infections among chronic hemodialysis patients. MMWR Recomm Rep 2001;50(RR-5):1–43.

9. Okoh EJ, Bucci JR, Simon JF, et al. HCV in patients with end-stage renal disease. Am J Gastroenterol 2008;103(8):2123–34.

10. Fabrizi F, Takkouche B, Lunghi G, et al. The impact of hepatitis C virus infection on survival in dialysis patients: meta-analysis of observational studies. J Viral Hepat 2007;14(10):697–703.

11. Liu CH, Kao JH. Treatment of hepatitis C virus infection in patients with end-stage renal disease. J Gastroenterol Hepatol 2011;26(2):228–39.

12. Mahmoud IM, Elhabashi AF, Elsawy E, et al. The impact of hepatitis C virus viremia on renal graft and patient survival: a 9-year prospective study. Am J Kidney Dis 2004;43(1):131–9.

13. Mathurin P, Mouquet C, Poynard T, et al. Impact of hepatitis B and C virus on kidney transplantation outcome. Hepatology 1999;29(1):257–63.

14. Al-Freah MA, Zeino Z, Heneghan MA. Management of hepatitis C in patients with chronic kidney disease. Curr Gastroenterol Rep 2012;14(1):78–86.

15. Bunchorntavakul C, Maneerattanaporn M, Chavalitdhamrong D. Management of patients with hepatitis C infection and renal disease. World J Hepatol 2015;7(2): 213–25.

16. Van Wagner LB, Baker T, Ahya SN, et al. Outcomes of patients with hepatitis C undergoing simultaneous liver-kidney transplantation. J Hepatol 2009;51(5):874–80.

17. Noureddin M, Ghany MG. Pharmacokinetics and pharmacodynamics of peginterferon and ribavirin: implications for clinical efficacy in the treatment of chronic hepatitis C. Gastroenterol Clin North Am 2010;39(3):649–58.

18. Berenguer M. Treatment of chronic hepatitis C in hemodialysis patients. Hepatology 2008;48(5):1690–9.

19. Bunchorntavakul C, Reddy KR. Ribavirin: how does it work and is it still needed? Curr Hepat Rep 2011;10:168–78.

20. Liu CH, Huang CF, Liu CJ, et al. Pegylated interferon-alpha2a with or without low-dose ribavirin for treatment-naive patients with hepatitis C virus genotype 1 receiving hemodialysis: a randomized trial. Ann Intern Med 2013;159(11):729–38.

21. Kidney Disease: Improving Global Outcomes (KDIGO). DIGO clinical practice guidelines for the prevention, diagnosis, evaluation, and treatment of hepatitis C in chronic kidney disease. Kidney Int Suppl 2008;(109):S1–99.

22. Pockros PJ, Reddy KR, Mantry PS, et al. Safety of ombitasvir/paritaprevir/ritonavir plus dasabuvir for treating HCV GT1 infection in patients with severe renal impairment or end-stage renal disease: the RUBY-1 study. J Hepatol 2015;62(Suppl 2): S257.

23. Yeh WW, Caro L, Guo Z, et al. Pharmacokinetics of co-administered HCV protease inhibitor MK-5172 and NS5A inhibitor MK-8742 in volunteers with end-stage renal disease on hemodialysis or severe renal impairment not on hemodialysis. Hepatology 2014;60(4 Suppl 1):1137A.

24. Roth D, Nelson D, Bruchfeld A, et al. Grazoprevir plus elbasvir in treatment-naive and treatment-experienced patients with hepatitis C virus genotype 1 infection and chronic kidney disease. J Hepatol 2015;62(Suppl 2):S263.

25. Westbrook RH, Dusheiko G. Natural history of hepatitis C. J Hepatol 2014;61(1 Suppl):S58–68.

26. Singal AG, Volk ML, Jensen D, et al. A sustained viral response is associated with reduced liver-related morbidity and mortality in patients with hepatitis C virus. Clin Gastroenterol Hepatol 2010;8(3):280–8, 288.e1.

27. van der Meer AJ, Veldt BJ, Feld JJ, et al. Association between sustained virological response and all-cause mortality among patients with chronic hepatitis C and advanced hepatic fibrosis. JAMA 2012;308(24):2584–93.

28. Saxena V, Manos MM, Yee HS, et al. Telaprevir or boceprevir triple therapy in patients with chronic hepatitis C and varying severity of cirrhosis. Aliment Pharmacol Ther 2014;39(10):1213–24.
29. Bunchorntavakul C, Reddy KR. Management of hepatitis C before and after liver transplantation in the era of rapidly evolving therapeutic advances. J Clin Transl Hepatol 2014;2:124–33.
30. Morgan RL, Baack B, Smith BD, et al. Eradication of hepatitis C virus infection and the development of hepatocellular carcinoma: a meta-analysis of observational studies. Ann Intern Med 2013;158(5 Pt 1):329–37.
31. Roche B, Samuel D. Hepatitis C virus treatment pre- and post-liver transplantation. Liver Int 2012;32(Suppl 1):120–8.
32. Hezode C, Fontaine H, Dorival C, et al. Triple therapy in treatment-experienced patients with HCV-cirrhosis in a multicentre cohort of the French Early Access Programme (ANRS CO20-CUPIC) - NCT01514890. J Hepatol 2013;59(3):434–41.
33. Gordon SC, Muir AJ, Lim JK, et al. Safety profile of boceprevir and telaprevir in chronic hepatitis C: real world experience from HCV-TARGET. J Hepatol 2015; 62(2):286–93.
34. Coilly A, Roche B, Duclos-Vallee JC, et al. Optimal therapy in hepatitis C virus liver transplant patients with direct acting antivirals. Liver Int 2015;35(Suppl 1):44–50.
35. Curry MP, Forns X, Chung RT, et al. Sofosbuvir and ribavirin prevent recurrence of HCV infection after liver transplantation: an open-label study. Gastroenterology 2015;148(1):100–7.e1.
36. European Association for Study of Liver. EASL clinical practice guidelines: management of hepatitis C virus infection. J Hepatol 2014;60(2):392–420.
37. Poordad F, Schiff ER, Vierling JM, et al. Daclatasvir, sofosbuvir, and ribavirin combination for HCV patients with advanced cirrhosis or post-transplant recurrence: ALLY-1 Phase 3 Study. J Hepatol 2015;62(Suppl 2):S261–262.
38. Charlton M, Everson GT, Flamm SL, et al. Ledipasvir and sofosbuvir plus ribavirin for treatment of HCV infection in patients with advanced liver disease. Gastroenterology 2015. [Epub ahead of print].
39. Manns M, Forns X, Samuel D, et al. Ledipasvir/sofosbuvir with ribavirin is safe and efficacious in decompensated and post-liver transplantation patients with HCV infection: preliminary results of the prospective SOLAR-2 trial. J Hepatol 2015;62(Suppl 2):S187–8.
40. Foster GR, McLauchlan J, Irving W, et al. Treatment of decompensated HCV cirrhosis in patients with diverse genotypes: 12 weeks sofosbuvir and NS5A inhibitors with/without ribavirin is effective in HCV Genotypes 1 and 3. J Hepatol 2015;62(Suppl 2):S190–1.
41. Jacobson IM, Poordad F, Firpi-Morell R, et al. Efficacy and safety of grazoprevir and elbasvir in hepatitis C genotype 1-infected patients with Child-Pugh class B cirrhosis (C-SALT part A). J Hepatol 2015;62(Suppl 2):S193–4.
42. Biggins SW, Bambha KM, Terrault NA, et al. Projected future increase in aging hepatitis C virus-infected liver transplant candidates: a potential effect of hepatocellular carcinoma. Liver Transpl 2012;18(12):1471–8.
43. Hatzakis A, Chulanov V, Gadano AC, et al. The present and future disease burden of hepatitis C virus (HCV) infections with today's treatment paradigm— volume 2. J Viral Hepat 2015;22(Suppl 1):26–45.
44. Gane EJ. The natural history of recurrent hepatitis C and what influences this. Liver Transpl 2008;14(Suppl 2):S36–44.
45. Watt K, Veldt B, Charlton M. A practical guide to the management of HCV infection following liver transplantation. Am J Transplant 2009;9(8):1707–13.

46. Forman LM, Lewis JD, Berlin JA, et al. The association between hepatitis C infection and survival after orthotopic liver transplantation. Gastroenterology 2002; 122(4):889–96.

47. Narang TK, Ahrens W, Russo MW. Post-liver transplant cholestatic hepatitis C: a systematic review of clinical and pathological findings and application of consensus criteria. Liver Transpl 2010;16(11):1228–35.

48. Coilly A, Roche B, Dumortier J, et al. Safety and efficacy of protease inhibitors to treat hepatitis C after liver transplantation: a multicenter experience. J Hepatol 2014;60(1):78–86.

49. Charlton M, Gane E, Manns MP, et al. Sofosbuvir and ribavirin for treatment of compensated recurrent hepatitis C virus infection after liver transplantation. Gastroenterology 2015;148(1):108–17.

50. Mantry PS, Kwo PY, Coakley E, et al. High sustained virologic response rates in liver transplant recipients with recurrent HCV genotype 1 infection receiving ABT-450/r/ombitasvir+dasabuvir plus ribavirin. Hepatology 2014;60(4 Suppl 1):298A–9A.

51. Pungpapong S, Aqel B, Leise M, et al. Multicenter experience using simeprevir and sofosbuvir with or without ribavirin to treat hepatitis C genotype 1 after liver transplant. Hepatology 2015;61(6):1880–6.

52. Gutierrez JA, Carrion AF, Avalos D, et al. Sofosbuvir and simeprevir for treatment of hepatitis C Virus infection in liver transplant recipients. Liver Transpl 2015; 21(6):823–30.

53. Forns X, Charlton M, Denning J, et al. Sofosbuvir compassionate use program for patients with severe recurrent hepatitis C after liver transplantation. Hepatology 2015;61(5):1485–94.

54. Alter MJ. Epidemiology of viral hepatitis and HIV co-infection. J Hepatol 2006; 44(1 Suppl):S6–9.

55. Sherman KE, Rouster SD, Chung RT, et al. Hepatitis C virus prevalence among patients infected with human immunodeficiency virus: a cross-sectional analysis of the US adult AIDS Clinical Trials Group. Clin Infect Dis 2002;34(6):831–7.

56. Sulkowski MS, Thomas DL. Hepatitis C in the HIV-infected patient. Clin Liver Dis 2003;7(1):179–94.

57. Sulkowski MS, Thomas DL. Hepatitis C in the HIV-infected person. Ann Intern Med 2003;138(3):197–207.

58. Kamal SM. Acute hepatitis C: a systematic review. Am J Gastroenterol 2008; 103(5):1283–97 [quiz: 1298].

59. Boesecke C, Rockstroh JK. Acute hepatitis C in patients with HIV. Semin Liver Dis 2012;32(2):130–7.

60. Weber R, Sabin CA, Friis-Moller N, et al. Liver-related deaths in persons infected with the human immunodeficiency virus: the D: A:D study. Arch Intern Med 2006; 166(15):1632–41.

61. Chen TY, Ding EL, Seage Iii GR, et al. Meta-analysis: increased mortality associated with hepatitis C in HIV-infected persons is unrelated to HIV disease progression. Clin Infect Dis 2009;49(10):1605–15.

62. Berenguer J, Alejos B, Hernando V, et al. Trends in mortality according to hepatitis C virus serostatus in the era of combination antiretroviral therapy. AIDS 2012; 26(17):2241–6.

63. Labarga P, Soriano V, Vispo ME, et al. Hepatotoxicity of antiretroviral drugs is reduced after successful treatment of chronic hepatitis C in HIV-infected patients. J Infect Dis 2007;196(5):670–6.

64. Rockstroh JK. Optimal therapy of HIV/HCV co-infected patients with direct acting antivirals. Liver Int 2015;35(Suppl 1):51–5.

65. Opravil M, Sasadeusz J, Cooper DA, et al. Effect of baseline CD4 cell count on the efficacy and safety of peginterferon Alfa-2a (40KD) plus ribavirin in patients with HIV/hepatitis C virus coinfection. J Acquir Immune Defic Syndr 2008;47(1): 36–49.
66. Sulkowski MS. Viral hepatitis and HIV coinfection. J Hepatol 2008;48(2):353–67.
67. European Association of the Study of the Liver. 2011 European Association of the Study of the Liver hepatitis C virus clinical practice guidelines. Liver Int 2012; 32(Suppl 1):2–8.
68. Fleischer R, Boxwell D, Sherman KE. Nucleoside analogues and mitochondrial toxicity. Clin Infect Dis 2004;38(8):e79–80.
69. Alvarez D, Dieterich DT, Brau N, et al. Zidovudine use but not weight-based ribavirin dosing impacts anaemia during HCV treatment in HIV-infected persons. J Viral Hepat 2006;13(10):683–9.
70. Rockstroh JK, Puoti M, Rodriguez-Torres M, et al. Sofosbuvir and ribavirin therapy for the treatment of HIV/HCV coinfected patients with HCV GT1-4 infection: the PHOTON-1 and -2 trials. Hepatology 2014;60(4 Suppl 1):295A–6A.
71. Osinusi A, Townsend K, Kohli A, et al. Virologic response following combined ledipasvir and sofosbuvir administration in patients with HCV genotype 1 and HIV co-infection. JAMA 2015;313(12):1232–9.
72. Sulkowski MS, Eron JJ, Wyles D, et al. Ombitasvir, paritaprevir co-dosed with ritonavir, dasabuvir, and ribavirin for hepatitis C in patients co-infected with HIV-1: a randomized trial. JAMA 2015;313(12):1223–31.
73. Wyles D, Ruane P, Sulkowski M, et al. Daclatasvir in combination with sofosbuvir for HIV/HCV coinfection: ALLY-2 study. Conference on Retroviruses and Opportunistic Infections (CROI). Seattle, WA, February 23-26, 2015.
74. Zeuzem S, Ghalib R, Reddy KR, et al. The phase 3 C-EDGE treatment-naive study of a 12-week oral regimen of grazoprevir/elbasvir in patients with chronic HCV genotype 1, 4, or 6 infection. J Hepatol 2015;62(Suppl 2):S213.

Hepatitis C: Issues in Children

Christine K. Lee, MD*, Maureen M. Jonas, MD

KEYWORDS

- Hepatitis C • Children • Perinatal transmission • Pegylated interferon • Ribavirin
- Direct acting antiviral

KEY POINTS

- Perinatal transmission is the most common mode of hepatitis C virus (HCV) acquisition in children.
- Progression to advanced liver disease is uncommon in childhood but has been reported.
- The principles of diagnosis and evaluation in children are the same as in adults.
- Unless clinically indicated, deferring treatment for chronic HCV in most children is suggested until interferon-free regimens are available.

INTRODUCTION

Hepatitis C virus (HCV) infection is an international health problem with an estimated prevalence of 64 to 170 million people around the world.[1,2] In the United States, approximately 2.3 million people have chronic HCV infection[3] Data from the National Health and Nutrition Examination Survey (NHANES) III for 1999 through 2002 suggest that approximately 0.17% of 6- to 11-year-olds are HCV antibody–positive (31,000) and 0.39% of 12- to 19-year olds are positive (101,000).[4] Of the children with HCV infection, it has been reported that approximately 75% to 80% become infected chronically.[5]

The leading source of HCV acquisition in children is perinatal transmission. The rate is thought to be about 5% from HCV viremic mothers and up to 10.8% in HCV and human immunodeficiency virus (HIV) coinfected mothers who are not receiving antiretroviral therapy.[6]

ACUTE INFECTION

Acute HCV infection is not commonly identified in children, unless associated with known outbreaks.[7] Patients should be monitored for 6 to 8 weeks for spontaneous resolution before treatment is considered. However, although direct-acting antiviral therapy is recommended for the treatment of acute HCV infection in adults, these agents are not yet approved for use in children.[8] Fulminant hepatitis C is uncommon in children, as in adults.

Division of Gastroenterology, Hepatology and Nutrition, Boston Children's Hospital, 300 Longwood Avenue, Boston, MA 02115, USA
* Corresponding author.
E-mail address: Christine.Lee@childrens.harvard.edu

Gastroenterol Clin N Am 44 (2015) 901–909
http://dx.doi.org/10.1016/j.gtc.2015.07.011
0889-8553/15/$ – see front matter © 2015 Elsevier Inc. All rights reserved.

NATURAL HISTORY

Liver disease from chronic HCV infection typically progresses slowly during the childhood years. Thus, the serious complications of advanced liver disease are rare.

For children infected during infancy by vertical transmission, HCV is spontaneously cleared in 20% to 45% of cases.[9–16] In a large series of 266 children with perinatally acquired HCV who were followed for a median of 4.2 years, approximately 20% cleared the infection at a median age of 15 months; 80% went on to have chronic infection.[17] Spontaneous resolution of perinatally acquired HCV is rare after age 3. HCV infection may be acquired later in childhood, because adolescents may acquire HCV through high-risk behaviors, such as intravenous/intranasal drug use and the use of shared tattoo equipment.[17]

Studies of HCV-infected children have demonstrated that hepatic fibrosis tends to increase with age, suggesting that the liver disease, although commonly mild, does progresses over time.[12,18,19] Advanced liver disease is uncommon before young adulthood.[10,11] However, there have been reports of decompensated cirrhosis in children as young as 4, 6, and 11 years,[19] and cirrhosis is well-described during childhood.[20,21] Factors associated with disease progression in children are immunosuppression (HIV infection or other etiologies), obesity, and likely viral factors.[22]

CASE IDENTIFICATION

Testing all children for HCV is not recommended. In a large study of children in an urban setting, only 1 child was positive for HCV out of the 1034 children screened.[23] A 2012 report demonstrated that the number of children identified with HCV in the United States was only a small proportion of the expected number.[24] Only 11.7% of cases had been identified in Florida between 2000 and 2009, and nationwide, this figure was only 4.9%. In addition, in Florida, only 1.6% of the identified children were receiving care for HCV infection and 2.8% had received care within the previous 5 years. Similar findings were reported in a 2015 Australian national surveillance study looking at the incidence of childhood hepatitis C from 2003 to 2007. This study reviewed the reports of new HCV infection in children younger than 15 years reported by Australian pediatricians. There were 45 confirmed cases reported over a 5-year period. In comparison, the reports of HCV infection made through another national disease surveillance system were 6-fold higher. However, even this is an underestimation, because the Australian national incidence as predicted by statistical modeling, is 125 to 250 HCV-infected children born yearly.[25]

Groups of children at high risk for HCV infection, for whom testing would be appropriate, are listed in **Box 1**.[21,26]

DIAGNOSIS

After the first 15 to 18 months of life, the approach to diagnosis of HCV infection in children is similar to that recommended for adults. Most infected individuals are seropositive for anti HCV; infection is confirmed with polymerase chain reaction testing for HCV RNA, and HCV genotyping is recommended to help guide future treatment. In general, liver biopsy is not required typically for either diagnosis or treatment decisions in children. However, biopsy could be considered if the:

- Degree of liver fibrosis would potentially influence treatment decisions, such as the decision to begin currently approved therapy or consider deferring treatment until new therapies are available; or

---

Box 1
Children at high risk for HCV infection

Evidence of hepatitis-elevated serum alanine aminotransferase and/or aspartate aminotransferase

Children whose mothers are HCV positive or have a history of intravenous drug use

- HCV antibody should be tested after 18 months of age. A positive result from earlier testing may reflect maternal antibody[27]

- HCV RNA testing may be done but infants with viremia may resolve spontaneously by age 3 years[6,28]

International adoptees or recent immigrants

- Especially children from high prevalence areas (Africa, China, Russia, Eastern Europe, Southeast Asia)

- Ability to assess adoptee children's risk factors for infection is difficult

Children with HIV infection

Victims of sexual assault or patients with history of multiple sexual partners

Injection or intranasal drug users

Children who have ever been on hemodialysis

Children who got a tattoo in an unregulated setting

Abbreviations: HCV, hepatitis C virus; HIV, human immunodeficiency virus.

- Patient has known or suspected other liver disease that would influence treatment decisions.

The histologic features of childhood HCV infection in children are similar to those found in adults. These include steatosis, portal lymphoid aggregates or follicles, and sinusoidal lymphocytes.[20,29] The severity of fibrosis tends to be less severe in general, although cirrhosis has been reported in children.[19–21]

Although serial monitoring of aminotransferases is often done in practice, it should be noted that serum aminotransferases do not always correlate with disease severity in children with HCV. In approximately one-third of children with HCV, aminotransferases are normal when there is biopsy evidence of inflammation.[22]

MALIGNANCY

Hepatocellular carcinoma is associated primarily with cirrhosis in HCV-infected patients. Because cirrhosis is not seen commonly in children, HCC is also rare in this population. Nonetheless, it is probably prudent to obtain liver ultrasounds and serum alpha fetoprotein annually in children with HCV-related cirrhosis.[30]

TREATMENT

The goal of treatment is to reduce mortality and HCV infection-associated health problems. As in adults, the primary treatment objective is a sustained virologic response (SVR), defined as an absence of detectable viral RNA 24 weeks after the cessation of therapy.

The development of direct-acting antiviral agents and combination drug regimens are major milestones in the treatment of HCV in adults. There are currently no published studies of these direct-acting antiviral agents in HCV-infected children. Although studies of the early protease inhibitors, telaprevir and boceprevir, were initiated in the pediatric population, these were halted with the prospect of highly effective, less toxic regimens. Clinical trials using direct-acting antiviral agents without interferon in children are currently enrolling.

Because of the ongoing trials of direct-acting antiviral agents in children, treatment for chronic hepatitis C in most children should be deferred until interferon-free regimens are available to this population. Because courses of treatment are typically brief, ranging from 12 to 24 weeks, data from pediatric trials should be forthcoming within 2 years. Deferring treatment for several years is often appropriate, because most children have mild liver disease that progresses slowly. However, in the following situations, using currently approved therapy, the combination of peginterferon and ribavirin, should be considered:

- Patient and family preference for immediate treatment.
- Patient has another medical condition that requires prompt treatment (eg, requirement for chronic immunosuppression because of the need for organ transplant).
- Signs of severe or progressive liver disease on liver biopsy. However, it should be noted that patients with cirrhosis do not respond as well and are at higher risk of adverse effects associated with interferon and ribavirin.
- Patient is in a medical system in which the availability of the direct-acting antiviral drugs will be limited or unlikely.

Direct-acting antiviral agents have been approved for use in adults in the United States, Canada, the European Union, Japan, and Russia. There are reports of ongoing efforts to expand production of these medications outside North America. In addition, the pharmaceutical companies have begun licensing agreements with numerous developing countries to expand access to these medications. Whether these drugs will be available for use in children in this expanded global marketplace, and the timeframe for that availability, is uncertain at this time.

CURRENTLY APPROVED TREATMENTS FOR CHILDREN
Pegylated Interferon and Ribavirin

The United States Food and Drug Administration approved the regimen of peginterferon alfa$_{2b}$ in 2008 for use in children with HCV who were 3 years and older with compensated liver disease. The use of peginterferon alfa$_{2a}$ in combination with ribavirin was approved in 2011 for children 5 years of age and older.

A metaanalysis examined the efficacy of peginterferon and ribavirin in 8 trials in children with HCV infection.[31] SVR was obtained in 58% of children with a low rate of relapse (7%). In addition, the rate of discontinuing treatment owing to virologic breakthrough was also low (4%). As in adults, the efficacy of peginterferon plus ribavirin was associated highly with viral genotype. Furthermore, as seen in adults, there is evidence that obesity in children with HCV infection is associated with a 12% decreased probability of achieving a SVR.[22]

Genotype 1

Based on the data in adults treated with direct-acting antiviral, it is advisable to consider deferring treatment for most children with genotype 1 HCV who do not have an indication for immediate treatment. This is particularly important because the currently approved regimens of peginterferon and ribavirin have a reported SVR rate of only 47% to 53%.[32,33] In adults, there are now 3 different recommended regimens with much greater efficacy. These regimens include (1) ledipasvir/sofosbuvir for 12 weeks or (2) paritaprevir/ritonavir/ombitasvir plus dasabuvir and ribavirin for 12 weeks (24 weeks in cirrhosis) or (3) sofosbuvir plus simeprevir with/without ribavirin for 12 weeks (24 weeks in cirrhosis). These regimens have been reported to induce SVR of 95% to 99% in adult patients with genotype 1 HCV.[8]

Genotypes 2 and 3

If treatment is desired soon, the only licensed therapy for children in the United States is a 24-week regimen of peginterferon with ribavirin, which has a reported SVR rate of 80% to 93%.[19,32] For most patients, we suggest deferring treatment to avoid the side effects of interferon. For adults with genotype 2, the current preferred treatment is the interferon-free regimen of sofosbuvir with ribavirin for 12 weeks (16 weeks in cirrhosis) with a reported SVR rate of 94%.[8] For adults with genotype 3, the same regimen is recommended for 24 weeks with a reported SVR of 84%.[8]

Dosing

Currently approved dosing for combination therapy with pegylated interferon and ribavirin for children are listed in **Box 2**. Interleukin-28B (*IL28B*)–associated single nucleotide polymorphisms have been strongly associated with the likelihood of achieving SVR with peginterferon and ribavirin in adults. There are preliminary studies showing a similar association in children.[34,35] *IL28B* genotype does not seem to be relevant when considering treatment with the new direct-acting antiviral regimens.

Adverse Effects

Peginterferon has many side effects, including:

- Pyrexia
- Headache

Box 2
Combination therapy with pegylated interferon and ribavirin for children

Pegylated interferon

- For children $\geq$ 3 years: peginterferon alfa$_{2b}$ 60 μg/m^2 subcutaneously weekly (maximum dose 1.5 μg/kg)

- For children $\geq$ 5 years: peginterferon alpha$_{2a}$ 180 μg/1.73 m^2 x Body Surface area subcutaneously weekly (maximum dose 180 μg)

Ribavirin

- 15 mg/kg/d orally with food, divided into 2 doses

- Available as 200 mg capsules and 40 mg/mL oral solution

Duration of therapy

- Genotype 1: 48 weeks

- Genotype 2 or 3: 24 weeks

- If the patient does not attain an early virologic response (a 2-log$_{10}$ decline in HCV RNA level at week 12), treatment should be discontinued

- In genotype 1 infection, the presence of detectable HCV at week 24 is an indication to discontinue therapy

Abbreviation: HCV, hepatitis C virus.

- Gastrointestinal symptoms
- Depression
- Weight loss, slow linear growth, and decreased body mass index during treatment
  - This typically returns to normal after cessation of therapy[36]
  - The effect on height can be noted up to 2 years after end of treatment
- Peginterferon$_{2a}$ is associated with retinopathy or uveitis in 2% to 3% of patients[37]
  - We recommend a baseline ophthalmologic examination and repeat examinations if symptoms develop
- Neutropenia can be marked, but clinical infections are uncommon

Ribavirin has side effects, including:

- Hemolytic anemia
- Teratogenicity
  - Pregnancy monitoring is recommended
  - Pregnancy is discouraged during and for 6 months after treatment

Contraindications to treatment with peginterferon and ribavirin include:

- Pregnancy
- Males with pregnant partners
- Autoimmune hepatitis
- Decompensated liver disease

Box 3
General care considerations for children with HCV

Household/school

- HCV is not transmitted by household contact (sharing utensils, food, water, touching, breastfeeding, etc) so no limitations are indicated
- Infected children should avoid sharing toothbrushes, nail clippers, and razors[41,42]
- Caretakers should use universal precautions to care for minor cuts/bruises
- Fresh/dried blood spills should be cleaned with 1 part bleach/10 parts water with protective gloves (www.cdc.gov)
- Transmission through saliva is low

Health maintenance

- Children with HCV should receive all age-appropriate vaccinations (including those for hepatitis A and B)
- HCV-infected children should avoid excessive weight gain/obesity
- School and sports participation should not be restricted

Adolescent counseling regarding risk behaviors

- Avoid alcohol
- Avoid high-risk behaviors (intravenous drug use, nasal cocaine)
- Avoid noncommercial self-tattooing and piercing with shared needles (commercial services are not associated with increased risk of transmission)
- Avoid sexual intercourse with multiple partners

Abbreviation: HCV, hepatitis C virus.

- Hemoglobinopathies
- Renal dysfunction

Prevention of Transmission

Focus should be placed on reducing perinatal transmission of HCV, because this is the primary source of new childhood infections. However, standard screening for HCV in pregnancy is not recommended because there are currently no proven strategies to reduce transmission (**Box 3**).

Established factors associated with an increased risk of vertical transmission are:

- Detectable HCV RNA during pregnancy/time of delivery
- Coinfection with HIV[15,38]
- Mothers who are intravenous drug users[39]

Possible risk factors of vertical transmission.

- Prolonged rupture of membranes of 6 hours or longer[40]
- Obstetric procedures (amniocentesis, scalp electrode monitoring)[40]

SUMMARY

Hepatitis C is a viral infection estimated to affect up to 170 million persons worldwide. Unfortunately, there is evidence that there are many more children infected than identified. Currently, perinatal transmission is the most common mode of acquisition during childhood. Chronic HCV infection progresses slowly during the childhood years. Thus, the serious complications of advanced liver disease rarely affect young patients. Since the introduction of direct-acting antiviral agents, treatment success for HCV infection in adults has improved significantly. Because progression to advanced liver disease is uncommon during the childhood years, treatment for chronic hepatitis C in children should be deferred until interferon-free regimens are available to this population. If treatment cannot be deferred, then peginterferon and ribavirin can be given to children with compensated liver disease. A strategy to reduce perinatal transmission will effectively prevent most new childhood HCV infections.

REFERENCES

1. World Health Organization. Hepatitis C- global prevalence (update). Wkly Epidemiol Rec 2000;75:18–9.
2. Gower E, Estes C, Blach S, et al. Global epidemiology and genotype distribution of the hepatitis C virus. J Hepatol 2014;61(1):45–57.
3. Ditah I, Ditah F, Devaki P, et al. The changing epidemiology of hepatitis C virus infection in the United States: national health and nutrition examination survey 2001 through 2010. J Hepatol 2014;60(4):691–8.
4. Armstrong G, Wasley A, Simard E, et al. The prevalence of hepatitis C virus infection in the United States, 1999 through 2002. Ann Intern Med 2006;144:705–14.
5. Alter MJ, Kruszon-Moran D, Nainan OV, et al. The prevalence of hepatitis C virus infection in the United States 1988-1994. N Engl J Med 1999;341:556–62.
6. Yeung LT, Kim SM, Roberts EA. Mother-to-infant transmission of hepatitis C virus. Hepatology 2001;34:223–9.
7. Jonas MM, Baron MJ, Bresee JS, et al. Clinical and virologic features of hepatitis C virus infection associated with intravenous immunoglobulin. Pediatrics 1996; 98:211.

8. AASLD/ HCV Guidelines Panel. Hepatitis C Guidance: AASLD-IDSA Recommendations for Testing, Managing, and Treating Adults Infected with Hepatitis C Virus. Hepatology 2015, in press.

9. Jhaveri R. Diagnosis and management of hepatitis C virus-infected children. Pediatr Infect Dis J 2011;30(11):983–5.

10. Minola E, Prati D, Suter F, et al. Age at infection affects the long-term outcome of transfusion-associated chronic hepatitis C. Blood 2002;99:4588–91.

11. Casiraghi MA, De Paschale M, Romano L, et al. Long-term outcome (35 years) of hepatitis C after acquisition of infection through mini transfusions of blood given at birth. Hepatology 2004;39:90–6.

12. Matsuoka S, Tatara K, Hayabuchi Y, et al. Serologic, virologic and histologic characteristics of chronic phase hepatitis C virus disease in children infected by transfusion. Pediatrics 1994;94:919–22.

13. Vogt M, Lang T, Frosner G, et al. Prevalence and clinical outcome of hepatitis C infection in children who underwent cardiac surgery before the implementation of blood-donor screening. N Engl J Med 1999;341:866–70.

14. Tovo PA, Pembrey LJ, Newell ML. Persistence rate and progression of vertically acquired hepatitis C infection. European Paediatric Hepatitis C infection. J Infect Dis 2000;181:419–24.

15. Mohan P, Colvin C, Glymph C, et al. Clinical spectrum and histopathologic features of chronic hepatitis C infection in children. J Pediatr 2007;150:168–74.

16. Matsuoka S, Tatara K, Hayabuchi Y, et al. Post-transfusion chronic hepatitis C in children. J Paediatr Child Health 1994;30:544–6.

17. European Paediatric Hepatitis C Virus Network. Three broad modalities in the natural history of vertically acquired hepatitis C virus infection. Clin Infect Dis 2005; 41:45–51.

18. Guido M, Bortolotti F, Leandro G, et al. Fibrosis in chronic hepatitis c acquired in infancy: is it only a matter of time? Am J Gastroenterol 2003;98:660–3.

19. Birnbaum AH, Shneider BL, Moy L. Hepatitis C in children. N Engl J Med 2000; 342:290–1.

20. Badizadegan K, Jonas MM, Ott MJ, et al. Histopathology of the liver in children with chronic hepatitis c viral infection. Hepatology 1998;28:1416–23.

21. Goodman ZD, Makhlouf HR, Liu L, et al. Pathology of chronic hepatitis C in children: liver biopsy findings in the Peds-C Trial. Hepatology 2008;47:836–43.

22. Delgado-Borrego A, Healey D, Negre B, et al. Influence of body mass index on outcome of pediatric chronic hepatitis C virus infection. J Pediatr Gastroenterol Nutr 2010;51(2):191–7.

23. El-Kamary SS, Serwint JR, Joffe A, et al. Prevalence of hepatitis C virus infection in urban children. J Pediatr 2003;143:54–9.

24. Delgado-Borrego A, Smith L, Jonas MM, et al. Expected and actual case ascertainment and treatment rates for children infected with hepatitis C in Florida and the United States: epidemiologic evidence from statewide and nationwide surveys. J Pediatr 2012;161:915–21.

25. Raynes-Greenow C, Polis S, Elliott E, et al. Childhood hepatitis C virus infection: an Australian national surveillance study of incident cases over five years. J Paediatr Child Health 2015. http://dx.doi.org/10.1111/jpc.12904.

26. Mack CL, Gonzalez-Peralta RP, Gupta N, et al. NASPGHAN practice guidelines. Diagnosis and management of hepatitis C infection in infants, children and adolescents. J Pediatr Gastroenterol Nutr 2012;54:838–55.

27. Ghany MG, Strader DB, Thomas DL, et al. Diagnosis, management and treatment of hepatitis C: an update. Hepatology 2009;49:1335–74.

28. Conte D, Fraquelli M, Prati D, et al. Prevalence and clinical course of chronic hepatitis C virus (HCV) infection and rate of HCV vertical transmission in a cohort of 15,250 pregnant women. Hepatology 2000;31:751–5.

29. Guido M, Rugge M, Jara P, et al. Chronic hepatitis C in children: the pathological and clinical spectrum. Gastroenterology 1998;115:1525–9.

30. Gonzalez-Peralta RP, Langham MR Jr, Andres JM, et al. Hepatocellular carcinoma in 2 young adolescents with chronic hepatitis C. J Pediatr Gastroenterol Nutr 2009;48:630–5.

31. Druyts E, Thorlund K, Wu P, et al. Efficacy and safety of pegylated interferon alfa-2a or alfa-2b plus ribavirin for the treatment of chronic hepatitis C in children and adolescents: a systematic review and meta-analysis. Clin Infect Dis 2013;56: 961–7.

32. Schwarz KB, Gonzalez-Peralta RP, Murray KF, et al. The combination of ribavirin and peginterferon is superior to peginterferon and placebo for children and adolescents with chronic hepatitis C. Gastroenterology 2011;140(2):450–8.

33. Wirth S, Ribes-Koninckx C, Calzado MA, et al. High sustained virologic response rates in children with chronic hepatitis c receiving peginterferon alfa-2b plus ribavirin. J Hepatol 2010;52:501–7.

34. Domagalski K, Pawlowska M, Tretyn A, et al. Impact of IL-28B polymorphism on pegylated interferon plus ribavirin treatment response in children and adolescents infected with HCV genotypes 1 and 4. Eur J Clin Microbiol Infect Dis 2013;32:745–54.

35. Shaker OG, Nassar YH, Nour ZA, et al. Single-nucleotide polymorphisms of IL-10 and IL-28B as predictors of the response of IFN therapy in HCV genotype 4-infected children. J Pediatr Gastroenterol Nutr 2013;57:155–60.

36. Jonas MM, Balistreri W, Gonzalez-Peralta RP, et al. Pegylated interferon for chronic hepatitis C in children affects growth and body composition: results from the pediatric study of hepatitis C (PEDS-C) trial. Hepatology 2012;56: 523–31.

37. Narkewicz MR, Rosenthal P, Schwarz KB, et al. Ophthalmologic complications in children with chronic hepatitis C treated with pegylated interferon. J Pediatr Gastroenterol Nutr 2010;51:183–6.

38. Benova L, Mohamoud YA, Calvert C, et al. Vertical transmission of hepatitis C virus; systematic review and meta-analysis. Clin Infect Dis 2014;59:765–73.

39. Resti M, Azzari C, Lega L, et al. Mother-to-infant transmission of hepatitis C virus. Acta Paediatr 1995;84:251–5.

40. Mast EE, Hwang LY, Seto DS, et al. Risk factors for perinatal transmission of hepatitis C virus (HCV) and the natural history of HCV infection acquired in infancy. J Infect Dis 2005;192:1880–9.

41. American Academy of Pediatrics. Hepatitis C. In: Pickering LK, editor. Red Book; 2015 report of committee on infectious diseases. 30th edition. Elk Grover Village (IL): American Academy of Pediatrics; 2015. p. 423–30.

42. Vegnente A, Iorio R, Saviano A, et al. Lack of intrafamilial transmission of hepatitis C virus in family members of children with chronic hepatitis C infection. Pediatr Infect Dis J 1994;13:886–9.

Index

Note: Page numbers of article titles are in **boldface** type.

Gastroenterol Clin N Am 44 (2015) 911–921
http://dx.doi.org/10.1016/S0889-8553(15)00113-2
0889-8553/15/$ – see front matter © 2015 Elsevier Inc. All rights reserved.

gastro.theclinics.com

United States Postal Service

Statement of Ownership, Management, and Circulation
(All Periodicals Publications Except Requestor Publications)

1. Publication Title	2. Publication Number									3. Filing Date
Gastroenterology Clinics of North America	0	0	0	-	2	7	7	9		9/18/15

4. Issue Frequency	5. Number of Issues Published Annually	6. Annual Subscription Price
Mar, Jun, Sep, Dec	4	$320.00

7. Complete Mailing Address of Known Office of Publication (Not printer) (Street, city, county, state, and ZIP+4®)

Elsevier Inc.
360 Park Avenue South
New York, NY 10010-1710

Contact Person
Stephen R. Bushing

Telephone (Include area code)
215-239-3688

8. Complete Mailing Address of Headquarters or General Business Office of Publisher (Not printer)

Elsevier Inc., 360 Park Avenue South, New York, NY 10010-1710

9. Full Names and Complete Mailing Addresses of Publisher, Editor, and Managing Editor (Do not leave blank)

Publisher (Name and complete mailing address)

Linda Belfus, Elsevier Inc., 1600 John F. Kennedy Blvd., Suite 1800, Philadelphia, PA 19103

Editor (Name and complete mailing address)

Kerry Holland, Elsevier Inc., 1600 John F. Kennedy Blvd., Suite 1800, Philadelphia, PA 19103-2899

Managing Editor (Name and complete mailing address)

Adrianne Brigido, Elsevier Inc., 1600 John F. Kennedy Blvd., Suite 1800, Philadelphia, PA 19103-2899

10. Owner (Do not leave blank. If the publication is owned by a corporation, give the name and address of the corporation immediately followed by the names and addresses of all stockholders owning or holding 1 percent or more of the total amount of stock. If not owned by a corporation, give the names and addresses of the individual owners. If owned by a partnership or other unincorporated firm, give its name and address as well as those of each individual owner. If the publication is published by a nonprofit organization, give its name and address.)

Full Name	Complete Mailing Address
Wholly owned subsidiary of	1600 John F. Kennedy Blvd., Ste. 1800
Reed/Elsevier, US holdings	Philadelphia, PA 19103-2899

11. Known Bondholders, Mortgagees, and Other Security Holders Owning or Holding 1 Percent or More of Total Amount of Bonds, Mortgages, or Other Securities. If none, check box ☐ None

Full Name	Complete Mailing Address
N/A	

12. Tax Status (For completion by nonprofit organizations authorized to mail at nonprofit rates) (Check one)
The purpose, function, and nonprofit status of this organization and the exempt status for federal income tax purposes:
☒ Has Not Changed During Preceding 12 Months
☐ Has Changed During Preceding 12 Months (Publisher must submit explanation of change with this statement)

PS Form 3526, July 2014 [Page 1 of 4 (Instructions Page 3)] (Instructions Page 3) PRIVACY NOTICE: See our Privacy policy in www.usps.com

---

13. Publication Title		14. Issue Date for Circulation Data Below
Gastroenterology Clinics of North America		September 2015

15. Extent and Nature of Circulation			Average No. Copies Each Issue During Preceding 12 Months	No. Copies of Single Issue Published Nearest to Filing Date
a. Total Number of Copies (Net press run)			748	625
b. Legitimate Paid and/Or Requested Distribution (By Mail and Outside the Mail)	(1)	Mailed Outside-County Paid/Requested Mail Subscriptions stated on PS Form 3541. (Include paid distribution above nominal rate, advertiser's proof copies and exchange copies)	233	187
	(2)	Mailed In-County Paid/Requested Mail Subscriptions stated on PS Form 3541. (Include paid distribution above nominal rate, advertiser's proof copies and exchange copies)		
	(3)	Paid Distribution Outside the Mails Including Sales Through Dealers And Carriers, Street Vendors, Counter Sales, and Other Paid Distribution Outside USPS®	163	195
	(4)	Paid Distribution by Other Classes of Mail Through the USPS (e.g. First-Class Mail®)		
c. Total Paid and/or Requested Circulation (Sum of 15b (1), (2), (3), and (4))		→	396	382
d. Free or Nominal Rate Distribution (By Mail and Outside the Mail)	(1)	Free or Nominal Rate Outside-County Copies included on PS Form 3541	93	90
	(2)	Free or Nominal Rate In-County Copies included on PS Form 3541		
	(3)	Free or Nominal Rate Copies mailed at Other classes Through the USPS (e.g. First-Class Mail®)		
	(4)	Free or Nominal Rate Distribution Outside the Mail (Carriers or Other means)		
e. Total Nonrequested Distribution (Sum of 15d (1), (2), (3) and (4))		→	93	90
f. Total Distribution (Sum of 15c and 15e)		→	489	472
g. Copies not Distributed (See instructions to publishers #4 (page #3))		→	259	153
h. Total (Sum of 15f and g)			748	625
i. Percent Paid and/or Requested Circulation (15c divided by 15f times 100)			80.98%	80.93%

* If you are claiming electronic copies go to line 16 on page 3. If you are not claiming Electronic copies, skip to line 17 on page 3.

16. Electronic Copy Circulation		Average No. Copies Each Issue During Preceding 12 Months	No. Copies of Single Issue Published Nearest to Filing Date
a. Paid Electronic Copies	→		
b. Total paid Print Copies (Line 15c) + Paid Electronic copies (Line 16a)	→		
c. Total Print Distribution (Line 15f) + Paid Electronic Copies (Line 16a)	→		
d. Percent Paid (Both Print & Electronic copies) (16b divided by 16c × 100)	→		

☐ I certify that 50% of all my distributed copies (electronic and print) are paid above a nominal price

17. Publication of Statement of Ownership
If the publication is a general publication, publication of this statement is required. Will be printed in the _December 2015_ issue of this publication.

18. Signature and Title of Editor, Publisher, Business Manager, or Owner

Stephen R. Bushing

Stephen R. Bushing – Inventory Distribution Coordinator

Date
September 18, 2015

I certify that all information furnished on this form is true and complete. I understand that anyone who furnishes false or misleading information on this form or who omits material or information requested on the form may be subject to criminal sanctions (including fines and imprisonment) and/or civil sanctions (including civil penalties).

PS Form 3526, July 2014 (Page 3 of 3)

Moving?

Make sure your subscription moves with you!

To notify us of your new address, find your **Clinics Account Number** (located on your mailing label above your name), and contact customer service at:

Email: journalscustomerservice-usa@elsevier.com

800-654-2452 (subscribers in the U.S. & Canada)
314-447-8871 (subscribers outside of the U.S. & Canada)

Fax number: 314-447-8029

Elsevier Health Sciences Division
Subscription Customer Service
3251 Riverport Lane
Maryland Heights, MO 63043

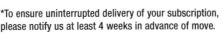

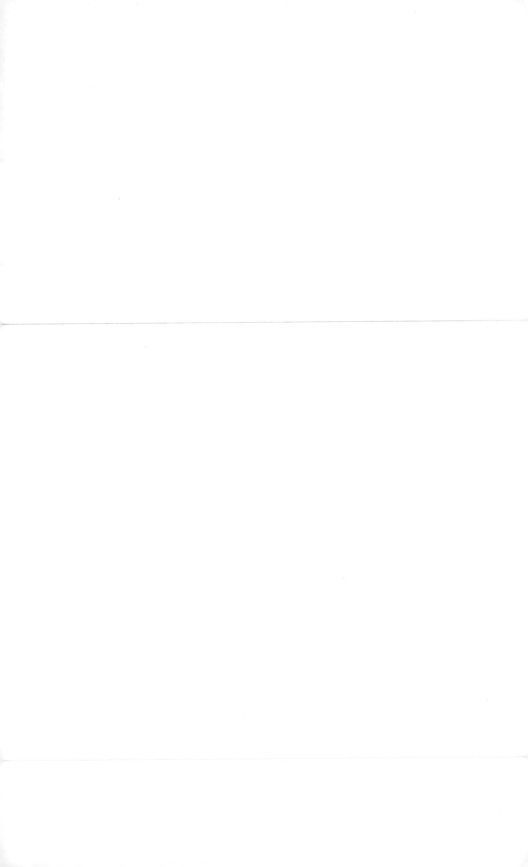